OXFORD MEDICAL PUBLICATIONS

Cancer clinical trials

methods and practice

Cancer clinical trials

methods and practice

Edited by

MARC E. BUYSE
MAURICE J. STAQUET
RICHARD J. SYLVESTER

European Organization for Research on Treatment of Cancer (EORTC) Data Center, Brussels, Belgium

OXFORD   NEW YORK   TORONTO
OXFORD UNIVERSITY PRESS
1984

Oxford University Press, Walton Street, Oxford OX2 6DP

London Glasgow New York Toronto
Delhi Bombay Calcutta Madras Karachi
Kuala Lumpur Singapore Hong Kong Tokyo
Nairobi Dar es Salaam Cape Town
Melbourne Auckland

and associates in
Beirut Berlin Ibadan Mexico City Nicosia

OXFORD *is a trade mark of Oxford University Press*

British Library Cataloguing in Publication Data

Cancer clinical trials—(Oxford medical publications)
1. Cancer—Treatment
I. Buyse, Marc E.   II. Staquet, Maurice, J.
III. Sylvester, Richard J.
616 99'406   RC270 8
ISBN 0-19-261357-X

Library of Congress Cataloging in Publication Data

Main entry under title:
Cancer clinical trials.
(Oxford medical publications)
Bibliography: p.
Includes index.
1. Cancer—Treatment—Evaluation—Addresses, essays, lectures. I. Buyse, Marc E. II. Staquet,
Maurice. III. Sylvester, Richard J. IV. Series. [DNLM: 1. Neoplasms—Drug therapy.
2. Antineoplastic agents—Therapeutic use. 3. Clinical trials—Methods. QZ 267 C2186]
RC270.8.C354   1983   616.99'406'0287   83-8090
ISBN 0-19-261357-X

Photoset by Cotswold Typesetting Ltd, Gloucester
Printed in Great Britain by the Thetford Press Ltd, Norfolk

Preface

Clinical trials have become one of the most widely accepted tools in the search for more effective cancer therapies. The last decade has shown a dramatic increase in the number of cancer clinical trials carried out with an accompanying advance in clinical trial methodology. Considerable methodoligical progress has been made recently and some excellent references are now available for trial organizers; yet a number of practical problems arise when one wishes to consult the literature.

First, the important contributions to trial methodology are widely scattered throughout both the medical and statistical literature. The purpose of this book is essentially to bring together in a single volume the fundamental concepts of trial design, planning, conduct, and analysis.

Secondly, papers are often fraught with statistical jargon (sometimes quite unnecessarily so) which will rebuff all except the highly motivated reader. This book is aimed at clinicians and statisticians alike; it is not meant to be a statistical textbook and all mathematical developments have been avoided.

Thirdly, many references are either too theoretical or too general in nature to answer the specific questions which trial organizers are likely to raise. With this in mind, the emphasis has been placed here not only on the principles involved but also on the practical aspects of carrying out a cancer clinical trial.

In short, this book is intended to provide all parties involved in cancer trials with a practical handbook summarizing the present state of the art. It will hopefully also be of interest to the experienced researchers, as some contributions include original results while most chapters give a fairly complete and up-dated list of references for further reading.

The book is divided into seven sections:

Section I deals with general considerations relevant to cancer trials, including the much debated issues of ethics and the quality of life of cancer patients.

Section II provides practical guidance in the planning and conduct of trials, with special emphasis on form design, data computerization, and quality control. A contribution is also devoted to the frequently overlooked problems related to protocol non-adherence.

Section III is devoted entirely to the reporting of treatment results and toxicities, both in solid and in non-solid tumours. The guidelines recommended in this section are already used by several co-operative groups and attempt at achieving a standardization in the publication of trial results.

Section IV gives a glimpse of pre-clinical and phase I trials, a very active field in which many hopes are vested.

Section V covers both the clinical and statistical aspects in the design and conduct of phase II trials.

Section VI reviews the issues at stake when designing phase III trials: design type, randomization and stratification, number of patients needed, and duration of the study. Alternative designs are also discussed.

Lastly, section VII introduces the fundamental statistical methods used in analysing phase III trial data, which basically entails comparing proportions and/or survival data. One contribution in this section addresses the important problem of interim analyses and early stopping rules, while the last two chapters discuss the importance of prognostic factors and the use of regression models.

It is hoped that this book will make researchers more aware of the proper techniques to be used in the design and analysis of clinical trials and will thus contribute to improving the overall standards of cancer research.

We wish to express our deep gratitude to all the contributors who have accepted to partake in this project.

We would also like to acknowledge the help of our colleagues in the preparation of this book, in particular S. Suciu, O. Dalesio, and M. Van Glabbeke for their review of some manuscripts, and A. Debaere and D. De Bel for their secretarial assistance.

Brussels   M.E.B., M.J.S., R.J.S.
February 1983

Acknowledgements

The EORTC Foundation will receive all royalties from sales of this book. The contributors freely gave their time and received no remuneration. The editors are extremely grateful to all of them.

Contents

Contributors

Alfred A. Bartolucci,
University of Alabama in Birmingham,
Birmingham,
Alabama 35294,
USA

Norman Breslow,
University of Washington,
Seattle,
Washington 98195,
USA

Byron W. Brown, Jr.,
Stanford University School of Medicine,
Stanford,
California 94305,
USA

Marc Buyse,
EORTC Data Center,
Brussels 1000,
Belgium

David P. Byar,
National Cancer Institute,
Bethesda,
Maryland 20205,
USA

Stephen K. Carter,
Bristol-Myers Company,
New York,
New York 10154,
USA

Gary M. Clark,
University of Texas Health Science Center,
San Antonio,
Texas 78284,
USA

Adèle L. Couzijn,
Dutch Cancer Institute,
Amsterdam 1066,
The Netherlands

Otilia Dalesio,
EORTC Data Center,
Brussels 1000,
Belgium

Marleen De Pauw,
EORTC Data Center,
Brussels 1000,
Belgium

Mark B. Edelstein,
Radiobiological Institute TNO,
Rijswijk 2280,
The Netherlands

Stephen L. George,
St. Jude Children's Research Hospital,
Memphis,
Tennessee 38101,
USA

Jay Herson,
Applied Logic Associates,
5615 Morningside, Suite 319,
Houston,
Texas 77005,
USA

Barth Hoogstraten,
Bethesda Hospital,
Cincinatti,
Ohio 45206,
USA

Boris Iglewicz,
Temple University,
Philadelphia,
Pennsylvania 19122,
USA

Daniel L. Kisner,
University of Texas Health Science Center,
San Antonio,
Texas 78284,
USA

John Kuhn,
University of Texas Health Science Center,
San Antonio,
Texas 78284,
USA

Stephen W. Lagakos,
Sidney Farber Cancer Institute,
Boston,
Massachussets 02115,
USA

Elisa T. Lee,
University of Oklahoma Health Sciences Center,
Oklahoma City,
Oklahoma 73190,
USA

Peter Lelieveld,
Radiobiological Institute TNO,
Rijswijk 2280,
The Netherlands

Corrie A. G. Linssen,
The Netherlands Cancer Institute,
1066 CX Amsterdam,
The Netherlands

Klim McPherson,
University of Oxford,
Oxford OX2 6HE,
England

Rodney B. Nelson, III,
127 Hamilton Street,
Geneva,
Illinois 60134,
USA

Julian Peto,
Institute of Cancer Research,
Division of Epidemiology,
Clifton Ave.,
Sutton,
Surrey,
England

Stuart J. Pocock,
Royal Free Hospital School of Medicine,
London NW3 2PN,
England

Harvey D. Preisler,
Roswell Park Memorial Institute,
Buffalo,
New York 14263,
USA

Richard Simon,
National Cancer Institute,
Bethesda,
Maryland 20205,
USA

Federico Spreafico,
Istituto di Ricerche Farmacologiche 'Mario Negri',
Milan 20157,
Italy

Maurice Staquet,
EORTC Data Center,
Brussels 1000,
Belgium

Richard Sylvester,
EORTC Data Center,
Brussels 1000,
Belgium

Henri J. Tagnon,
Institut Jules Bordet,
Brussels 1000,
Belgium

Frits S. A. M. van Dam,
The Netherlands Cancer Institute,
1066 CX Amsterdam,
The Netherlands

Daniel D. Von Hoff,
University of Texas Health Science Center,
San Antonio,
Texas 78284,
USA

Robert Zittoun,
Hôtel Dieu de Paris,
Paris 75181,
France

Part I
General issues

1 Cancer trials: pseudoscience or situation science?

Rodney B. Nelson, III

Do not make gold, make medicine. Paracelsus (Pachter 1951)

From the Renaissance beginnings of scientific inquiry new ideas have met with criticisms and ridicule. Today the new becomes the orthodox in a few short years. Still, doctrine needs the dialectic if science is to progress. Few writers have advanced scientific medicine by quarrelling with it. Yet the man who brought science to therapeutics at about the time Copernicus removed the earth from the centre of the universe was one of those few.

Aureolus Theophrastus Bombastus, or Paracelsus, rejected Hippocrates, Galen, and the orthodox. He argued that diseases had specific causes and could have specific chemical cures. By introducing mercurials for syphilis he quite literally fulfilled the alchemists' dream of turning mercury into gold, as metal traders scrambled to corner the market on mercury. So Paracelsus taught the alchemists something of the economics of medicine. The bombastic Paracelsus was wrong about nearly everything except his insistence on free inquiry. He also taught that academic dogma was: 'Orthodoxy defending the citadel of ignorance.'

More recently, another scientist and physician faced scorn and ridicule for announcing discoveries. Robert Koch soared from humble country doctor to director of the heavily endowed Koch Institute in a few short years. He endured, and sarcastically rebutted, attacks on his claim that he had discovered the agent responsible for tuberculosis. Some thought the supposed bacilli were bits of fibrin, others could not stain the organism themselves and therefore claimed that no one could.

The Kaiser had mandated a war on tuberculosis, and Koch was under tremendous pressure to produce a victory ahead of the rival French. When Koch announced in 1890 at the International Congress in Berlin that he had discovered tuberculin and that it was a cure for tuberculosis, tuberculin became gold. Andrew Carnegie was so impressed he gave Koch $100 000. The substance itself sold for $1000 per vial (Brown 1935).

Ethics, economics, politics, and science have always influenced the practice of medicine. For example, in a single recent issue of the most widely circulated US daily newspaper, two pieces on clinical research appeared. In one, the dramatic price run-up of the stock of a major drug firm was explained to be on the basis of favourable results from a Scandinavian clinical trial of one of the firm's new drugs (Anon 1981a). In the other, a noted clinical investigator was said to be facing censure and withdrawal of governmental grant funding because of alleged, illicit genetic experiments conducted on human subjects in Italy (Anon 1981b).

Yet the practitioners and investigators of every era have declared themselves independent of economic and political influence. The time has come to acknowledge that multiple and complex forces are mixed into the crucible of scientific inquiry. Keen governmental interest in the politics and economics of science led to the death of Gallileo and forced Paracelsus into a nomadic lifestyle similar to that of some present-day scientific iconoclasts. (Paracelsus ultimately succumbed to the after-effects of a tavern brawl.) Thus, any contemporary examples that may be cited in this essay are for illustration only!

A University of California geologist gave a convincing argument for the integration of politics and science during a lecture at the Fermi Laboratory, the largest nuclear laboratory in the US. He described the methodology employed for predicting earthquakes in two cultures: the United States and China. The geologist related that in the US prediction was attempted by a few experts who devised an elaborate and expensive method of bouncing laser beams over long distances so that movements of land masses along a fault could be plotted with millimetre accuracy. In China, on the other hand, every village elected a 'barefoot' geologist who plotted movements by triangulation using primitive surveying equipment, and then forwarded the data to regional centres for analysis.

Now it turns out that neither method is much good for predicting earthquakes. But a huge difference exists in political and economic impact. When an unexpected earthquake hits the US, the populace looks for an expert to tar and feather, and votes to reduce research spending. In China, after an earthquake, the people look at each other and say: 'Well that method didn't work. We'd better innovate and increase our commitment to a solution.' Perhaps the US approach illustrates what Erwin Chargaff, the molecular biologist was referring to when he wrote about knowledge without wisdom (Chargaff 1980).

The question of what treatment to choose for a cancer patient comes down to a question of evaluation. Evaluation has become the 'buzz' word of the decade among educators, corporate executives, health-care planners, and politicians. Of course the evaluation of evidence has always been the business of scientific physicians. The evaluation literature abounds with references to response evaluation, connoisseurship, goal-free evaluation, and on and on. Groups of experts are convened to arrive at a consensus on cancer treatment based on something called the Delphi Method (Special report 1980; Linestone and Turoff 1975).

Scientific physicians sit back rather smugly knowing that their evaluations rest on the bed-rock of the scientific method. For many cancer physicians the scientific method of evaluation is a process called the clinical trial. Too often, however, the clinical trial evaluation is pseudoscience. This is so because the experimental rules are bent or broken so that results can appear to satisfy arbitrary standards of proof, or the results are presented after adjustments to the data that magnify the apparent benefit. This is not to be construed as an argument in favour of rigid rule making. Clinical treatment decisions should not be based on pseudoscience. Rather, these decisions should be based on situation science.

Joseph Fletcher, the dean of American bioethicists, wrote a classic monograph in 1956 entitled *Situation Ethics*. He argued that three approaches to decision-making exist: the legalistic, the antinomian, and the situational. His argument can be extended to decision-making in cancer treatment.

With the legalistic approach 'one enters every decision making situation encumbered with a whole apparatus of prefabricated rules and regulations. Not just the spirit, but the letter of the law reigns.' The rules and paraphernalia of inferential statistics frequently become the law for clinical trials. The penalty for servile obedience to these laws is the stifling of creativity. Mendel's statistics may have been too perfect to be stochastically believable, but his was a descriptive science, not an inferential one. He may have been guilty of 'cleaning up' his data.

The antinomian (literally 'against law') approach to decision making is the polar opposite of the legalistic. One enters each decision with no laws, maxims, or guidelines whatsoever. The existentialism of Sartre demands that one decide only on the basis of the moment. Thus, any collection of data, either prospective or retrospective, becomes irrelevant to the antinomial cancer therapist, who says: 'this case is too unique to invoke any rules, no matter how complex and stratified the data upon which such rules are based'.

The third approach is the situational. The situational therapist enters each decision armed with as many data-based rules as he can muster. But as Fletcher has pointed out, the situationalist is empirical, data conscious, and inquisitive. His decisions are all hypothetical, never categorical. So cancer treatment decisions should be based on situation science. To recommend such an approach is hazardous since Richard Nixon attempted to justify some of the activities of his administration by invoking situation ethics. But just as in wine drinking, abuse should not be an argument against proper use.

'Polecat' (i.e. skunk), 'polemic' (i.e. the art of disputation), and 'polestar' (i.e. guiding principle) are consecutive entries in the Merriam–Webster Dictionary (1974). Science is the pursuit of the third, not the practice of the second for purposes of accusing investigators of being the first. None the less, situation science does have a place for adversarial evaluation

(Levine 1974), though situation science would never be restricted to that process. The major advantage of adversarial judicial evaluation has been summarized: 'The judicial model demands that the evaluation focus on relevant and significant issues as determined by a broad variety of persons involved in or affected by the program.' Science is largely based on rules of evidence, which in turn are based on logic. Cancer therapeutics must be pragmatic, so rules governing clinical trials must be guidelines not laws. Or as William James wrote in *On Pragmatism:* 'The true, to put it briefly, is only the expedient in our way of thinking, just as the right is only the expedient in our way of behaving' (James 1976).

The evaluation of a clinical trial design is deceptively simple on the surface. All that is needed is to focus on five key elements: the hypotheses to be tested; the description of the trial population; the 'events' or outcomes to be tabulated; the difference in outcome felt to be clinically important to detect (that is the 'delta'); the false positive, type I, or 'alpha error risk' (that much worshipped p of less than 0.05); and the false negative, type II, or 'beta error risk'. But if the process is so simple, why does so much controversy exist? Everyone seems to agree that the evils of chance and the evils of bias must both be carefully controlled in any scientific experiment. The evils of chance are relatively easy to master through legalistic statistical rules (though precisely what methods should be used remains a situational decision). But, to borrow from the nosology of the hepatologists, it is the non-alpha, non-beta errors that plague the cancer clinical trial literature, and these situational errors all relate to the evils of bias.

Mark Twain remarked about science in general what many have felt about cancer clinical trials: 'There is something fascinating about science. One gets such wholesale returns of conjecture out of such a trifling investment of fact' (Twain 1876). All too frequently retrospective conjecture is woven almost imperceptively into the fabric of the methods and results sections of a cancer clinical trial. The legalistic rules that relate to the stochastic handling of clinical trial data cannot 'control' the fertile minds of innovative investigators who fit their data to the situation. Situation science is needed to control the 'tyranny of N' and to prevent the creation of an illusion of objectivity based on numbers and probabilities.

There are at least five ways by which the 'tyranny of N' can distort the truth in clinical trials, without the published numerical data in any way reflecting that tyranny directly. Subtle situational decisions must be made consciously or unconsciously by investigators and editors at many points in the design, conduct, and reporting of clinical trials. These unspecified decisions are what made Sir Peter Medawar decide that many scientific papers are fraudulent (Medawar 1964).

The first problem with 'N' arises for the reader of a trial report when he wonders if the '37 patients with stage III gigacytomas studied' were selected from an eligible population of 37, 137, or 1037. Authors face a more serious quandary. Most authors, to a greater or lesser extent, would like the reader to believe that their sample is a random sample of all patients with a carefully described set of characteristics. (Legalistically, this may work to their disadvantage since $n-1$ must be the divisor for their variance instead of the more powerful n (Feinstein 1973)). If authors document carefully throughout a lengthy methods section the path that their trial population took as it emerged from the universe of all possible patients, their paper will be rejected as too verbose by reviewers, who also express 'serious reservations about the sampling methodology'.

Worse still, if their paper does come to rest in some obscure journal the results will be rejected by vocal critics because of the 'carefully selected patient population'. (Note the innuendo in the use of the word 'carefully'.) As a result, few successful authors make much of an attempt to describe the transitions traversed by the final population. Thus enters an unseen non-alpha, non-beta risk: transition bias (Feinstein 1971).

Secondly, the published 'N' may have been subjected to some curious 'censoring' by well-meaning investigators who attempt to 'clean up' the data. This practice seems innocent enough, but as will be seen later, it can effect important distortions. *Post facto* selective censoring usually involves treating a dead person as still alive but 'lost'. The rationale for this is that the person died of a 'competing risk' (that is a disease other than the one being studied). Of course, anyone who has ever filled out a death certificate knows the difficult judgement calls that must be made. The concept of competing risks is simple enough, though the statistical methods for dealing with them can become complex (Prentice and Kalbfleisch 1978). The reader always wonders whether this decision to 'censor' was part of the original design.

The word 'censoring' itself when used in this context (not to be confused with the censoring that occurs when a patient is truly still alive at the time of analysis) is a quaint eccentricity of clinical investigators. Bench researchers refer to a similar practice as 'throwing out the outliers' (that is ignoring as spurious data points lying far from the mean). Mendel may have used this statute to 'impose' the Hardy–Weinberg Law on his peas.

Perhaps not surprisingly, it appears authors may even confuse themselves when they censor their data. For example, the ten-year summary report of the NCI MOPP experience for advanced Hodgkin's Disease states: '... for patients who achieve complete remission, the probability of surviving beyond five years is 82 per cent and for ten years is 73 per cent' (DeVita, Simon, Hubbard, Young, Berard, Moxley, Frei, Carbone and Canellos 1980). They apparently forgot that they had censored (that is treated as lost) 23 patients known to be dead from other causes. The real survival probability was not given, but would be about 55 per cent at ten years.

Even less surprising is the fact that readers can be misled. An eminent cancer researcher quoted (from the ever dangerous abstract—DeVita, Cannellos, Hubbard, Chabner, and Young 1976) the same erroneous figures in a widely read review (Kaplan 1980). Such is the potential for confusion when concepts like 'tumour mortality', 'disease-free survival', etc. creep in unnoticed. The NCI MOPP report does give considerable detail about the censoring, and the authors' use of situation science is apparent to any careful reader. Another MOPP series of similar magnitude apparently would have us believe that no patients died from the competing risks of trauma, infection, vascular accidents, suicide, etc. (Farber, Proxnitz, Cadman, Lutes, Bertino, and Fischer 1980). Similar unreported censoring has lead to a major controversy surrounding the Anturane Myocardial Infarction Trial (Relman 1980). The time has come to censure selective censoring unless it is explicit.

A third way the 'tyranny of N' can creep into treatment evaluation is by retrospective stratification. Again, many situations make this attractive, if not completely legal. While retrospective censoring can lead to adjustments in the numerators of compared proportions, retrospective stratification can permit adjustment of the denominators. With a small digital computer and a fertile imagination an investigator can test several scenarios in a few minutes. The abstract then can read 'nebulomycin improves disease-free survival ($p = 0.05$) in pre-menopausal women with breast cancer who have grey hair and six or seven nodes positive'.

An interesting example of stratifying retrospectively by adherence to a treatment was provided by the Coronary Drug Project Clofibrate Trial (Coronary Drug Project Research Group 1980). When patients who adhered to the clofibrate regimen were compared with the strata that admitted to non-adherence, the clofibrate adherence strata seemed to have improved survival. Yet exactly the same phenomenon was noted between adherers and non-adherers to the placebo! Readjustment of the Milan CMF adjuvant breast data has been done by dose, with the conclusion that the treatment was effective in prolonging relanse-free survival among post-menopausal patients who tolerated close to full dose (Bonadonna 1981). Here no placebo control exists, and it is possible certainly that the dose was critical. But doubt lingers.

Fourthly, when 'N' is discussed in the initial stages of planning a trial, the question usually is: 'How many patients will be needed to detect the predetermined delta at the specified alpha and beta risks?' But the question is not so simple. More appropriate might be: 'How many events (for example deaths) will have to occur?' Stochastic tests can be easily applied to proportions created by dividing the number of events (such as deaths) by the number of patients. But this would 'waste' any information contained in the time of the events.

Most modern clinical trials are analysed by an elegant 'non-parametric' test known as the log-rank test or one of its variants. (The choice of test may be important, and there are parametric, and 'semi-parametric' options available (Green 1974).) The log-rank test utilizes two measurements on each patient: whether he dies and when (if he has not died when the trial is being analysed he is censored and his survival time is credited to his treatment arm).

Unfortunately, the 'power' of the trial will depend to a far greater extent on the number of events than on the number of patients (Peto, Pike, Armitage, Brewlow, Cox, Howard, Mantel, McPherson, Peto, Smith 1977). So if 1000 patients are readily available for your trial, but only 1 per cent are expected to die or otherwise fail the treatment each year, even with a postulated 50 per cent delta between treatments, you might ask your statistical consultant: 'Will I still be alive when enough events have occurred?' After all, you have your curriculum vitae to consider.

Since events and their timing are both important in determining 'N', your planning must consider the shape and magnitude of the 'risk function', or 'hazard function'. Some interesting problems emerge from such a consideration. Many biological hazard functions have a graph shaped like a longitudinal slice of a bath tub (Gross and Clark 1975). A patient is at great risk the night before his radical surgery or just prior to his remission induction chemotherapy. If he survives the first few days or weeks his risk falls and levels off along the bottom of the curve. If several patients achieve this low plateau and the residual risk can be attributed to unrelated competing risks, a proportion of patients are said to be 'cured'. ('Cure' is another of those words simple in concept but complicated in practice (Frei and Gehan 1971; Osgood 1958).) Eventually though, the risk will go up again, if for no other reason than because of all the 'competing risks' that come with old age.

Of course, the shape of the hazard function may resemble a fish hook or a straight line, etc. Just as the Gaussian curve is not a law of nature when it comes to 'normality' (Elveback, Guiller, and Keating 1970), neither is any particular risk function always applicable.

The analysis of early, highly censored results may obscure a more important long-range effect by providing no information on the distance to and shape of the far end of the risk function. Worrying about the far end of the curve while planning an 'N' for a non-oat-cell lung cancer trial is currently quite absurd. The proximal end of the risk function is too high in an absolute sense and does not fall very rapidly, if at all, with any known treatment other than curative surgery. But the initial height and shape of the hazard function may be more important to patients than many cure-oriented physicians think. A treatment that improves 5-year survival when compared with a placebo may not be accepted by patients if the initial risk is too high (McNeil, Weichselbaum, and Pauker 1978).

On the other hand, with shallow hazard functions with long flat bottoms the distance to and shape of the far end may become the critical factor. In treatment of ovarian cancer with alkylating agents, for example, there is a sixtyfold increase in risk of acute leukaemia at two years (Reimer, Hoover, Fraumeni, and Young 1977). As these agents are applied more frequently in lower risk adjuvant settings, analysis of early returns, even in trials with huge numbers of patients, may be seriously misleading. This is particularly so if the results are based on censored 'disease-free' analyses. Multi-modality treatment of early seminoma, a disease of younger men, has become so successful that controversy has arisen over the risks and benefits of achieving high initial remission rates versus 'allowing' a proportion of early failures who can be salvaged later (Hubbard and Macdonald 1982). Problems such as this will be fruitful areas for the Bayesian decision analysts (Weinstein and Fineberg 1980).

A fifth tyranny of 'N' relates to a different number: the number of trials in progress. All trials are probably not equal in regard to their probability of publication or in their impact on opinion. Certainly the epidemiology of abstracts indicates a high rate of fatality prior to final publication (Goldman and Loscalzo 1980). Consider that you are an editor of a large prestigious journal. In a year 1200 small (that is fewer than 25 events) trial reports are submitted to you for publication. Assume that you 'know' that in 1000 of these trials no difference between the compared treatments exists. For the other 200 you 'know' that when 50 per cent of patients on one treatment are dead, only 33 per cent of the other group will be dead. Fifty of the 1000 trials where no difference exists will show a misleading 'significant' difference by chance alone (reflecting the alpha risk of 0.05), and only about 50 of the 200 trials where a true difference exists will result in a correct significant result (reflecting the very high beta, or false-negative risk of small trials (Freiman, Chalmers *et al.* 1978).

Thus, 200 of the trials will have misleading statistical conclusions, and only 100 will give 'significant' results (though half of these will be wrong). All this assumes no multiple peeks, retrospective stratification, or creative censoring. As the editor, which of the 1200 reports will you accept? You must attempt to grapple with the non-alpha, non-beta risks and make a situational decision.

The legalistic approach will not put an end to the tyranny of 'N', nor will it ensure objectivity. Perhaps what is needed is a re-emphasis of the 'bio' portion of biostatistics. New 'events' may be needed that may be difficult to measure, but more revealing (Sackett and Gent 1979). Staging systems based on clinical rather than anatomical considerations seem to have utility, at least for some cancers (Feinstein 1968). Preliminary attempts to use such 'events' as weight loss and deterioration in performance status have been made (Lad, Nelson, Diecamp *et al.* 1981). These may be particularly useful in assessing non-curative treatments, though formidable problems in ensuring objectivity remain.

The situation scientist neither accepts the 'curse of Kelvin' (Feinstein 1971; 'If you can't express it in numbers you don't understand it'), nor does he ridicule those who attempt to measure with the cynical comment of 'if you can't measure it, measure it anyway'. Indeed, the situation scientist would acknowledge that there may be a situation in which the 'milli-Helen' (that quantity of female beauty that is sufficient to launch exactly one ship) is the best objective measurement available.

Perhaps cancer therapists can borrow something of the methodology of the enologists (Amerine and Roessler 1976). They all start with the premise that the quality of the wine is in the glass, but this has not paralysed them into accepting the notion that objectivity is impossible (Gale 1975). They have defined their terms precisely, and standardized their judges. If a judge deems a wine 'too acetic' his threshold for that determination is known to be about 0.07 grams per 100 millilitres. This objectivity says nothing about whether people may or may not like their wines acetic. The enologists have also recognized the polarizing effect that group discussion can have, and that a few dominant people can sway opinion and destroy objectivity (Meyers and Lamb 1975).

Claude Bernard's *caveat* that a physician 'never makes experiments to confirm his ideas, but simply to control them' (Bernard 1956) is as applicable today as it was a hundred years ago. Fifty years ago people asked 'Is the statistical method of any value in medical research?' (Greenwood 1923). To speak of a possible tyranny of 'N' is not to denigrate the contributions of men like Mainland, Berkson, and Bradford Hill. If today people ask 'Is the clinical trial method of any value in cancer research?', we should remember the advice given by Bradford Hill twenty-five years ago: 'One must go seek more facts, paying less attention to technique of handling the data and far more to the development and perfection of methods of obtaining them' (Bradford Hill 1953). If this essay contains criticism of some current methods, that adversarial evaluation is only intended as what John Dewey put so succinctly: 'The end of criticism is the re-education of the perception of the work of art' (Dewey 1934).

Elsewhere in this volume experts have set down their solutions to many of the problems with cancer clinical trial methods. The stakes are high and situations vary, so all should recall the wisdom of Alfred North Whitehead: 'The simple-minded use of the notions "right or wrong" is one of the chief obstacles to the progress of understanding' (Whitehead 1968).

REFERENCES

Amerine, M. A. and Roessler, E. B. (1976). *Wines: their sensory evaluation.* Freeman, San Francisco.
Anon. (1981*a*). Merck clears hurdle in effort to market new medicine. *Wall St. J.* 29 *May*, 18.
—— *US* (1981*b*). Health panel urges disciplining of blood researcher. *Wall St. J.* 29 May, 18.
Bernard, C. (1956). *Introduction to experimental medicine.* Dover Reprint, New York.
Bonadonna, G. and Valagussa, P. (1981). Dose–response effect of adjuvant chemotherapy in breast cancer. *New Engl. J. Med.* **304**, 10–15.
Bradford Hill, A. (1953). Observation and experiment. *New. Engl. J. Med.* **248**, 995.
Brown, L. (1935). Robert Koch, an American Tribute. *Ann. med. Hist.* **7**, 385.
Chargaff, E. (1980). Knowledge without wisdom. *Harper's Magazine* May.
Coronary Drug Project Research Group. (1980). Influence of adherence to treatment

and response of cholesterol on mortality in the Coronary Drug Project. *New Engl. J. Med.* **303**, 1038.

DeVita, V. T., Cannellos, G., Hubbard, S. M., Chabner, B. and Young, R. (1976). Chemotherapy of Hodgkin's Disease with MOPP: a ten year progress report. *Proc. Am. Soc. clin. Oncol.* **17**, 269 (abstract).

—— Simon, R. M., Hubbard, S. M., *et al.* (1980). Curability of advanced Hodgkin's Disease. *Ann. intern. Med.* **92**, 587–95.

Dewey, J. (1934). *Art as experience.* Morton Balch, New York.

Elveback, L. R., Guiller, C. L., and Keating, F. R. (1970). Health, normality and the ghost of Gauss. *J. Am. med. Ass.* **211**, 69–75.

Farber, L. R., Prosnitz, L. R., Cadman, E. C., Lutes, R., Bertino, J. R., and Fischer, D. B. (1980). Curative potential of combined modality therapy for advanced Hodgkin's Disease. *Cancer* **46**, 1509–17.

Feinstein, A. R. (1968). A new staging system for cancer and a reappraisal of early treatment and cure by radical surgery. *New Engl. J. Med.* **279**, 747.

—— (1971*a*). Clinical biostatistics. X. Sources of transition bias in cohort statistics. *Clin Pharmac. Ther.* **12**, 704.

—— (1971*b*). On exorcizing the ghost of Gauss and the curse of Kelvin. *Clin Pharmac. Ther.* **12**, 1003.

—— (1973). Clinical biostatistics. XXIV: The role of randomization in sampling, testing, allocation, and credulous idolatry. *Clin Pharmac. Ther.* **14**, 1035.

Fletcher, J. (1956). *Situation ethics.* Westminster Press, Philadelphia.

Frei, E. and Gehan, E. A. (1971). Definition of cure for Hodgkin's Disease. *Cancer Res.* **31**, 1826–33.

Freiman, J. A., Chalmers, T. C., Smith, H. Jr., and Kuebler, R. R. (1978). The importance of beta, the type II error and sample size in the design and interpretation of the randomized control trial. *New Engl. J. Med.* **299**, 690–4.

Gale, G. (1975). Are some aesthetic judgements empirically true? *Am. phil. Q.* **12**, 341–8.

Goldman, L. and Loscalzo, A. (1980). Fate of cardiology research originally published in abstract form. *New Engl. J. Med.* **303**, 255–9.

Green, S. B. (1981). Randomized clinical trials: design and analysis. *Sem. Oncol.* **8**, 417–23.

Greenwood, M. (1923). Is the statistical method of any value in medical research? *Lancet* **ii**, 153–8.

Gross, A. J., and Clark, V. A. (1975). *Survival distributions.* Wiley, New York.

Hubbard, S. M., and MacDonald, J. S. (1982). An introduction to current controversies in cancer management: stage I testicular cancer—a case in point. *Cancer Treat. Rep.* **66**, 1–5.

James, W. (1976). *On pragmatism.* Harvard University Press, Cambridge, Massachusetts.

Kaplan, H. S. (1980). Hodgkin's Disease: unfolding concepts concerning its nature, management, and prognosis. *Cancer* **45**, 2439–74.

Lad, T., Nelson, R., Diecamp, D., Kukla, L. J., Sarma, P. R., Larson, C. S., Aurvie, E. T., Chawla, M. S., Tichler, T., Zavila, P., and McGuire, W. P. III. (1981). Immediate versus postponed combination chemotherapy for unresectable non-oat cell lung cancer. *Cancer Treat. Rep.* **65**, 1087, 973–8.

Levine, M. (1974). Scientific method and the adversary model. *Am. Psychol.* September, 666–77.

Linestone, H. A., and Turoff, M. (1975). *The Delphi Method: techniques and applications.* Addison–Welsley, Reading, Massachusetts.

McNeil, B. J., Weichselbaum, R., and Pauker, S. (1978). Fallacy of the five year survival in lung cancer. *New Engl. J. Med.* **299,** 1397–401.

Medawar, P. (1964). Is the scientific paper fraudulent? *Sat. Rev.* **47,** 42–3.

Merriam–Webster Dictionary. (1974). Springfield, Massachusetts.

Meyers, D. G., and Lamm, H. (1975). The polarizing effect of group discussion. *Am. Scient.* **63,** 297–303.

Osgood, E. E. (1958). Methods for analysing survival data illustrated by Hodgkin's Disease. *Am. J. Med.* **21,** 40–7.

Pachter, H. M. (1951). *Magic into science: the story of Paracelsus.* Henry Schuman, New York.

Peto, R., Pike, M., Armitage, P., Breslow, N. E., Cox, D. R., Howard, S. V., Mantel, N., McPherson, K., Peto, J., and Smith, P. G. (1977). Design and analysis of randomized clinical trials requiring prolonged observations of each patient. II. Analysis and examples. *Br. J. Cancer* **35,** 1–35.

Prentice, R. and Kalbfleisch, J. (1978). The analysis of failure times in the presence of competing risks. *Biometrics* **34,** 541–54.

Reimer, R. R., Hoover, R., Fraumeni, J. F. Jr. and Young, R. C. (1977). Acute leukemia after alkylating-agent therapy of ovarian cancer. *New Engl. J. Med.* **297,** 177–81.

Relman, A. S. (1980). Sulfinpyrazone after myocardial infarction: no decision yet. *New Engl. J. Med.* **303,** 1476.

Sackett, D. L. and Gent, M. (1979). Controversy in counting and attributing events in clinical trials. *New Engl. J. Med.* **301,** 1410–12.

Special Report. (1980). NIH consensus-development statement: adjuvant therapy of breast cancer. *New Engl. J. Med.* **303,** 831–2,

Twain, M. (1876). *Life on the Mississippi.* American Publishing Co., Cambridge, Massachusetts.

Weinstein, M. C., and Fineberg, H. V. (1980). *Clinical decision analysis.* Saunders, Philadelphia.

Whitehead, A. N. (1968). *Modes of thought.* The Free Press, Glencoe, Illinois.

2 Ethical considerations in controlled clinical trials

Henri J. Tagnon

INTRODUCTION

The French writer Paul Claudel used to say that the judgement between right and wrong as prescribed by moral law is ordinarily a simple matter with no perplexing alternatives although the practice of it may be difficult. This seems to be true of the moral principles which should govern the practice of medicine and in this instance the conduct of controlled clinical trials. Moral principles applied in a profession like medicine are usually called ethical principles or ethics, but the change in name does not change what is designated. Simply expressed the moral law of medicine is that the human being as an individual deserves first consideration, society exists for the individual and not the individual for society. This concept is acknowledged if not always applied in our type of civilization. The philosopher Kant (1848) has enunciated two principles which are the guidelines of what is considered moral behaviour: the first says : 'A person, yourself or someone else, should never be treated as a means to an end, but always as an end in himself.' The second is as important: 'Always act in every situation in such a way that your behaviour becomes a maxim of universal application.' Kant called these two principles 'categorical imperative', and he meant that the obligation they prescribe is compelling. To avoid controversy, we can perhaps consider these principles not only as prescriptions of conscience but more simply their observance as the very condition for civilized life as we understand it, their rejection leading inexorably and sometimes very quickly to the horrors of Nazi Germany, concentration camps, torture chambers, gulags, and other forms of profound and lethal diseases of society. Medicine and medical research exist for the betterment of health and should never become contributors to this moral disorder.

However there is a prescript of the special ethics of medicine which deserves careful consideration: it is the general obligation of the medical profession to advance medical knowledge in order to increase our means of curing disease. This obligation is particularly compelling for those of us who work in institutions supported by taxpayers' money and in university hospitals. Most patients rightly expect a research attitude and an optimistic outlook in their doctor. The students are entitled to receiving the stimulation from an intellectually active teacher who introduces them to the hope of a better future. These expectations create corresponding ethical obligations for the clinician and the teacher, and force him to consider how he can best discharge them and, at the same time, respect the general principles of moral behaviour.

COMPARATIVE CLINICAL TRIALS

Consider now the ethical question created by the therapeutic clinical trial and especially the comparative trial in which two or more treatments are compared, one of which is the standard treatment. Such comparisons are *scientifically* justified by the fact that in oncology only a slight improvement can usually be expected from a new treatment. It is uncommon that a new treatment will be strikingly superior to the standard treatment. Oncological therapeutic research progresses in small steps and the only method to demonstrate the superior effectiveness of a new treatment is the comparative clinical trial.

They are *ethically* justified provided the patient entered in the trial can reasonably expect or hope to derive a benefit from the experimentation and this condition results in the following three situations. Firstly, patients for whom existing treatments are ineffective are entitled to receive a new, experimental treatment, provided of course this new treatment has been adequately tested in the laboratory of experimental pharmacology or physiology. Secondly patients not responding well to the standard treatment of their disease should be given the opportunity represented by a potentially better treatment to be tested in comparison with the usual treatment. Thirdly, and in contrast with the previous situations, the physician should be very reserved about testing a new treatment of a disease which can be cured in a large proportion of cases with existing methods.

Simple examples of these three situations and the application of these rules are familiar to all oncologists. We know that the treatment of non-small-cell bronchial carcinoma is very unsatisfactory. Given this situation, it is ethically permissible and even recommended to enter patients with this diagnosis in clinical trials in order to fulfil the hope of the physician as well as of the patient to develop a better treatment. This same concept of the need for improvement should be extended to the group of patients whose disease responds favourably to treatment in a sizeable but still insufficient percentage of cases. For instance, 70 per cent of patients with breast cancer, all stages combined, eventually die of their disease. This is not acceptable.

Under these conditions, it can be considered unethical for the oncologist not to engage in clinical studies destined to improve the outlook. In this situation, the unjustified fear of experimenting with new methods would lead to an ethically improper inaction. Comparative randomized trials in generalized breast cancer have slowly improved the outlook for an increasing number of patients, and similar comparative randomized trials have brought about adjuvant treatments which are sometimes postponing recurrence of the disease and prolonging life. In this case also, a confident reliance on a sterile tradition is a disservice to the patient and represents an unethical attitude. The third situation is represented by Hodgkin's Disease. Although occasional remissions sometimes of long duration were obtained with older methods, imaginative, and ethically commendable experimentation has improved the prognosis of this disease to the point where experimentation has now become hazardous since further amelioration of the present results appears difficult. Yet there is still room for progress and new and better treatments should be tested on the small group of non-responders or resistant patients.

A most important condition should be observed in therapeutic research in humans: especially in the field of oncology, research should be sophisticated with up-to-date methodology and with the considerable logistic and statistical support often required in comparative trials. Clinical research cannot be ethical if it is not scientifically acceptable. Particular care should be taken in the planning and execution of the project to arrive at a scientifically valid conclusion with the smallest possible number of patients. Inadequate experimentation leading to results that cannot be interpreted forces a repetition of the trial. Thus a larger than necessary number of patients become involved and interpretation of new results is rendered more difficult. New and sometimes formidable ethical problems are created by scientific failure. A good example of the exposure of an unnecessarily large number of patients to experimental therapy is represented by the numerous inconclusive trials of the effect of anticoagulation on myocardial infarctions (Chalmers, Matta, Smith, and Kunzler 1977).

McGuire (1980) rightly says of medical practice in general: 'For the practice of medicine to be ethical it must be scientific . . . Unscientific medicine . . . is deceitful and immoral.' This statement is true also in the case of the comparative clinical trial. I have stated the same view at a meeting in Brussels: 'One of the ethical exigencies of human therapeutic research is that it should be of high scientific standard. Bad research is always unethical; only good research can be ethical. Scientific morality is part of general morality' (Tagnon 1975).

RANDOMIZED TRIALS

Randomization of patients between two or more treatments for purposes of comparison and control has been discussed abundantly in the literature. Certain investigators have disputed the necessity of randomization and asserted that historical controls, taken from past publications or past unpublished observations may be adequate for comparison under certain conditions. The two opposing views were presented in great detail in a symposium organized by Lortat-Jacob, Mathé and Servier (1978). Gehan

(1978) favours historial controls from selected past studies for practical and ethical reasons, although his position is not absolute. He quotes Atkins (1966) who states that a randomized clinical trial may be considered ethical if the statistician would be willing to have himself or a close member of his family entered into it. However this is not necessarily a sound basis for judgement, as reassuring to the statistician as it may be. The ethical evaluation of a comparative trial should be based on objective criteria. The evolution of ideas on medical practice and experimentation is in the direction of gradually replacing purely subjective attitudes by reasonably assessed moral values which include feelings and emotions among the many other elements of judgement.

Another opinion underlines the diversity of attitudes: Israël (1978) thinks that randomized trials 'are an outdated tool no longer adapted to what is known about cancer today'. However the majority of investigators are in favour of the randomized trial. Although the methodology of clinical trials is not the subject of this chapter, it is impossible to dissociate scientific from ethical considerations and different methods of evaluation carry different ethical problems. This is clearly shown in the studies on anticoagulation and mortality from myocardial infarction, some of which used historical controls and some randomized controls. The reader is referred to the original text of Peto (1978) for this discussion.

If one uses historical controls, all patients under investigation receive the new treatment. If this turns out to be less active or more toxic than the standard treatment, all patients will receive the inferior treatment. On the other hand, in a randomized study of a new inferior treatment only one-half of the patients will receive the less active or more toxic treatment. The ethical choice seems to be in favour of the randomized trial in this case. Other considerations have been added in favour of randomization; they are excellently expressed by Cochrane, St. Léger, and Sweetnam (1979). The comparative clinical trial is of particular value when the new treatment is only slightly superior (or inferior) to the standard treatment. In this case the design of the trial is scientifically and ethically important for the demonstration of this difference and an unbiased evaluation can only be obtained by randomizing patients between the two treatments. When a new treatment is clearly and obviously superior to its predecessors, then randomization is unnecessary and should not be done. But this is an uncommon occurrence.

In controlled clinical trials, the control treatment is represented by the best available standard treatment of the disease under study. It is not permissible ethically to deprive a fraction of patients with potentially lethal or irreversibly invalidating diseases from an effective treatment. Therefore the use of *placebos* as control treatment is prohibited except under certain conditions, for instance in research on the treatment of pain when this is not too severe and not associated with a disabling disease. It is well known that a placebo may be an effective treatment of certain types of pain in certain patients and this fact justifies the use of placebos in this type of study. The use of placebos is necessary and ethically acceptable also as control treatment in the study of adjuvant therapy in the form of chemotherapy or radiotherapy administered after the local treatment of the primary tumour. An adjuvant treatment is justified for tumours in which the primary treatment is notoriously insufficient to cure a majority of the patients. This is the case for breast cancer patients, the majority of whom eventually die of their disease, regardless of the type of primary treatment they received (Mueller, Ames, and Anderson 1978). But adjuvant treatment does not seem justified for tumours which are curable by the primary treatment or whose rare recurrences are easily and effectively treated when they appear: this is the case for testicular tumours at all stages. Adjuvant chemotherapy has unpleasant and potentially toxic side-effects which should not be inflicted without a clear necessity, and the definite hope that the patients will benefit from it. Thus adjuvant treatment consists of drugs or therapeutic procedures which have proved effective in producing regressions of established metastases of the tumour under study. For instance, the adjuvant treatment of breast cancer consists of the administration of either melphalan or the combination endoxan-methotrexate-5-fluorouracil with or without tamoxifen, because each of these two treatments are effective in the treatment of established metastatic breast disease. Untested innovative chemotherapy has no place in a programme of adjuvant therapy.

Double-blind technique

This does not introduce special ethical problems provided the results obtained in the randomized double-blind study are regularly reviewed by a committee of physicians not participating in the study, and who are able to evaluate toxic or other undesirable effects and to issue warnings to the investigators during the course of the trial.

TESTING ESTABLISHED TREATMENTS

A special case is represented by the testing in a comparative trial of a treatment which has been in general use for some time and is part of current general practice. Such testing should be done. All presently employed but untested treatments should be progressively re-evaluated using up-to-date method-ology. There are now several examples of generally accepted treatments administered to thousands of patients which have been found by objective testing to be ineffective or even harmful. Such was the case for the high dosage of synthetic oestrogens used in cancer of the prostate (Veterans Administration Cooperative Urological Research Group 1967). Another more recent example is the controlled trial of clofibrate which produced disturbing results, demonstrating an increase in mortality which was not anticipated (Committee of Principal Investigators 1978). There are many others and this makes one wonder whether the concern about the ethics of present-day medical practice should not be shifted from the controlled clinical trial to the everyday practice of medicine, in the private office or the hospital. No doubt physicians will feel more and more ethically involved when they administer untested treatments which still represent a very sizeable part of present-day therapeutics. This increased sense of responsibility is certainly the result of the widespread use of comparative clinical trials which have given the ethics of medicine a new dimension.

PROTOCOL ADHERENCE

Granted that the randomized controlled trial is more ethical there are a few questions in need of an answer. For instance, what is to be done when moderately strong, but not decisive, evidence begins to emerge in the course of the trial in favour of one treatment? Should one stop the comparative trial? Actually the investigators are not supposed to know the partial results collected during the course of the trial. On the other hand, few physicians would acccept to continue giving a new treatment without having information on its favourable or unfavourable effects. The way out of this difficulty is to appoint a small committee of competent physicians not participating in the trial, but having access to the results at any time during the trial. They are given the task of ruling that the trial be continued or interrupted.

However, stopping a trial before a statistically significant result is obtained, and on the basis of a trend which could become reversed with a continuation of the trial, is not an ethically indifferent decision. The lack of a firm conclusion will lead to new trials and the involvement of more patients receiving an untested treatment. There are deplorable examples of such a chain of events (Chalmers *et al.* 1977) confirming the ethical obligation, with some restrictions, to conduct a comparative trial to a firm conclusion with the smallest possible number of patients.

The restrictions are that it is impossible and undesirable to ignore the feelings of a physician participating in a trial. If, despite the fact that he is a co-author of the protocol of treatment, he feels that a particular patient should receive another treatment than the one scheduled for him by the randomiz-ation, then the patient should be withdrawn from the trial and receive whatever treatment his physician thinks best. The decision to give a patient a treatment out of protocol must be obeyed even if it is irrational. We have had the experience in a comparative trial on squamous-cell bronchial cancer of a physician who refused to omit the administration of corticoids, an omission clearly recommended in the protocol. His reason was that he was 'convinced' that corticoids are beneficial, this in the face of evidence provided by a recently terminated excellent trial which showed the lack of benefit from the administration of corticoids in this condition. Physicians with irrational requirements of this kind should probably not participate in clinical trials or should be admitted in the group as non-participating observers until they mature sufficiently to become active participants. It goes without saying that a patient should never be denied a clearly indicated treatment when circumstances not anticipated in the protocol command it. Disruption of the protocol can never be invoked against this decision which belongs entirely to the responsible physician.

INFORMED CONSENT

Informed consent is differently understood in different countries. Patient care in a controlled clinical trial which benefits the individual patient does not, in my opinion, require a different relationship between doctor and patient than the one prevalent in ordinary medical practice. The modern everyday practice of medicine is moving toward a less authoritarian and a more confiding relationship between physician and patient, and it has become acceptable and customary to explain a treatment to the patient and obtain his agreement. In the case of a novel treatment, for instance in a controlled clinical trial, this mutual confidence should come into play and because of the novelty, the doctor should obtain the patient's agreement as required by good general practice. It is wise also when applying such novel treatment alone to ask the opinion of experienced colleagues on the advisability of testing this new treatment on this particular patient. These considerations apply also in the case of patients treated experimentally under a protocol of treatment by a group of physicians.

One of the functions of the detailed protocol of treatment used in every clinical trial is to describe without ambiguity the therapeutic procedures and methods of evaluation of results, thereby avoiding uncertainty in the conversation with the patient. The mode of production of a protocol, by an open discussion in a group of investigators is a solid if not perfect guarantee that ethical requirements will be taken into account. This consideration strongly suggests that new treatments should be a group undertaking rather than an individual's initiative and the patient should probably be made aware of this.

The Medical Research Council (1962) has published an excellent and short report on the *Responsibility in investigations on human subjects*. This report also discussed the ethical and legal implications of procedures applied to an individual when not of potential benefit to him. It correctly points out that the benefit to humanity or posterity would afford no defence in the event of legal proceedings. There is some question in my mind whether informed consent, if obtained in this situation, makes this type of procedure ethically acceptable and whether an individual's consent gives permission to the investigator to carry out an experiment not of potential benefit to the patient. The report of the Medical Research Council suggests that it does. However I think that if the procedure is dangerous or potentially disabling, informed consent does not relieve the investigator of his responsibility. Therefore particular attention should be paid to the possible consequences of procedures not of direct benefit to the individual and abstention is advised when there is the least doubt about the consequences. The Medical Research Council does not take a firm stand on the question of informed consent. It adopts the common-sense attitude that good medical practice implies a frank and open discussion of the treatment with the patient whether the treatment is experimental or not.

Many clinicians are of the opinion that informed consent cannot be a general rule in therapeutic investigative medicine. The surgical unit at St. Mary's Hospital in London writes: 'When the relative frequency of death is the arbiter of success or failure, and this result can only be applied to future generations of patients, then the need for a randomized controlled trial should be established beyond doubt and, if it is, then the nature of informed consent should not necessarily involve the patient in the decision making' (Fielding, Blesovsky, and Stewart-Brown 1979).

Peto (1978) is more outspoken about informed consent and calls it a 'legalistic trick to devolve what should properly be the doctor's responsibilities onto the patient. It may serve a useful purpose in warding off American lawyers, but in less litigious countries it is not necessary *unless the doctor concerned feels it to be so*' (my italics).

In contrast with the above considerations, the Code of Federal Regulations (1978) entitled *Protection of human subjects* make it mandatory for all recipients or prospective recipients of DHEW[2.1] support to obtain informed consent from all patients included in clinical trials. The mode and form of obtaining and recording informed consent is described in every detail in this Code which should be consulted by all investigators to whom it applies. Since this is a Code of Federal Regulations and therefore has the meaning of a law, investigators are under obligation to observe it although this has been recently disputed (Durant 1981).

Zelen (1979), a statistician with a wide experience in the organization of clinical trials, analyses the factors which make randomized trials the most effective form of clinical investigation of therapy. He also reviews the reasons which make investigators and patients sometimes reluctant to participate in such trials, one of the reasons being the obligation of informed consent and of informing the patient about all risks and benefits, the alternative treatments available, and the patient's right to withdraw at any time. If the patient has to be informed of the choice by randomization of the treatment he receives, he may interpret this as 'a treatment by a computer'. The patient's physician knows that randomization is ethical only if he believes that all treatments under study are potentially equally effective but he finds it difficult to tell his patient that he does not know which treatment is best. For these and other reasons Zelen thinks that 'there is a serious concern that the federal

[2.1] Department of Health, Education, and Welfare, USA.

regulations governing informed patient consent may be unrealistic in practice'. He proposes a new way to plan randomized clinical trials. The original article should be read for the details of this new method which does not directly concern our ethical preoccupation. However, Zelen discusses in detail the ethical implications of this and other forms of randomization, and this discussion is pursued in editorial comments in the same issue of the *New England Journal of Medicine*. In one of the editorials the author reaffirms the often forgotten notion that entering a patient in a randomized trial is permitted only if a proved method of treatment is not withheld from the patient. In other terms the two or more forms of treatment under scrutiny should be potentially of approximately equal effectiveness and one of them, the control, should be the best standard treatment (Curran 1979).

In another editorial (Fost 1979), the author concludes that consent is often no more than a ritual function, leaving the patient no more informed or autonomous than he would have been if no information had been disclosed. Yet efforts should be continued in order to find a solution and keep the patient informed without making his life as a patient difficult, or even intolerable.

My position is that the physician should evaluate the amount of information each individual patient can tolerate and how much responsibility in the decision he is able to assume without excessive anxiety and fear. Whatever the patient cannot assume should be taken by the physician upon himself. In other words, the emotional impact of decisions about disease and treatment should not be transferred too lightly from the physician to the patient under the pretext of obtaining informed consent. The impact should be shared, and the physician's participation should be greater whenever the patient's emotional conformation lessens his possibilities of participating. This duty is exacting for the doctor but to be a physician is to accept such obligations. There are physicians of great professional competence but unable themselves to emotionally withstand the distress of their patients. These physicians should probably not participate in controlled clinical trials. Obviously, when the law or an administrative regulation requires informed consent in clinical trials, the physician has no choice and should obey the regulation.

The physician's obligation in medical practice and in clinical research has been best expressed by Francis Weld Peabody (1930), a famous physician: 'The secret of the care of the patient is to care for the patient'. There is probably no better answer to the ethical questions posed by medical practice.

SOME TRENDS IN THE PRESENT DAY EVALUATION OF MEDICAL ETHICS

The introduction of controlled clinical trials on a large scale in the last twenty, and especially the last ten years represents a revolution in clinical investigation and has altered considerably the study of clinical pharmacology and the mode of introduction of new methods of treatment. This has been striking particularly in therapeutic oncology but it has affected all sections of medical practice. As a result there has developed an increasing interest in the ethical problems associated with this type of clinical investigation (Fried 1974). This is certainly a welcome development, but one may wonder why such ethical preoccupation was less prevalent in the practice of medicine before or outside controlled clinical trials. In the office or hospital practice of medicine where no research is carried out, the opportunities for ethical infractions could be more numerous than in the practice of a group of physicians carrying out a controlled clinical trial following a carefully prepared protocol and able to watch each other in open discussion. Certainly the honest but isolated physician, by the very fact of his isolation encounters less opposition to his administration of useless, if not harmful, medication than if he were in a group. I am not here indicting the private practice of medicine, but just mentioning that probably patients have never enjoyed as much protection and good care based on the science of medicine as the patients entered in clinical trials. Therefore the ethical preoccupation with these trials is quite legitimate, but a similar preoccupation should be extended to the other forms of medical practice with the same interests and passions that are addressed to the controlled clinical trials, whatever the method of control is.

Medical ethics is not a new invention. It is just the old morality applied to a situation—medical research—which is in fast evolution and presents us with puzzling circumstances. Among these are the controlled clinical trials but these are less puzzling than many others like abortion, the new genetics, euthanasia, etc. We oncologists are lucky, our problem is relatively simple (Clouser 1975; Dunphy 1976).

Some of the new trends in the increasing interest in medical ethics are listed in Fox (1974). Her article contains an extensive bibliography of the bioethical literature. Another useful survey of the recent literature on the ethics of medicine has been performed by Jonsen, Cassel, Lo, and Perkins (1980). It is remarkable that these problems are no longer entirely within the jurisdiction of the medical profession but involve sociologists, philosophers, theologians, lawyers, religious ministers, and also the public at large. This may be a desirable development if kept within reasonable bounds in order to allow the physicians and health personnel to continue to assume responsibility for the care of the patients. A noteworthy initiative has been the study of public judgements regarding ethical issues in medical research by the Center for the Study of Drug Development, at the University of Rochester Medical Center, which published a progress report in August 1978. This study's main conclusion is that the public is very interested by clinical trials for the improvement of the treatment of diseases and has maintained its confidence in the medical profession.

Finally, Freireich (1981) has advocated novel methods for conducting trials and has pointed out that the method for doing clinical research is itself an area of research. His department is active in studying the possibilities offered by new methods. The last word obviously has not been said on the scientific methodology of clinical research and, just as obviously, it has not been said on its ethical aspects.

REFERENCES

Atkins, H. (1966). Conduct of a controlled clinical trial. *Br. med. J.* **ii,** 377.

Center for the Study of Drug Development, University of Rochester Medical Center, Rochester, New York. Report August 1978.

Chalmers, T. C., Matta, R. J., Smith, H., and Kunzler, A. M. (1977). Evidence favouring the use of anticoagulants in the hospital phase of acute myocardial infarction. *New Engl. J. Med.* **302,** 351.

Clouser, K. D. (1975). Medical ethics: some uses, abuses and limitations. *New Engl. J. Med.* **293,** 384–7.

Cochrane, A. L., St. Léger, A. S., and Sweetnam, P. (1979). Letter to the Editor. *Br. med. J.* **1,** 486.

Code of Federal Regulations. (1978). *45 CFR 46 and certain other related laws and regulations on protection of human subjects,* revised 11 January. PPR Reports, DHEW.

Committee of Principal Investigators. (1978). A cooperative trial in the primary prevention of ischaemic heart disease using clofibrate. *Br. heart J.* **40,** 1069–118.

Curran, W. J. (1979). Reasonableness and randomization in clinical trials: fundamental law and governmental regulation. *New Engl. J. Med.* **300,** 1273–5.

Dunphy, J. E. (1976). On caring for the patient with cancer. *New Engl. J. Med.* **295,** 313.

Durant, J. R. (1981). Science, ethics and due process. *Ann. Intern. Med.* **95,** 116–17.

Fielding, L. P., Blesovsky, L., and Stewart-Brown, S. (1979). Letter to the Editor. *Br. med. J.* **2,** 486–7.

Fost, N. (1979). Consent as a barrier to research. *New Engl. J. Med.* **300,** 1272–3.

Fox, R. C. (1974). Ethical and existential developments in contemporaneous American medicine: their implications for culture and society. *Melbank Mem. Fund Q. Health Soc.* (Fall) 445–83.

Freireich, E. J. (1981). *Presidential address.* ASCO Minutes 17th Meeting 1 May. Washington DC.

Fried, C. (1974). *Medical experimentation: personal integrity and social policy.* North Holland, Amsterdam.

Gehan, A. (1978). Comparative clinical trials with historical controls: a statistician's view. *Biomedicine* (Special Issue) **28,** 13–18.

Israël, L. (1978). Practical and conceptual limitations of best conceived randomized trials. *Biomedicine* (Special Issue) **28,** 36–9.

Jonsen, R. A., Cassel, C., Lo, B., and Perkins, H. S. (1980). The ethics of medicine: an annotated bibliography of recent literature. *Ann. intern. Med.* **92,** 136–41.

Kant, E. (1848). *Critique de la raison pratique,* pp. 58, 71. Lagrange, Paris.

Lortat-Jacob, J. L., Mathé, G., and Servier, J. (1978). International meeting on comparative therapeutic trials. *Biomedicine* (Special issue) **28,** 2–63.

Medical Research Council Report. (1962). *Responsibility in investigations on human subjects.* Cmnd. 2382, pp. 21–5. Medical Research Council, London.

McGuire Jr., H. H. (1980). Letter to the Editor. *New Engl. J. Med.* **302,** 351.

Mueller, C. B., Ames, F. and Anderson, G. D. (1978). Breast cancer in 3558 women:

age as a significant determinant in the rate of dying and causes of death. Surgery **83,** 123–33.

Peabody, F. W. (1930). *Doctor and patient.* MacMillan, New York.

Peto, R. (1978). Clinical trial methodology. *Biomedicine* (Special Issue) **28,** 24–35.

Tagnon, H. (1975). L'expérimentation en médecine: aspects éthiques. *Belgian Society of Medical Ethics and Morality. Proceedings of a meeting in March 1975*, pp. 27–30. Imprimerie Médicale et Scientifique, Brussels.

Veterans Administration Cooperative Urological Research Group. (1967). Treatment and survival of patients with cancer of the prostate. *Surgery Gynec. Obstet.* **124,** 1011–17.

Zelen, M. (1979). A new design for randomized clinical trials. *New Engl. J. Med.* **300,** 22, 1242–5.

3 Evaluating 'quality of life' in cancer clinical trials

Frits S. A. M. van Dam, Corrie A. G. Linssen, and Adèle L. Couzijn

Quality . . . you know what it is, yet you don't know what it is. But that's self-contradictory. But some things *are* better than others, that is, they have more quality. But when you try to say what the quality is, apart from the things that have it, it all goes *poof!* There's nothing to talk about. (Pirsig 1976)

INTRODUCTION

The Achilles' heel of many trials is possibly to be found in the criteria used in the evaluation of the trial's outcome. In clinical studies, too much accent is placed on success criteria that have been developed in the laboratory using experimental animals: passive recipients of a drug (Rose 1976). However the situation is different when human beings are involved. As Rose put it, 'We should describe therapies as part of a system which includes the drug, the doctor prescribing it, the individual taking it, and his or her environment.' And Bleehen (1980) states in a review article on the management of non-small-cell lung carcinoma by radio therapy and chemotherapy: 'Even when used appropriately by skilled practitioners, adverse effects can occur. It is therefore important to assess the value of all such treatments not only in conventional terms of survival, which is usually short, but also in terms of palliation of existing symptoms and the general quality of life.' If this is taken seriously, we should reconsider the way data are analysed, and use techniques by means of which it is possible to judge the outcome of a trial on a broad range of criteria—biochemical, physiological, and behavioural.

The central concept used in connection with behavioural indices is 'quality of life'. Bardelli and Saracci (1978) conducted a literature survey concerning the frequency with which 'quality of life' was measured in six major cancer journals. Their conclusion was that 'quality of life' is taken into account only rarely. The way the term 'quality' is used suggests that it refers to an investigation of a consumers' organization in which certain products are evaluated; in this case 'life'. However absurd it may seem, it may not be such an inadequate analogue. Let us have a look at how a consumers' organization defines the quality of products. Recently in The Netherlands an investigation of the quality of breast prostheses was carried out. Prostheses were evaluated with regard to the number of sizes available, comfort in wearing, figure correction, durability, skin irritation, etc. The various aspects were given a different weight and together led to a final conclusion. Obviously nothing in general can be said about breast prostheses, only something about their attributes. In other words, one defines the value of an object by defining its attributes. Let us go back now to the concept 'quality of life'. As prostheses in general cannot be evaluated, 'life' in general cannot be evaluated. The best one can do is to evaluate a number of aspects of a patient's life. Which aspects depend very much on the research questions at hand, the group of patients, and the kind of therapy. Besides, certain aspects are more important for one group than for another. Just think of the problems of patients with a colostomy which specifically pertain to stoma care and social and sexual problems, as compared with the problems of patients with advanced breast cancer who are being treated with cytostatic drugs.

It is not very surprising that Jansen (1979), scanning the literature from a computer search (revealing about one hundred articles published between 1974 and 1979, with the concept 'quality of life' as a keyword) concluded that the concept 'quality of life' is quite polymorphous. It refers to such varied topics as physical and psychological complaints, feelings of well-being, sexual functioning, and general activities (for example going to work or school); and each author claims that that particular area represents 'quality of life'. It seems prudent to abandon this term altogether to permit precision in discussion.

We thus agree with Alexander and Willems (1981) who state that to obtain an accurate indication of 'quality of life', the measurements must include quantifiable indices of what people do, where they do it, with whom they do it, and how they do it. Measurements of this sort constitute the minimum requirements for assessing 'quality of life'. The best one can say about the concept 'quality of life' is that it indicates an important field of enquiry, but to use it in research is rather misleading.

MEASUREMENT PROBLEMS

A starting point in this review is the notion that in measuring psychosocial consequences of cancer therapies, the nomothetic approach is required. Nomothetic measurement simply means the measurement of the same property in all subjects. Obviously the same attribute must be measured in all subjects regardless of the treatment arm. The nomothetic approach is in contrast to the idiographic approach, the study and interpretation of the particular individual, which is of course of great value as a source of ideas, as a reminder of the complexity of the individual personality (for example, how he copes with his illness and treatment). In clinical trials we are interested in patients in general or in patients of a particular kind. The study of the individual cannot be an end in itself but only a means to a larger objective (Fiske 1971).

In his paper 'Evaluation of toxicity: statistical considerations', Herson (1980) poses a number of questions with regard to the evaluation of 'somatic' toxicity in phase III trials which also pertain to psychosocial toxicity. He differentiates between general and specific toxicity. While the general questions are the same for all trials, the specific questions depend upon the design of the trial. With regard to general toxicity a further difference is made between the description of toxicity and the aetiology of toxicity. He also makes a plea for the use of a toxicity index as, for example, white blood cell count as an index for leukopenia. He formulates several requirements an index should meet, such as: an index should be relatively uncorrelated with other toxicity indices, indices should be robust to occasional missing data and occasional extreme values, etc.

Fiske (1971) makes a strong plea for the use of indices in psychosocial research. He defines an index as follows: a quantity or score assigned to a person on the basis of several responses and taken to represent the degree to which he possesses an attribute. Much of the confusion in psychosocial oncology research would be solved if we could develop several psychosocial indices, generally applicable in a large number of trials. Besides those indices individual researchers could then create measures suited for specific trials.

The term 'measure' as used here refers to a data-collecting device to assist in the process of obtaining observations in a manner that allows for quantification, e.g. a questionnaire, a paper and pencil test, an interview, an observation protocol, a rating scale or a mechanical instrument (Ward 1977).

In contrast to the medical sciences, the social sciences have not yet produced measures valid, reliable, and feasible enough to be used routinely in cancer clinical trials. Also no data are available on other groups of patients or on non-patient groups with which the scores of cancer patients may be compared. Therefore, the routine application of behavioural measures in clinical trials is, as yet, met with many problems. What can and must be done is to use clinical trials in developing these measures, something which is possible only in close co-operation with clinicians. What follows will be not so much an overview of what has been accomplished thus far, which is rather meagre indeed (Schmale 1980), but a kind of inventory of problems to be solved before behavioural measures can be applied in clinical trials and, more important still, before clinicians can draw conclusions from these measures concerning the therapies they give.

Validity

Given that we are interested in measuring anxiety or malaise in a trial, how do we know whether we are actually measuring anxiety or malaise? This kind of question pertains to 'validity'. Validity may thus be defined as: 'the extent to which a test measures the variable or concept it is intended to measure' (Fiske 1971). Questions regarding validity are considered as crucial in the behavioural sciences; therefore a lot of work is done to find indications of the validity of measures in the behavioural sciences. An example of the laborious work in validating a measure is given below.

At the Dutch Cancer Institute a so-called 'complaint questionnaire' has been in use now for several years. From research (Linssen, Hanewald, and van Dam 1981) it appeared that patients treated with different kinds of chemotherapy or radiotherapy, who reported many complaints, also indicated that they felt more ill, needed to rest more during the day, were hindered more in their daily activities, and used more kinds of medicine than those patients reporting fewer complaints on this questionnaire. It is of importance to find out whether an instrument actually measures the expected differences between groups and points of measurement. As to the 'complaint questionnaire' it has been shown that this list differentiates well between patients treated with chemotherapy and controls. Also periods of rest can be clearly discerned from injection periods. It is also important to know that an instrument does not correlate with variables it is not supposed to measure. In a study of 20 patients with advanced testicular cancer (Couzijn, Bokkel Huinink, van Dam, and Hanewald 1982), treated with combination chemotherapy, only a very slight correlation was found between the complaints and a neuroticism score. This may be regarded as an indication that this questionnaire measures something other than neuroticism. Also no correlation existed between the number of complaints and social class.

There is a problem in cancer research with regards to existing instruments. Most of the instruments have not been validated for cancer patients and certainly not for cancer patients receiving treatment. As we are not dealing with psychiatric patients but with 'normal' people under heavy stress, most instruments do not apply. For instance, Beck's depression inventory does not take into account the physical complaints cancer patients have due to their illness and treatment, therefore, in order to get a proper idea of depression in cancer patients, items which pertain to complaints, such as fatigue and anorexia (Plumb and Holland 1977) should be omitted. Stewart (1980) states: 'As in depression, it is preferable to assess anxiety in terms of affect so as not to confound it with symptoms of illness. This means that almost all anxiety scales have to be adapted or new ones have to be developed if one is interested in measuring anxiety in cancer patients.'

As Barofsky (1981) concluded: 'Assessment instruments which include components that could yield false-positive responses (responses to items that may involve disease-dependent bodily dysfunctions) have the potential to be confounded when used to assess the psychiatric, psychological or social status of the cancer patient.'

For a more extensive discussion on validity one is referred to some of the excellent textbooks available (for example Cronbach 1970; Fiske 1971; Anastasi 1976).

Reliability

Reliability refers to the extent to which scores derived by a specific instrument, can repeatedly be obtained over time and/or across raters. It is essential to have some idea of the reliability of measures, otherwise no generally applicable conclusions can be drawn. In the social sciences reliability is a topic which takes as central a place in measurement problems as does validity.

The observation scale most currently in use in cancer research, the Karnofsky rating scale, has low reliability coefficients (Hutchinson, Boyd and Feinstein 1979; Yates, Chalmer, and McKegney 1980) and should be used only if its users are properly trained and controlled. In contrast, the reliability of self-assessment instruments seems to be quite satisfactory. For the 'complaint questionnaire' in use at the Dutch Cancer Institute, 88 per cent of the items of the questionnaire, completed at two (similar) points of measurement, were scored identically. Priestman and Baum (1976) found test–retest correlations for their test of 0.73. Pecararo, Inui, Chen, Plorde, and Heller (1979) found test–retest agreement of 90 per cent.

Norms

A score on a test only has significance as compared with other test scores; in itself it is meaningless. In cancer research one would have to know (a) at which point in treatment the measure was used, (b) how patients with the same disease, without treatment do on the same test, and possibly (c) what the scores are of a similar population (age, sex) but without any disease. It would be of great help if we had the scores of a number of patient groups, under different therapeutic regimens on the tests we apply in trials. Unfortunately little such data are available at present.

In the case of phase II trials it might be useful to work with so-called difference scores to obtain an estimation of the changes brought about by the treatment, even though from a psychometric point of view the use of difference scores is controversial. However, in the case of randomized trials it will not be necessary to use pre-treatment measurements and difference scores (although it might be very useful to have an idea of pre-treatment levels) as it may be assumed that pre-treatment levels are equal in all arms of a randomized trial.

Time span

Herson (1980) states that in order to evaluate toxicity it is important to be precise about the treatment periods. He states that a trial should be divided into time periods which correspond to important treatment events. One of the fundamental challenges would be to summarize toxicity during each period. This has serious implications for the time period to which the questions the patients are asked apply. For instance, in almost every course of chemotherapy two periods generally can be distinguished: a period during which the immediate effects of the drug are at hand—nausea, fatiguability, etc.—and a period of rest during which a patient recovers from these short-term effects.

There are several arguments to limit the time period over which one is questioning the patient. Asking questions over the last month, even the last week, will certainly lead to confusion on the part of the patient over which period exactly he is reporting. Research concerning the difference between vague and clear questions gives further support to limit the time-span over which one is questioning. When asked a vague question like: 'how tired were you in general, or during the last two or four weeks?', it has been shown that what is obtained from the subjects is a tendency to complain. If one looks closely into questionnaires which measure neuroticism, that is the one thing they all have in common: they give the subjects the opportunity to complain (van den Aardweg 1981). The more precisely that the question is phrased, the smaller the chance that neuroticism or a tendency to complain is measured. Since in most trials we are not so much interested in measuring neuroticism as we are in the nature of psychosocial toxicity, it is of the utmost importance to put the questions as clear as possible. Hence our plea to limit the time-span of the questions to one day preferably. Of course there are some disadvantages in using one day only. Firstly one may be capitalizing too much on accidental events which took place that day (that day usually being the day before going to the hospital for treatment) although haphazard events will generally be the same for the groups compared in the trial if these groups are large enough. Secondly certain topics are not relevant when questioned over one day, for example attitude towards illness.

As an illustration, the reader is advised to do a brief experiment in order to appreciate the difference and importance of being accurate about time-spans, namely to try to answer for himself questions like 'how tired were you?', 'did you have a headache?', 'did you feel miserable?', over several time periods.

Feasibility

In most articles which have appeared on measuring 'quality of life', no mention is made of the difficulties encountered in the practical application of measures. The following observations, made at the Dutch Cancer Institute, possibly apply in general.

1. Co-operation of patients. Standardized psychosocial measures are uncommon in almost all hospitals. Therefore, in our experience, a specially trained medical secretary or nurse should take care whenever a patient is to be

tested, that, for example, the questionnaires are available, that they are actually completed and handed in, etc.

2. We have found hardly any patients to have trouble taking a test due to neuropsychological complications. Barofsky (1981) states: 'In studies of most types of cancer the psychomotor or intellectual functioning of cancer patients should not impair the validity of standardized assessment instruments.'

3. Measures should not be too extensive, otherwise patients will become annoyed. In our experience a frequently applied test should certainly take no longer than 15 to 20 minutes.

4. Frequency of measuring should not be too high, since otherwise the patients will become careless in completing the test. A frequency of once a week should be considered too high. We found once every 4 or 5 weeks to be feasible.

5. The purpose of the measure or test must be explained carefully: in the first place because patients have a right to know why they are asked to complete a test, secondly because patients may get the idea that the test is used to decide upon their therapy and therefore they will possibly fake for the good, for example by listing fewer complaints than they actually have.

6. Quite a number of patients are not accustomed to filling out a paper and pencil test and become uneasy about it. If possible a nurse or secretary should be present while the patient is completing the test. Also it is advisable that the test be devised in such a way that it can be answered verbally instead of in writing. Alexander and Willems (1981) state that recent work demonstrates that data can be obtained reliably by having patients record their own behaviour in a diary-like format or by means of a structured interview, either face to face or by telephone. Irwin, Gottlieb, Kramer and Danoff (1982) concluded that equal or even better results are obtained by telephone surveys as compared with personal interviews, while being far less costly. They successfully conducted the majority of their interviews on 'quality of life' after radiotherapy, by telephone.

7. The test should be devised in such a way that it is easy to check immediately after the patient has completed it, whether any mistakes have been made, questions omitted, etc.

8. There should be a check on who actually completed the test. If the patient is supposed to complete it, it is important to know that he actually did so. (A small study (Couzijn *et al.* 1982), in which the wives of the patients were asked to complete the test as they thought applied to their husbands, showed that in about 25 per cent of the cases there was considerable disagreement between the patients and their wives regarding the number and kind of complaints.)

9. The content of the tests, questionnaires, or interviews should be phrased carefully to avoid undue anxiety. This applies especially when the prognosis is involved, but also in talking about other factors such as sexuality. Patients may then become uneasy and refuse further co-operation.

10. And last but not least: there are not only negative effects due to psychosocial research with cancer patients. We have often heard patients remark that they were pleased that finally someone paid attention to their circumstances and emotions. Often a long talk ensued. Therefore, it is imperative to have the possibility to refer patients to a social worker, psychologist, or psychiatrist.

METHODS OF INQUIRY

There are various methods by means of which data about patients may be obtained.

Clinical observation

The Karnofsky Performance Status Scale (KPS) (Karnofsky and Burchenall 1949), an 11-point observation scale, is often used in clinical trials. Despite the problems of the KPS regarding its reliability, its validity seems to be robust. Aisner and Hansen (1981) write: 'In nearly every investigation in which performance status has been considered, it has been found to be one of the most, if not the most, important prognostic factor in determining survival for patients with non-small-cell lung cancer.' A related scale has been developed by Zubrod, Schneidermann, Frei, Brindley, Gold, Schnider, Oviedo, Gorman, Jones, Johnson, Colsky, Chalmers, Ferguson, Derick, Holland, Selawry, Regelson, Lasagna, and Owens (1960). Another similar instrument is Carlens Vitagram (Nou and Aberg 1980). To our knowledge there are no studies which have compared these different observation scales. Wood, Cooper and Sartorius (1981) validated the KPS by comparing it with some accepted physical therapy assessment techniques. They concluded that these latter techniques appeared to offer no advantage over the KPS as an evaluation tool for studies. Spitzer, Dobson, Chesterman, Levi, Shepherd, Battista, and Catchlove (1981) developed a Quality of Life Index. It has five items (activity, daily living, health, support, outlook) and its range of scores is 0–10. Its psychometric properties have been scrutinized extensively and seem satisfactory: so far no clinical trials have been published which use this scale.

The problems with observation scales in clinical research are by no means easily solved, one of the main problems being the difficulty of adequately training the ever-changing medical personnel and the lack of control of the way these rating scales are applied. Also there is the possible bias on the part of the doctor using an observation scale: for example, for certain trials a specific score on the Karnofsky scale has to be reached before the patient is allowed to enter; also a doctor may consider a given trial too burdensome for a patient and this may consciously or unconsciously influence his observation.

Clinical interviews

Various kinds of interviews may be discerned: structured interviews in which the wording, sequence of questions, and possible answers are fixed in advance, and guidelines are given for the interviewer about how to (re)act; semi-structured interviews in which the interviewer has more freedom, for example in changing the wording, and open interviews in which the wording and sequence is left largely to the discretion of the interviewer. Group interviews as a means of obtaining information from cancer patients are not mentioned in the literature. However, like the open interview this can be a fruitful method in an exploratory phase.

Open interviews

There is an abundance of literature in which clinicians give their impressions of the 'quality of life' of their patients, based on medical (open) interviews (Jansen 1979). Such data are hardly comparable, and thus useless in clinical trials.

Semi-structured interviews

There are several thoroughly tested methods of interviewing leading to comparable data, although for the process of data gathering trained interviewers are indispensable. To our knowledge there are four sets of interviews used in cancer research, on the basis of which patients are assigned a score with regard to various areas of psychosocial functioning.

—The Present State Examination (Wing *et al.* 1974) applied by Maguire, Tait, Brooke, Thomas, and Sellwood (1980) in a study of patients with breast cancer.

—The Current and Past Psychopathology Scales (Endicott and Spitzer 1972), applied by Plumb and Holland (1981) in an investigation of patients with advanced cancer.

—Gordon, Freidenbergs, Diller, Hibbard, Wolf, Levine, Lipkins, Ezrachi, and Lucido (1980) carried out an extensive and sophisticated investigation into the efficacy of intervention programmes for various groups of cancer patients. They modelled their interview after that of Burdoch and Hardesty (1968).

—The Psychosocial Adjustment to Illness Scale (PAIS) (Derogatis 1976), applied in a study of patients with Hodgkin's Disease (Morrow, Chiarello, and Derogatis 1978).

All these scales have been scrutinized with regard to their reliability and validity. However, they take some time to apply, varying from 20 to 30 minutes to over an hour, requiring varying degrees of training and experience of the interviewers in handling the instrument. The method to be preferred is hard to say, as this depends on the research questions. The PAIS seems to be a scale with some advantages over the other scales as it takes relatively little time and does not seem to require a great amount of training on the part of the interviewers; furthermore, a self-report form has been derived from it (Derogatis 1977a). On the other side the PAIS does not take into account psychopathology, which the Present State Examination does. The latter also has the advantage of having been tested in cross-cultural research: an advantage in international multi-centre cancer research.

Self report by the patient: questionnaires

A number of self-report devices are available which might be of some use in clinical cancer trials.

An outstanding instrument is the SCL-90 (Derogatis 1977b). It has been applied in an adjuvant chemotherapy trial of the Eastern Cooperative Oncology Group. The instrument consists of 90 questions with five possible answers, ranging from 'not at all distressed by the complaint' to 'extremely distressed by the complaint'. Subscores may be derived, for example general neurotic feelings, somatic symptoms, fear, depression, and problems in functioning. One drawback may be the inclusion of many somatic items, which complicate the interpretation of some of the questionnaires subscales and somewhat limit its use in cancer research.

Priestman and Baum (1976) asked patients to indicate on a 10 centimetre line how much they were troubled by a number of complaints; at each end of the line descriptions are given of extremes of each complaint. They found rather satisfying test–retest reliabilities (0.73) and also some indication of the predictive validity of this instrument. Padilla, Presant, Grant, Metter, Baer, and Finnie (1980) used Priestman's method and also found rather satisfying test–retest reliabilities. They also found some indication with regard to the instrument's construct validity.

Besides these instruments quite a number of questionnaires for special purposes have been developed by several investigators. None of them have been investigated sufficiently to warrant recommendation at this moment. The description given by McCorkle (1981) is a good example of how to proceed in the development of questionnaires.

Instruments which have not been tested for cancer patients but which look promising are the Personal Functioning Index, combining self-care, mobility, and physical activities, and the Role Functioning Index, combining role activities and general limitations. These scales can be completed by the patient in five to ten minutes. They have been studied quite extensively with regard to their psychometric properties and norms are available for the general (American) population (Stewart, Ware, and Brook 1981). High priority should be given to research with different groups of cancer patients under different therapeutic regimens to test the validity and the sensitivity to change of these scales. Meenan, Gertman, and Mason (1980) devised, by means of an eclectic approach, an instrument for measuring health status in arthritis patients. This instrument (a self-administered questionnaire) consisting of nine subscales (mobility, physical activity, dexterity, social role, social activity, activities of daily living, pain, depression, and anxiety) meets high psychometric standards and could perhaps be used in oncology after adapting some of its subscales.

There are a number of difficulties in regard to self-ratings (response-tendency, etc.) but these seem surmountable (Locker and Dunt 1978) if proper instructions are given.

Other sources of information

There are hardly any data about patients from sources such as relatives or general practitioners, and there are certainly no instruments for obtaining this information from them. For some research questions it may be worthwhile to use data from medical records (for example the number of times patients have to see the doctor, etc.), data about general functioning (at work, at school) (Craig, Comstock and Geiser 1974) and data about financial support (Funch and Mettlin 1982).

Specific issues

For certain groups of patients specific questionnaires have to be developed in order to be able to evaluate their problems, for example for colostomy patients (Wirsching, Drünerm, and Herrmann 1975), laryngectomies Brouwer, Snow, and van Dam 1979), patients with head and neck cancer (David and Barrett 1977) and patients with carcinoma of the oesophagus (Stoller, Samer, Toppin, and Flores 1977). Excellent reviews on problems in measurement concerning patients with breast cancer (the kind of cancer which has, until now, received the most attention of behavioural scientists), can be found in Meyerowitz (1980) and Morris (1979). For reviews of problems of patients with gynaecological cancer one is referred to Bush (1979) and Newton (1979). The reader is referred to Melzack (1975) for a description of a questionnaire developed to gain insight into the problems of measuring pain. A fatigue scale has been applied in a study of patients receiving localized radiotherapy (Haylock and Hart 1979). A 'fear of recurrence scale' (an important area in psychosocial oncology) has been developed by Northouse (1981). Another area in which measurement is of great importance is nausea (Penta, Poster, Bruno, and Macdonald 1981; Sallan, Cronin, Zelen, and Zinberg 1981). Little attention has been paid to the psychometric properties of instruments in this field (Poster, Penta, and Bruno 1981).

Depending on the research questions, standard psychological tests may be applied. Silberfarb, Philibert, and Levine (1980) applied a cognitive and affective test in search of cognitive impairment of cancer patients.

An area often unjustly neglected is that of positive affect. Almost all the interviews and questionnaires used in cancer research probe into complaints and negative affects of patients. Fontana, Marcus, Dowds, and Hughes (1980) state: 'If people are to report on their own psychological well being, both positive and negative affect should be included in order to obtain a complete account. Exclusive focus on negative affect will provide information regarding psychological impairment, and will yield little indication of psychological health.' Another argument is that patients sometimes become annoyed and depressed by the very wording of the questions. They object to never being asked whether anything goes well. Again, depending on the research questions at hand, it might be useful to include questions about positive affect. In this regard one is referred to the work of Andrews and Withey (1976) and to that of Huisman (1981) who has written a survey of methods for measuring positive affect. Another important argument for including both positive and negative affect is the fact that they are virtually uncorrelated (Chalmer and Yates 1978). However, there are problems in interpreting these data since traumatic events, for example cancer and its associated therapy, can lead to relatively higher levels of perceived well being (Irwin *et al.* 1982). In short, including negative affects only (as is now usually the case) gives but a limited view on the patient's adaptation to his illness.

Choosing the appropriate instrument

Meenan *et al.* (1980), referring to Miller (1973) who stressed the point that a multi-dimensional health-status index should meet a number of criteria, stated: 'First, it should be practical: the costs and time to collect the data should be small and the qv'stions should be comprehensible. Second it should be simple: the index ought to contain a limited number of reasonably discrete scales and the results should be easy to score and interpret. Third, it should be dependable: the results must meet accepted standards of reliability, scalability and validity. Finally, it should be useful: the index ought to be applicable to the population and questions being studied and useful for problems of patient management and resource allocation.'

When choosing an instrument one should also keep in mind that the instrument ought to be sensitive enough to detect changes within individuals over time. Jette (1980) emphasizes this as an important property of an instrument.

Another kind of consideration is that in most hospitals very few people are available with sufficient training in conducting interviews. In most cases this means that one should rely on self-assessment procedures. However, the forms should be devised in such a way that the patients can also answer the questions verbally in case they are not accustomed to completing questionnaires.

Before a measure is used in a different society, considerable research should be carried out with regard to its value in another language and another culture

(Sartorius 1979). A concise review of the problems in psychological measurement in cross-cultural research can be found in Lonner (1981).

EVALUATION OF OUTCOMES

The aim of implementing psychosocial measures is, of course, to influence decisions about trials. The problem then becomes one of the way decisions are made.

Multiple indices

If more than one index (a score for an attribute) is used the problem of the inter-relationship between these indices arises. In a study of the effects of various rehabilitation programmes it turned out that multiple indicators of physical functioning intercorrelated reasonably well, but that low correlations existed between assessments of social functioning on the one side and physical functioning on the other (Albrecht and Higgins 1977). The question then becomes how to handle divergent outcomes. Jette (1980) points to similar problems concerning health status indicators.

Levels of enquiry

Rose (1976) points very cogently to the fact that there are many levels at which one can describe and explain biological phenomena. He describes a hierarchy of explanation and description in which the following levels can be discerned:
1. physical;
2. chemical;
3. anatomical-biochemical;
4. physiological (units);
5. physiological (systems);
6. psychological;
7. social-psychological;
8. social.

Each of these descriptions and explanations may be complete in their own right, yet which one is relevant depends upon the purpose of the description. In order to clarify Rose's view, the following example is frequently used: music can be described by a physical scientist using words like frequency and pitch; a music critic will describe the music as he experiences it, the way he interprets the music. Both describe the same phenomenon, but although the descriptions cannot be derived from one another, both of the descriptions are legitimate.

Most of the outcome criteria for evaluating treatment are on the anatomical-biochemical level (3): response of tumours to various treatments, survival rates at some fixed points in time, survival curves. What is requested by both doctors and patients is an addition, namely outcome criteria on the psychological, social-psychological, or social level. Which outcome criteria are chosen and at which level one measures depends very much on the purpose of the trial. If we are interested in brain damage of children under various therapeutic regimens, we should use a neuropsychological test battery, and we are clearly measuring at level 6, the psychological level. If the purpose of the trial is the comparison of breast-conserving therapy versus breast amputation, and we want to know the impact of the two therapies on the body image of the patient and on the relationship with her husband, we are measuring at level 6 and level 7. And if the purpose of our trial is to measure the effect of maintenance therapy in treating testicular cancer, we should include, for example, an outcome criterion from which we may conclude how the daily life of the patient and his family is affected (levels 7 and 8). Naturally, outcome criteria on the biochemical and anatomical level remain of the utmost importance.

In short, it depends very much on the trial at hand which level of enquiry is to be chosen and which measures are to be used. It is useful to note that only correlational relationships exist between the various levels and no causal relationships. It is never justified to conclude from an effect on the anatomical-biochemical level that it causes an effect on, for example, the psychological level, or vice versa as is often done in psychosomatic research. There may be good reasons to suppose that such a relationship exists, but it remains to be proven.

What is needed then is a theory in which a divergence of outcomes is accounted for and which orders them according to their relevance for the problem at hand (Van Heerden 1977). McNeil, Weichselbaum, and Pauker (1980) have made a beginning, but as long as we do not have a theory that can handle these data adequately, we cannot but rely on the most deceptive of our senses: common sense.

CONCLUSION

The concept 'quality of life' is becoming increasingly popular in both the medical and general press. From the way this term is used it apparently denotes an important field of enquiry but is in itself too vague to be used for the evaluation of psychosocial side-effects of cancer therapies.

Research in this area is evaluative enquiry, as Smith, Glass and Miller (1980) state: 'it involves obtaining information to judge the worth of a program, product or procedure'. It would be very much exaggerated to state that there is a choice of data-gathering instruments suitable for use in cancer trials, scrutinized with respect to their validity, reliability, and feasibility. Therefore, we cannot advise any one instrument for routine implementation in trials. However, there are a number of promising developments: psychiatrists and psychologists are working closely together with oncologists in various (inter)national groups. For instance, a Study Group on Quality of Life has recently been created within the European Organization for Research on Treatment of Cancer (EORTC). It is of the utmost importance that these groups co-ordinate their efforts in the search of high quality data-gathering instruments. For, concluding with Brashear (1978): 'Without specific definitions or qualifications, quality of life or quality of survival should not be given decision making relevance.'

ACKNOWLEDGEMENT

This article has been written within the framework and with financial support of the World Health Organization.

REFERENCES

Aisner, J. and Hansen, H. H. (1981). Commentary: current status of chemotherapy for non-small cell lung cancer. *Cancer Treat. Rep.* **65**, 979–86.

Albrecht, G. L. and Higgins, P. C. (1977). Rehabilitation success: the interrelationships of multiple criteria. *J. Health soc. Behav.* **18**, 36–45.

Alexander, J. L. and Willems, E. P. (1981). Quality of Life: some measurement requirements. *Archs physiol. med. Rehabil.* **62**, 261–5.

Anastasi, A. (1976). *Psychological testing.* Collier MacMillan International Editions, New York.

Andrews, F. M. and Withey, S. B. (1976) *Social indicators of well-being.* Plenum Press, New York.

Bardelli, D. and Saracci, R. (1978) *Measuring the quality of life in cancer clinical trials: a sample survey of published trials.* UICC Technical Report Series, Geneva.

Barofsky, I. (1981). Issues and Approaches to the psychosocial assessment of the cancer patient. In *Medical psychology, contribution to behavioral medicine* (eds. Ch. K. Prokop, and L. A. Bradley). Academic Press, New York.

Bleehen, N. (1980). Management of inoperable squamous cell, adeno- and large cell carcinoma. In *Lung Cancer* (eds. H. H. Hansen and M. Rørth), Exerpta Medica, Amsterdam.

Brashear, R. E. (1978). Should asymptomatic patients with inoperable bronchogenic carcinoma receive immediate radiotherapy? NO. *Am. Rev. resp. Dis.* **117**, 411–13.

Brouwer, B., Snow, G., and van Dam, F. S. A. M. (1979). Experiences of patients who undergo laryngectomy. *Clin. Otolaryngol.* **4**, 109–18.

Burdoch, E. and Hardesty, A. (1968). Psychological test for psychopathology, *J. Abnorm. Psychol.* **73**, 62–9.

Bush, R. (1979). *Malignancies of the ovary, uterus and cervix.* Edward Arnold, London.

Chalmer, B. and Yates, J. (1978). Evaluation of 'quality of life' in patients with advanced cancer. Paper presented at the *Sixty-Ninth Annual Meeting of the American Association of Cancer Research*, Washington DC.

Couzijn, A., Bokkel Huinink, W. W., van Dam, F. S. A. M., and Hanewald, G. J. F. P. (1982). Chemotherapy for disseminated testicular cancer; experience of patients and their partners, *Ned Tijdschrift v. Geneeskunde.* **126**, 1854–7.

Craig, T. J., Comstock, G. W., and Geiser, P. B. (1974). The quality of survival in breast cancer: a case-control comparison. *Cancer* **33**, 1451–7.

Cronbach, L. J. (1970) *Essentials of Psychological testing*, Harper, New York.

David, D. J. and Barrett, J. A. (1977). Psychosocial aspects of head and neck cancer surgery. *Aust. NZ J. Surg.* **47**, 584–9.

Derogatis, L. R. (1976). *Scoring and procedures manual for PAIS, clinical and psychometric research*. Johns Hopkins University Press, Baltimore, Maryland.

—— (1977a). *PAIS S. R. Self Report*. Johns Hopkins University Press, Baltimore, Maryland.

—— (1977b). *The SCL - 90 Manual*. Johns Hopkins University Press, Baltimore, Maryland.

Endicott, J. and Spitzer, R. L. (1972). Current and past psychopathology scales (CAPPS). *Archs gen. Psychiat.* **27**, 678–87.

Fiske, D. W. (1971). *Measuring the concept of personality*. Aldine, Chicago.

Fontana, A. F., Marcus, J. L., Noel Dowds, B., and Hughes, L. A. (1980). Psychological impairment and psychological health in the physically ill, *Psychosom. Med.* **42**, 279–88.

Funch, D. P. and Mettlin, C. (1982). The role of support in relation to recovery from breast surgery. *Soc. Sci. Med.* **16**, 91–8.

Gordon, W. A., Freidenbergs, I., Diller, L., Hibbard, M., Wolf, C., Levine, L., Lipkins, Ezrachi, O., and Lucido, D. (1980). Efficacy of psychosocial intervention with cancer patients, *J. consult. clin. Psychol.* **48**, 743–59.

Haylock, P. J. and Hart, L. K. (1979). Fatigue in patients receiving localized radiation. *Cancer Nursing* 461–7.

Herson, J. (1980). Evaluation of toxicity: statistical considerations. *Cancer Treat. Rep.* **64**, 463–7.

Huisman, S. (1981). Het Meten van Positieve Aspecten van Welzijn bij Kankerpatiënten. MA Thesis, Psychological Laboratory, University of Amsterdam.

Hutchinson, T. A., Boyd, N. F., Feinstein, A. R. (1979). Scientific problems in clinical scales, as demonstrated in the Karnofsky Index of Performance Status. *J. chron. Dis.* **32**, 661–6.

Irwin, P. H., Gottlieb, A., Kramer, S., and Danoff, B. (1982). Quality of life after radiation therapy: a study of 309 cancer survivors. *Soc. Indicators Res.* **10**, 187–210.

Jansen, A. M. (1979). De Kwaliteit van het Leven en de Kankerpatiënt. MA Thesis, Psychological Laboratory, University of Amsterdam.

Jette, A. M. (1980). Health and status indicators: their utility in chronic disease evaluation research. *J. chron. Dis.* **33**, 567–79.

Karnofsky, D. A. and Burchenall, J. H. (1949). The clinical evaluation of chemotherapeutic agents in cancer. In *Evaluation of chemotherapeutic agents* (ed. M. C. Macleod) pp. 199–205. Columbia University Press, New York.

Linssen, A. C. G., Hanewald, G. F. P., and van Dam, F. S. A. M. (1981) The development of the 'complaint questionnaire' at the Netherlands Cancer Institute. In *Proceedings of the First Workshop EORTC study group on quality of life*. Antoni van Leeuwenhoek Ziekenhuis, Amsterdam.

Locker, D. and Dunt, D. (1978). Theoretical and methodological issues in sociological studies of consumer satisfactions with medical care. *Soc. Sci. Med.* **12**, 283–92.

Lonner, W. J. (1981). Psychological tests and inter-cultural counseling. In *Counseling across cultures* (eds. P. P. Pedersen, J. G. Draguns, W. J. Lonner, and J. E. Trimble). Revised edn The University Press of Hawaii.

Maguire, P., Tait, A., Brooke, M., Thomas, C., and Sellwood, R. (1980). Effect of counselling on the psychiatric morbidity associated with mastectomy. *Br. med. J.* **281**, 1454–5.

McCorkle, R. (1981). Non-obtrusive measures in clinical nursing research. In *Cancer*

Nursing update, proceedings of the 2nd Int. Cancer Nursing Conference (ed. R. Tiffany). Baillière Tindall, London.

McNeil, B. J., Weichselbaum, R., and Pauker, S. G. (1981). Speech and survival: tradeoffs between quality and quantity of life in laryngeal cancer. *New Engl. J. Med.* **305,** 982–7.

Meenan, R. F., Gertman, P. M., and Mason, J. H. (1980). Measuring health status in arthritis: the arthritis impact scales. *Arthritis Rheum.* **23,** 146–52.

Melzack, R. (1975). The McGill pain questionnaire: major properties and screening methods. *Pain* **1,** 277–99.

Meyerowitz, B. E. (1980). Psychological correlates of breast cancer and its treatments. *Psychol. Bull.* **87,** 108–31.

Miller, J. E. (1973). Guidelines for selecting a health status index. In *Health status indexes* (ed. R. L. Berg), pp. 243–51. Hospital Research and Education Trust, Chicago.

Morris, T. (1979). Psychological adjustment to mastectomy. *Cancer Treat. Rev.* **6,** 41–61.

Morrow, G. R., Chiarello, R. J., and Derogatis, L. R. (1978). A new scale for assessing patients' psychosocial adjustment to medical illness. *Psychol. Med.* **8,** 605–10.

Newton, M. (1979). Quality of life for the gynecologic oncology patient. *Am. J. Obstet. Gynec.* **134,** 866–9.

Northouse, L. L. (1981). Mastectomy patients and the fear of cancer recurrence. *Cancer Nursing* **4,** 213–20.

Nou, E. and Aberg, T. (1980). Quality of survival in patients with surgically treated bronchial carcinoma. *Thorax* **35,** 255–63.

Padilla, G. V., Presant, C., Grant, M. M., Metter, G., Baer, Ch., and Finnie, P. (1980). *Quality of life instrument for patients with cancer.* Department of Nursing Research, City of Hope National Medical Center, Duarte, California. (Pre-publication.)

Pecoraro, R. E., Inui, Th.S., Chen, M. S., Plorde, D. K., and Heller, J. L. (1979). Validity and reliability of a self-administered health history questionnaire. *Publ. Hlth. Rep.* **94,** 231–8.

Penta, J. S., Poster, D. S., Bruno, D. S., and Macdonald, J. S. (1981). Clinical trials with antiemetic agents in cancer patients receiving chemotherapy. *J. clin. Pharmac.* **21,** 11S–21S.

Pirsig, R. M. (1976). *Zen and the art of motorcycle maintenance.* Transworld, Buffalo, New York.

Plumb, M. M. and Holland, J. (1977). Comparative studies of psychological function in patients with advanced cancer. I. Self-reported depressive symptoms. *Psychosom. Med.* **39,** 264–76.

—— (1981). Comparative studies of psychological function in patients with advanced cancer. II. Interviewer-rated current and past psychological symptoms, *Psychosom. Med.* **43,** 243–54.

Poster, D. S., Penta, J. S., and Bruno, S. (1981). *Treatment of cancer chemotherapy-induced nausea and vomiting.* Masson, New York.

Priestman, T. J., and Baum, M. (1976). Evaluation of quality of life in patients receiving treatment for advanced breast cancer. *Lancet* **i,** 899–901.

Rose, S. (1976). *The Conscious brain.* Vintage Books, New York.

Sallan, S. E., Cronin, C., Zelen, M., and Zinberg, N. E. (1980). Antiemetics in patients receiving chemotherapy for cancer: a randomized comparison of delta-9-tethrahydrocannabinol and prochloroperazine. *New Engl. J. Med.* **302,** 135–8.

Sartorius, N. (1979). Crosscultural Psychiatry. In *Psychiatrie der Gegenwart*, Bd.I/1 2.Aufl., Springer, Berlin.

Schmale, A. H. (1980). Clinical trials in psychosocial medicine: methodologic and statistical considerations. Part I Introduction. *Cancer Treat. Rep.* **64**, 441–3.

Smith, M. L., Glass, G. V., and Miller, T. I. (1980). *The benefits of psychotherapy*, Johns Hopkins University Press, Baltimore.

Silberfarb, P. M., Philibert, D., and Levine, P. M. (1980). Psychosocial aspects of neoplastic disease. II. Affective and cognitive effects of chemotherapy in cancer patients. *Am. J. Psychiat.* **137**, 597–601.

Spitzer, W. O., Dobson, A. J., Chesterman, E., Levi, J., Shepherd, R., Battista, R. N., and Catchlove, B. R. (1981). Measuring the quality of life of cancer patients. A concise QL-index for use by physicians. *J. chron. Dis.* **34**, 585–97.

Stewart, A. L., Ware, J. E., and Brook, R. H. (1981). Advances in the measurement of functional status: construction of aggregate indexes. *Med. Care* **19**, 473–88.

Stewart, A. L. (1980). *Coping with serious illness.* P-6640, The Rand Corp. Santa Monica, California.

Stoller, J. I., Samer, K. J., Toppin, D. I., and Flores, A. D. (1977). Carcinoma of the esophagus: a new proposal for the evaluation of treatment. *Can. J. Surg.* **20**, 454–9.

van den Aardweg, G. M. H. (1981). Klagen, een 'huisarts' over een psychologisch onderwerp, *De Psycholoog*, **16**, 142–5.

van den Heerden. (1977). Convergerende operatie. Problemen en verwachtingen, *Ned. Tijdschr. voor de Psychologie*, **32**, 187–94.

Ward, M. J. and Lindemann, C. (eds.) (1977). *Instruments for measuring nursing practice and other health care variables 1.* US Department of Health, Education and Welfare, Hyattsville, Maryland.

Wing, J. K., Cooper, J. E., and Sartorius, N. (1974). *Measurement and classification of psychiatric symptoms.* Cambridge University Press.

Wirsching, M. Drünerm, H. U., and Herrmann, G. (1975). Results of psychosocial adjustment to long-term colostomy. *Psychother. Psychosom.* **26**, 245–56.

Wood, C. A., Anderson, J., and Yates, J. (1981). Physical function assessment in patients with advanced cancer using the Karnofsky Performance Status, Med. Ped. Oncol. **9**, 129–32.

Yates, J. W., Chalmer, B., and McKegney, P. (1980). Evaluation of patients with advanced cancer using the Karnofsky Performance Status. *Cancer* **45**, 2220–4.

Zubrod, C. G., Schneidermann, M., Frei, E., III, Brindley, C., Gold, L. G., Schnider, B., Oviedo, R., Gorman, J., Jones, R., Jr., Johnson, U., Colsky, J., Chalmers, T., Ferguson, B., Derick, M., Holland, J., Selawry, O., Regelson, W., Lasagna, C., and Owens, A. H., Jr. (1960). Appraisal of methods for the study of chemotherapy of cancer in man: comparative therapeutic trial of nitrogen mustard and triethylene thio phosphoramide. *J. chron. Dis.* **11**, 7–33.

Part II
Planning and conduct

4 Planning cancer clinical trials

Richard Sylvester

INTRODUCTION

The importance of proper planning, organization, and design of cancer clinical trials along with the need for a clear and detailed protocol cannot be overemphasized since these factors are crucial in determining the eventual success of a study. A poorly run study is not only a waste of time and money, but it may also do harm by providing an incorrect answer to an important question. The purpose of this chapter is to present some of the basic principles inherent in the planning of a cancer clinical trial and in the design of a protocol. As many papers have been written on these topics, an extensive bibliography will be given so that the reader may pursue the topics discussed in this chapter in more detail than is possible here.

PLANNING A CLINICAL TRIAL

What is a clinical trial?

A clinical trial may be defined as a carefully designed, prospective medical study which attempts to answer a precisely defined set of questions with respect to the effects of a particular treatment or treatments. A prerequisite for any clinical trial is a good idea which is worth testing. A clinical trial should attempt to answer the most important questions that can be raised concerning the disease under study, obtain the correct results, and be able to convince others of the validity of the outcome. It should be designed to answer a limited set of clear, concise and well-defined questions and must not have so many objectives, or be so ambitious or so complex that it cannot be reliably carried out by its participants. A clinical trial is a major undertaking which requires considerable money, personnel, facilities, time, and effort. Thus the need for the study, its value, and its potential impact on the medical community must all be carefully considered to ensure that the interest of the question justifies the time and expense necessary to carry it out.

The protocol

The most important document pertaining to any clinical trial is the protocol, a self-contained description of the rationale, objectives, and logistics of the study. Just as a well-written protocol does not in itself justify carrying out an otherwise poor study, a poorly designed protocol with insufficient attention paid to the trial's methodology may not allow one to provide a definitive answer to an important question. The protocol must be detailed and precisely worded so that the study is uniformly carried out by all its participants. The topics that should be included in a typical protocol are presented in Table 4.1. Detailed guidelines for the preparation of cancer clinical trial protocols have been published elsewhere (Staquet, Sylvester, and Jasmin 1980; Gore 1981; Sylvester, Machin, and Staquet 1982) and will not be discussed here.

Table 4.1. *Protocol contents*

1. Title page
2. Background and introduction
3. Objectives of the trial
4. Patient selection criteria
5. Trial design and schema
6. Therapeutic regimens, dose modification and toxicity
7. Required clinical evaluations, laboratory tests and follow-up
8. Criteria of evaluation
9. Registration and randomization of patients
10. Forms and procedures for collecting data
11. Statistical considerations
12. Administrative responsibilities
13. Informed consent
14. References
15. Appendices

A committee of scientists representing each of the different disciplines involved in the study should be appointed to plan, design, and write the protocol. In planning a clinical trial there must be a close contact between the clinicians involved in the trial and the statisticians from the very beginning. More than just simply calculating the number of patients required for the study and its expected duration, the statistician should be involved in all phases of protocol planning and trial design (Breslow 1978; Ederer 1979). One should not be too anxious to start patient entry in the trial without allowing sufficient time for the protocol to be designed, written, revised, and eventually reviewed by an external review board.

Definition of trial objectives

The first steps in planning a clinical trial are to define the objectives of the study and to determine the type of trial which should be carried out, that is, whether a phase I trial, phase II trial or a phase III trial is appropriate (Fig. 4.1). A phase I trial is essentially a toxicity screening study where after testing in animals, a new drug is administered for the first time in man in order to determine the maximum tolerated dose (Von Hoff, Kuhn, and Clark 1983). Several patients are treated at each of a series of increasing dosage levels in order to determine which level should be tested in a phase II trial. Once a maximum tolerated dose is determined from a phase I study, the drug is screened for potential anti-tumour activity in a phase II trial in a limited number of patients with advanced measurable disease (Carter 1983). The purpose of a phase II trial is to determine whether or not the drug has sufficient activity at an acceptable level of toxicity to warrant further testing in a larger number of patients. A phase II study is not an absolute test of the drug's efficacy but rather a screen of the drug at a given dose in a given group of patients. For example a drug may initially be tested in twenty patients and rejected from further study if no responses are observed. If at least one response is recorded then additional patients will be treated in order to obtain a more precise estimate of the response rate.

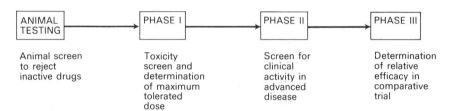

Fig. 4.1. Steps in testing a new drug.

If the phase II trial proves positive, the next step is to test the relative efficacy of the drug in a comparative phase III study where the drug may be compared with either placebo or the best available conventional treatment, either alone or in combination with other drugs. A phase III trial is a considerable investment in time and money and should not be undertaken unless adequate preliminary phase I and phase II trials have been carried out.

It is of the utmost importance to define the objectives of the study and the hypothesis to be tested in as unambiguous a manner as possible. It is better to limit the protocol to a few very precise questions that can be easily answered than to pose too many questions and to wind up not being able to adequately answer any of them. The type of questions posed and the resulting end-points will, of course, depend on whether you are trying to show that the treatment has an anti-tumour effect in patients with advanced disease or whether it will delay the time to recurrence and/or death among patients who are apparently disease-free after curative treatment of the primary tumour.

Review of the literature

Once the general objectives of the trial have been agreed upon, it should be verified whether or not the trial, or a similar one, has already been carried out or is in the process of being carried out elsewhere. The US National Institutes of Health (1982) have published a summary of over 2000 phase II and phase III cancer clinical trials currently being conducted throughout the world. This information is extracted from CLINPROT, a computerized data base which is available to researchers through the MEDLARS System of the US National Library of Medicine. Other sources of ongoing or recently completed cancer clinical trials include CANCERLINE, a computerized cancer research data bank maintained by the US National Cancer Institute, summaries published by the International Union Against Cancer (UICC 1978) and the European Organization for Research on Treatment of Cancer (EORTC 1983), Excerpta Medica (1982) and the yearly proceedings of the American Association for Cancer Research and the American Society of Clinical Oncology (AACR and ASCO 1982), and the European Society for Medical Oncology (ESMO 1981). In addition the Oncology Information Service at the University of Leeds in England publishes a monthly bulletin of recent references covering over 1700 journals and books on 18 different cancer topics. Other more general reference sources include the *Science Citation Index*, the *Index Medicus*, *Current Contents* (*Life Sciences*) and MEDLINE, a computerized medical reference file of the US National Library of Medicine.

The next step is to make a complete review of the literature for the results of previous trials of interest which have a direct bearing upon the proposed trial. Only in this manner can the trial be placed in its proper perspective. An excellent starting-point for this search is the book edited by Staquet (1978) which reviews by tumour site the contributions provided by randomized clinical trials. At the same time the most important prognostic factors related to the disease under study must be identified in order to establish subgroups of patients with similar or differing prognoses. These factors can then be used to determine patient selection criteria and stratification variables. Knowledge of patient prognosis is also required for determining the number of patients required in the study, its duration, and aids in the selection of the appropriate end-points for evaluating treatment efficacy.

Definition of patient population

Patient-entry criteria should be as detailed and precise as possible in order to accurately define the patient population under study. Frequently a staging system based on the TNM classification is employed to describe the patient's disease characteristics (TNM 1978; American Joint Committee 1977). While the entry criteria should not be so restrictive that an insufficient number of patients will be eligible for entry into the study, the patient population should be reasonably homogeneous so that all patients have a similar type of disease and prognosis. One should avoid including in the trial small subgroups of patients who have a potentially different prognosis from the others. There will not be enough of these patients to analyse them separately and including them in the analysis may weaken the overall treatment comparison. While liberal patient-entry criteria will result in entering the required number of patients in a shorter period of time, there may be a loss of power in one's ability to detect a difference in treatment efficacy. The inclusion of patients who are more likely to respond or fail on both of the treatments provides no information in the comparison of relative treatment efficacy. Because it is not usually possible to determine if the relative efficacy of the treatments differs in the various subgroups of patients entered due to small patient numbers, the overall results will apply to this mixture of patients entered and not to any well-defined group. On the other hand, if the patient-entry criteria are too strict, patient accrual will become a problem and the results may be valid only for a very small percentage of the overall patient population.

Evaluation of treatment efficacy

One of the most critical aspects of any trial is the precise definition of the end-points and the criteria used to assess treatment efficacy. Otherwise one cannot ensure that the correct follow-up examinations will be done and that the proper data will be recorded. The *WHO Handbook for Reporting Results of Cancer Treatment* (WHO 1979), the contents of which have also been published in *Cancer* (Miller, Hoogstraten, Staquet, and Winkler 1981), is a document which should be consulted not only when publishing trial results, but also when planning the trial, since it provides detailed guidelines for the definition of most of the usual end-points adopted in cancer trials and also covers the problem of grading toxicity. Kisner and Sylvester (1980) have published a companion article which deals with the reporting of results specifically in the realm of cancer clinical trials. It is very important that all patients, even those in an untreated control group, be followed up at the same frequency and evaluated using the same techniques in order to avoid bias when comparing treatments. If not, then patients in one group may appear to have a longer duration of remission simply because they have been evaluated less frequently. If possible the evaluation of treatment response should be made by someone who is unaware of the treatment assigned using parameters which are objective in nature. It should be remembered that the determination of a patient's response to treatment is subject to a non-negligible measurement error (Moertel and Hanley 1976). Any important laboratory investigations should, whenever possible, be performed by a central laboratory.

In the design of a phase III trial there are two principal types of trials that must be considered: trials studying adjuvant treatment in patients clinically disease free after a 'curative' primary treatment, and trials in patients with advanced disease.

The goal of the adjuvant study is usually to compare the duration of remission (disease-free interval), disease-free survival, or survival in two or more treatment groups among patients who may potentially be cured by the primary treatment. In designing the study, one should standardize the primary treatment which patients receive so that valid inferences concerning the adjuvant treatment can be drawn. It should also be remembered that the number of patients required for an adjuvant trial is not based simply on the number of patients entered, but on the number of patients for whom the end-point (relapse or death) will be observed during the course of the follow-up. For some tumour types a long follow-up period may be needed to observe the required number of failures. Patients who are cured by the primary treatment contribute no information concerning the efficacy of the adjuvant treatment. Thus very large numbers of patients may be required in order to carry out an adjuvant study if a non-negligible proportion of the patients are expected to remain disease free during the course of the study.

While the initial analysis will be based on the disease-free interval and acute toxicity, later analyses must also consider the overall duration of survival and chronic toxicity after an extended period of follow-up (Carter 1978). Since late relapses may significantly change the initial preliminary findings, a long follow-up period is usually necessary.

The use of the duration of remission or disease-free interval in an adjuvant study as the primary end-point has the advantage that this information is available sooner than the date of death, and that patients normally receive only the treatment assigned by the protocol during this time period. If the duration of survival is correlated with the duration of remission, then the duration of remission is in itself a meaningful end-point. However, if the patients who relapse after chemotherapy are refractory to further treatment and die quickly, whereas patients who relapse after no chemotherapy respond to chemotherapy at the time of relapse, then it may not be true that the duration of remission is correlated with the duration of survival. Patients may also die due to side-effects or toxicity resulting from the treatment. The duration of survival would be the ideal end-point except for the fact that not all patients may die due to their disease, death may take a long time to observe and a patient's ultimate duration of survival may be influenced by what treatment is given at the time of relapse. If the duration of survival is retained as a criteria of evaluation, then one should standardize whenever possible the treatment given upon relapse.

In studies of advanced disease, the primary end-point used to assess treatment activity is often taken to be the percentage of responders or the response rate. This end-point has the advantage of being assessable more quickly than the duration of response or survival. Depending on the percentage of responders, it may or may not be meaningful to compare the treatments with respect to the duration of response. As the time to death will usually be observed during the course of the trial in a large percentage of the patients entered, an analysis of the duration of survival is usually appropriate and will generally require less patients and a shorter follow-up time than the corresponding analysis for an adjuvant study. Since in advanced patients the duration of survival is often short after progression of the disease, standardization of the treatment after progression is less critical here than in adjuvant studies. In general, studies of advanced disease require fewer patients than adjuvant studies and can be completed in a shorter period of time.

The choice of the proper end-point is often crucial to the success or failure of the study. In advanced prostate cancer for example the choice of the end-point for evaluation of treatment efficacy is by no means a simple one. The primary lesion is notoriously difficult to measure while successive bone scans can be difficult to interpret. Thus the determination of a response to treatment may be associated with considerable measurement error. On the other hand, most patients with this disease are very old and many will die of unrelated diseases so that survival is also a poor end-point. In this case the most appropriate end-point is probably the time to progression as measured by new hot spots on the bone scan and X-ray or the appearance or increase in size of measurable lesions.

Whatever end-points are finally chosen to assess the treatment efficacy, one should not forget to also include a measure of the patient's quality of life as one of the parameters studied.

Calculation of sample size

When planning comparative trials one must take into consideration the fact that cancer patients tend to be very heterogeneous and that differences in therapeutic effect are usually smaller than differences due to prognostic factors. In order to obtain correct results and to be able to convince others of their validity, large randomized trials are usually required to detect small but medically important treatment differences while, at the same time, reducing the risk of error or bias to a minimum. The treatments must be given to a sufficiently large and representative sample of the patients under study so that valid inferences can be drawn concerning their effectiveness for the target population.

Using the primary end-point of interest, the required sample size is calculated based on the smallest difference in treatment efficacy which is important enough to detect, and on α and β, the size of the type I and type II errors, respectively. The number of patients required for the study increases as the difference to be detected becomes smaller and also as the error rates are set lower. The values for these parameters should be fixed prior to undertaking the sample-size calculation. They should not be thought of as variables whose values can be changed as one sees fit, simply to arrive at a smaller sample size. In practice, error rates of $\alpha = 0.05$ and $\beta = 0.10$ or 0.20 are often employed. Too large an increase in any of these parameters will seriously damage the trial's capability of providing a meaningful result. In most settings the number of patients should be calculated based on a two-sided hypothesis test. Further details are provided by George in Chapter 18 of this book.

Choice of error rates

It is important to consider the eventual consequences that an incorrect conclusion will have on the future treatment of the disease under study. In phase II trials it is customary to set the probability of a false-negative conclusion (type II error) at $\beta = 0.01$ or 0.05 since if an effective drug is found to be negative in a phase II trial, it is unlikely that the drug will be retested at a later date and an effective drug will have been missed. In phase III trials, it is normally the type I error, α, or the probability of a false-positive error which is preset to some specified low level, usually 0.05 or less. However the choice of whether α or β is to be fixed should depend upon the type of study and type of treatments to be compared and should be reconsidered for each new trial.

Usually one attempts to detect a certain degree of difference between the treatments. If one were to compare two treatment regimens of equal toxicity and cost, and which were otherwise similar except perhaps with respect to treatment efficacy, then it would be appropriate to fix the β error at a low level. In this case one wishes to maximize the probability of detecting a difference in treatment efficacy if a difference does indeed exist. A false-positive conclusion is not damaging since the two treatment regimens are in fact similar from all points of view. If, on the other hand, one were to compare a new more toxic or more costly regimen against a standard control treatment, one would not want to say that the new treatment is better than the control unless it can be shown definitively to be superior in efficacy. In this case it is the type I error, α, which must be minimized. If for example a new toxic chemotherapy was being compared with an untreated control group in an adjuvant study where a certain percentage of patients may be cured by the primary treatment, one would not want to conclude that the treated group fared better than the untreated group unless one could be reasonably confident that the conclusion was correct. The chemotherapy must be proved effective beyond a reasonable doubt to justify its use in a patient who has possibly been cured by the primary treatment.

In the case of the comparison of a new conservative treatment with a standard treatment, one wishes to show in some sense that the two treatments are equivalent. In this case one can only rule out a given difference in therapeutic effect with a certain degree of confidence and one must be very careful in the choice of α and β since a false-negative conclusion in this setting can have very serious consequences (Makuch and Simon 1978*a*).

More generally α and β should also be chosen so as to maintain at an acceptable level the false-positive and false-negative rates in a sequence of trials (Staquet, Rozencweig, Von Hoff and Muggia 1979; Simon 1982).

Trial design

The choice of the proper trial design is important to the eventual success of the protocol. The simplest design involves randomization between two different treatment regimens to answer one specific question. If one wishes to study two separate and unrelated questions, then a 2×2 factorial design should be envisaged in order to make optimal use of the patients who are available (Peto 1978). This would be the case for example if one wished to simultaneously study the effects of both chemotherapy and hormonal therapy in an adjuvant setting, or to study different induction and maintenance therapies in leukaemia trials (two separate randomizations). Often factorial designs can be used to answer simultaneously two different questions in the same protocol without appreciably increasing the number of patients required as compared with a two-arm study. Three-arm trials tend to be inefficient, especially if centres may choose to randomize to a subset of the treatments due to a lack of agreement on which treatments should be studied (Makuch and Simon 1978*b*). If a three-arm multi-centre trial is planned, then all participants should agree to randomize between the three treatment choices and should not be allowed to randomize to a subset of them. If a three-arm study is being considered, it should be investigated whether a four-arm 2×2 factorial design can be implemented which will require fewer patients than the three-arm trial.

The number of treatments that can be compared realistically in a clinical trial depends on the patient-entry rate, but in general two-arm trials are to be preferred (or perhaps four arms if a factorial design can be implemented), as these studies are generally easier to carry out and can be completed in the shortest length of time with the fewest number of patients. All comparative trials should include a control group receiving the standard treatment, otherwise the results of the trial may not allow one to place the treatment regimens in their proper perspective upon the trial's completion. The treatments to be compared should be sufficiently dissimilar to provide a realistic chance of finding a significant difference between them. In general a simple two-arm trial with the treatments being as different as possible gives one the greatest chance of detecting a significant difference between the treatment groups. In this manner a negative result will also be meaningful since two extremes will have been studied. In any case the trial must be designed in such a manner that negative results will be meaningful since, in practice, a large percentage of trials conducted do provide a negative conclusion.

Trial feasibility

Even a well-written protocol which attempts to answer a very important question will not achieve its objectives if the trial is not feasible. The trial should be kept as simple as possible so that it can be carried out by all participants in a reasonable length of time and without numerous protocol violations. Treatment regimens, follow-up schedules, and evaluations must not be so difficult or demanding that they are a continual source of protocol violations or result in frequent missing data. Any special studies not directly related to the principal question of interest should be made optional in order not to discourage potential participants. The data forms should not be so long or so complex that clinicians are dissuaded from filling them out. One must also be certain that the treatments to be tested are available in sufficient supply and at a low enough cost to permit their application during the entire course of the study.

Clinical trials can be very expensive to carry out and the question of funding for the trial must not be taken too lightly, especially if there is an administrative staff to pay for the trial's co-ordination and for processing and analysis of the data. One should ascertain at an early stage whether or not the funding of the trial is likely to pose a problem and, if so, if there is a possibility of obtaining a grant from a governmental agency or perhaps, for certain trials, financial assistance from a pharmaceutical company, either in the form of a grant or a free supply of drugs.

One of the biggest stumbling blocks to the successful completion of a cancer clinical trial is the lack of a sufficient patient accrual from which to observe the required number of events during the course of patient follow-up. If one is comparing the time to death for two different treatments for example, then several hundred patients will have to be entered in order to observe the 75 to 100 deaths that will be required on each arm just to detect an increase of about 50 per cent in the median duration of survival (George and Desu 1974). Many trials do not achieve a sufficient number of evaluable patients to provide a scientifically convincing assessment of treatment effectiveness. It is a waste of time, manpower, and money to start a clinical trial by attempting to detect only unrealistically large treatment differences, simply because an insufficient number of patients are available to detect smaller more likely differences. Clinical trials with inadequate sample sizes will have a low probability of detecting clinically significant differences and are thus doomed to failure before they start. A negative result in such a trial will generally be meaningless since an insufficient number of patients will have been treated to have a reasonable chance of detecting small but important differences. There exist too many examples in the literature of small trials in which it is impossible to draw valid conclusions.

Freiman, Chalmers, Smith, and Kuebler (1978) studied the results of 71 negative trials and found that most of these studies included too few patients to provide a reasonable assurance that a clinically meaningful difference would not be missed. In particular, 94 per cent of the trials had a greater than 10 per cent risk (β) of missing a true 25 per cent improvement in therapeutic efficacy. The number of patients entered was generally too small to detect realistic treatment differences and thus resulted in the inevitable conclusion that there were no significant treatment differences.

A survey by Pocock, Armitage, and Galton (1978) of fifty trials registered with the UICC Information Office also illustrated the widespread nature of low patient accrual and found that investigators were often overly optimistic in estimating the potential patient accrual rate. Many of the trials surveyed failed to achieve the required number of patients and/or lasted excessively long. The median accrual rate was only 33 patients per year with the median time necessary to achieve the required accrual being over 4 years.

The lack of a sufficient number of patients to adequately carry out the study may be due either to poor planning prior to the start of the trial or to overestimating initially the expected patient accrual rate. Although the number of patients available per year for the study should be ascertained during the planning stage, this figure is often grossly overestimated, especially in multi-centre trials, and must often be reduced by a factor of two or more to obtain a more accurate estimate. In addition, one should always allow for the fact that some patients entered may be ineligible while others may not be adequately treated in accordance with the protocol. Thus, in calculating the required number of patients and the expected duration of patient entry and follow-up, more patients than estimated will be required in order to obtain an adequate number of eligible and properly treated patients (George 1983).

A sufficient number of patients must be available so that the entry of patients in the trial can be terminated after a period of at most 2 to 3 years. After this time interest in the protocol usually begins to wane, the entry rate may decrease and one may be tempted to make important changes in the protocol which can compromise the study. If the trial runs too long other more promising therapies may appear in the meantime and the question under study may no longer be of interest when the results finally become available. When designing the study a change in the primary end-point of interest may often result in a considerable decrease in the number of patients required for the trial, for example comparing the percentage of complete responders rather than just the percentage of responders, or taking the time to progression instead of the response rate. Also, since what is important is not so much the number of patients entered in a trial but rather the number of end-points observed, one should consider taking the earliest occurring valid end-point for the purpose of treatment comparison. Collins, Bingham, Weiss,

Williford, and Kuhn (1980) present some adaptive strategies that one might adopt if faced with the problem of an inadequate patient accrual.

Multi-centre trials

For many types of tumours the establishment of a multi-centre trial will prove necessary in order to achieve the required number of patients in a shorter period of time. Meinert (1980; 1981) and Staquet (1976) discussed some of the organizational aspects to be considered in setting up and running multi-centre trials, while Machin, Staquet, and Sylvester (1979) presented an overview of the advantages and disadvantages of such trials from both administrative and statistical points of view. While multi-centre trials increase the heterogeneity of the patients entered and the heterogeneity of treatment application and response assessment, they are a more reliable real-world evaluation of the treatments under study and their results are more readily accepted by the medical community as a whole. In addition the results from a multi-centre trial are more readily generalizable to the overall population of patients with the disease in question.

One should restrict participation in a multi-centre trial to those centres thought most likely to co-operate seriously for the period of the trial and who will provide more than just an occasional patient from time to time (Sylvester, Pinedo, De Pauw, Staquet, Buyse, Renard, and Bonadonna 1981). If participants in a multi-centre trial do not enter all their eligible patients, then accrual may be no faster than in a single centre trial and the sample of patients entered may not be representative of the population of interest. This may occur for example if an investigator is not fully committed to the trial due to conflicts with local studies.

If all attempts to recruit the required number of patients in a reasonable length of time fail, then the trial should be abandoned rather than continuing indefinitely, and one should attempt to participate in another trial studying the same or a similar question. Only through more realistic planning, a true collaboration where all centres enter all their eligible patients, and a more accurate appraisal of the patient entry rate can these problems be overcome.

The co-ordinating office and data centre

An essential part of any clinical trial is the establishment of the necessary medical support committees, review groups and data processing facilities. A clinician closely connected to the study (such as the principal author of the protocol) should be appointed as study co-ordinator and assume overall responsibility for the trial. His task is to assure that the trial runs smoothly and that the various aspects of the trial are properly co-ordinated. He should also set up an extramural review committee to review all case records with respect to patient eligibility, evaluability, and response to treatment. As appropriate other subcommittees dealing with treatment policy, X-ray review, and pathology review should also be established. In addition to the medical support committees it is imperative that the proper administrative and data processing facilities be set up. A general overview of the functions of a co-ordinating centre are presented in a series of articles in the September 1980 issue of *Controlled Clinical Trials*. Staquet, Sylvester, Machin, Van Glabbeke, De Grauwe, Wennerholm, Tyrrell, Renard, De Pauw, Eeckhoudt, Tyrrell, and Tagnon (1977) review the structure of the EORTC Data Center which is designed to service multi-centre trials while Bonadonna and Valagussa (1978) describe their experience in organizing and carrying out single centre trials.

An experienced and adequately trained staff of medical secretaries, data managers, computer analysts, and statisticians must be available to handle the day to day work involved with trial design, and with the processing and analysis of the data. This includes design of the data forms and the randomization log, the registration and randomization of patients (Herson, 1980), the review, correction, and processing of the data forms, their computerization, and the preparation of administrative and statistical reports. In order to be able to quickly and efficiently process and analyse large quantities of complex data, all studies, except for perhaps small pilot studies, should be placed on the computer. The data forms should be designed jointly by the study co-ordinator, data manager, computer analyst, and statistician involved in the study. In general, forms should contain complete data on the patient's characteristics at entry to the study and then only the minimal follow-up data necessary for the evaluation of the end-points of interest. The forms should be tested in practice on the initial patients entered in the trial prior to their final adoption and printing. A more detailed account of the design of data forms can be found in the following chapter.

In any type of trial carried out, whether single centre or multi-centre, comparative or not, it is important that a centralized randomization or registration be carried out. A randomization log is generally employed and provides a random series of treatment assignments which are allocated in strict sequence to patients as they enter the trial. There are three important advantages to a centralized randomization:

1. One can verify that the randomization or registration has been impartially carried out without bias. A system of envelopes can be too easily abused to ensure an unbiased entry of patients.

2. With a centralized randomization it is known at all times exactly how many patients have been entered in the study and their identity.

3. Missing or overdue forms can be requested for *all* patients entered in the study since the identity of all patients entered will be known.

A straightforward and easy to implement randomization scheme is generally to be preferred to more complex schemes which cannot be quickly and easily carried out when an investigator calls. Stratification by institution and the one or two most important prognostic factors may also be employed to ensure that the treatment groups are comparable with respect to the most important prognostic factors.

FURTHER READING

There are many good books and papers which treat in more detail the aspects of planning a clinical trial. In addition to the references previously cited in the text, the following bibliography provides a list of recommended references and a starting-point for further reading.

Books

1. Burdette, W. J. and Gehan, E. A. (1970). *Planning and analysis of clinical studies.* Charles C. Thomas, Springfield, Illinois.
2. Friedman, L. M., Furberg, C. D., and De Mets, D. L. (1981). *Fundamentals of clinical trials.* John Wright, PSG, Inc., Boston.
3. Johnson, F. N. and Johnson, S. (eds.) (1977). *Clinical trials.* Blackwell Scientific Publications, London.

Book chapters

4. Gehan, E. A. and Schneiderman, M. A. (1973). Experimental design of clinical trials. In *Cancer medicine*, (eds. J. Holland and E. Frei), pp. 499–519. Lea and Fibiger, Philadelphia.
5. George, S. L. (1976). Practical problems in the design, conduct and analysis of cooperative clinical trials. In *Proceedings of the 9th International Biometric Conference*, Vol. 1, pp. 227–44. The Biometric Society, Raleigh, North California.
6. Simon, R. (1979). Heterogeneity and standardization in clinical trials. In *Controversies in cancer: design of trials and treatment* (eds. H. J. Tagnon and M. J. Staquet), pp. 37–49. Masson Publishing USA, Inc., New York.
7. Zelen, M. (1975). Aspects of the planning and analysis of clinical trials in cancer. In *A survey of statistical design and linear models.* (ed. J. N. Srivastava), pp. 629–46. North Holland Publishing Company, Amsterdam.

Papers

8. Carter, S. K. (1980). Clinical considerations in the design of clinical trials. *Cancer Treat. Rep.* **64,** 367–71.
9. Chalmers, T. C., Smith, H., Blackburn, B., Silverman, B., Schroeder, B., Reitman, D., and Ambroz, A. (1981). A method for assessing the quality of a randomized trial. *Cont. clin. Trials* **2,** 31–49.
10. Hammond, D. (1980). The training of clinical trial statisticians: a clinician's view. *Biometrics* **36,** 679–85.
11. Mosteller, F., Gilbert, J. P., and McPeek, B. (1980). Reporting standards and research strategies for controlled trials: agenda for the Editor. *Cont. clin. Trials* **1,** 37–58.
12. Peterson, A. V. and Fisher, L. D. (1980). Teaching the principles of clinical trials design and management. *Biometrics* **36,** 687–97.

13. Peto, R., Pike, M. C., Armitage, P., Breslow, N. E., Cox, D. R., Howard, S. V., Mantel, N., McPherson, K., Peto, J., and Smith, P. G. (1976). Design and analysis of randomized clinical trials requiring prolonged observation of each patient. I. Introduction and design. *Br. J. Cancer* **34**, 585–612.
14. Pocock, S. J. (1979). Allocation of patients to treatment in clinical trials. *Biometrics*, **35**, 183–97.
15. Proceedings of the Second International Symposium on Long-Term Clinical Trials. (1981). In *Cont. clin. Trials* **1**, 4.

Finally, 'Statistics in Question', a series of articles by S. Gore and published in the *British Medical Journal* in weekly installments from 16 May to 8 August 1981, provides an informal and non-technical discussion of many of the aspects of planning and assessing clinical trials, and is highly recommended reading.

CONCLUSIONS

This chapter provides a very basic introduction to the principles involved in planning cancer clinical trials. Further details concerning many of the topics touched upon can be found elsewhere in this book with the references in the recommended reading list and bibliography providing a relatively complete coverage of the topic.

All these guidelines are for nought, however, if a convincing answer to the questions posed by the protocol is not possible due to an insufficient number of patients having been entered in the study. An insufficient patient entry rate is probably the most frequent reason for a trial's failure to adequately answer the questions it set out to study. Thus when planning a study, it is of the utmost importance that the trial's feasibility be carefully evaluated with respect to both the number of patients that will be required and the estimated duration of time necessary to enter these patients. Hopefully a more realistic appraisal of this information will reduce the number of studies which do not provide a scientifically convincing result.

ACKNOWLEDGEMENTS

This work was supported by grant number 2 UIO CA 11488–13, awarded by the National Cancer Institute, Department of Health, Education, and Welfare, USA.

REFERENCES

AACR and ASCO (1982). *Proceedings of the American Association for Cancer Research and American Society of Clinical Oncology* (ed. P. N. Magee), Vol. 23. Cancer Research Inc., Waverly Press, Baltimore.
American Joint Committee (1977). *Manual for staging of cancer*. American Joint Committee for Cancer Staging and End Results Reporting, Chicago.

Bonadonna, G. and Valagussa, P. (1978). The logistics of clinical trials. *Biomedicine* (Special Issue) **28**, 43–8.

Breslow, N. (1978). Perspectives on the statician's role in cooperative clinical research. *Cancer* **41**, 326–32.

Carter, S. (1978). The analysis of adjuvant trials. *Cancer Treat. Rev.* **5**, 1–5.

——. (1983). Clinical aspects in the design and conduct of phase II trials. In *Cancer clinical trials: methods and practice* (eds. M. Buyse, M. Staquet, and R. Sylvester), pp. 223–38. Oxford University Press.

Collins, J. F., Bingham, S. F., Weiss, D. G., Williford, W. O., and Kuhn, R. M. (1980). Some adaptive strategies for inadequate sample acquisition in veteran's administration co-operative clinical trials. *Control. clin. Trials* **1**, 227–48.

Ederer, F. (1979). The statistician's role in developing a protocol for a clinical trial. *Am. Statist.* **33**, 116–19.

EORTC (1983). *EORTC: organization and current research* (ed. M. J. Staquet). EORTC, Brussels.

ESMO (1981). *Book of Conference Abstracts, European Society for Medical Oncology*. Swiss Cancer League, Geneva.

Excerpta Medica (1982). *Cancer*. Excerpta Medica, Amsterdam.

Freiman, J. A., Chalmers, T. C., Smith, H., and Kuebler, R. R. (1978). The importance of beta, the type II error and sample size in the design and interpretation of the randomized control trial. *New Engl. J. Med.* **299**, 690–4.

George, S. (1983). The required size and length of a phase III clinical trial. In *Cancer clinical trials: methods and practice* (eds. M. Buyse, M. Staquet, and R. Sylvester) pp. 287–310. Oxford University Press.

——and Desu, M. M. (1974). Planning the size and duration of a clinical trial studying the time to some critical event. *J. chron. Dis.* **27**, 15–24.

Gore, S. (1981). Assessing clinical trials—protocol and monitoring. *Br. med. J.* **283**, 369–71.

Herson, J. (1980). Patient registration in a cooperative oncology group. *Control. clin. Trials* **1**, 101–10.

Kisner, D. and Sylvester, R. (1980). *Guidelines for reporting cancer clinical trials*. Colloque INSERM/Direction de la Pharmacie, Evaluation des Medicaments. INSERM, Paris **96**, 477–88.

Machin, D., Staquet, M. J., and Sylvester, R. J. (1979). Advantages and defects of single-center and multi-center clinical trials. In *Controversies in cancer: design of trials and treatment* (eds. H. J. Tagnon and M. J. Staquet), pp. 7–15. Masson, New York.

Makuch, R. and Simon, R. (1978a). Sample size requirements for evaluating a conservative therapy, *Cancer Treat. Rep.* **62**, 1037–40.

—— (1978b). Note on the design of multi-institution three-treatment studies. *Cancer clin. Trials* **1**, 301–3.

Meinert, C. L. (1980). Toward more definitive clinical trials. *Control. clin. Trials* **1**, 249–61.

—— (1981). Organization of multicenter clinical trials. *Control. clin. Trials* **1**, 305–12.

Miller, A. B., Hoogstraten, B., Staquet, M., and Winkler, A. (1981). Reporting results of cancer treatment. *Cancer* **47**, 207–14.

Moertel, C. G. and Hanley, J. A. (1976). The effect of measuring error on the results of therapeutic trials in advanced cancer. *Cancer* **38**, 388–94.

Peto, R. (1978). Clinical trial methodology. *Biomedicine* (Special Issue) **28**, 24–36.

Pocock, S. J., Armitage, P., and Galton, D. A. G. (1978). The size of cancer clinical trials: an international survey. In *Methods and Impact of controlled therapeutic trials in cancer*, UICC Technical Report Series, Vol. 36, pp. 5–32. UICC, Geneva.

Simon, R. (1982). Randomized clinical trials and research strategy. *Cancer Treat. Rep.* **66,** 1083–7.

Staquet, M. (1976). The practice of cooperative clinical trials. *Eur. J. Cancer* **12,** 241–3.

—— (ed.) (1978). *Randomized trials in cancer: a critical review by sites.* EORTC Monograph Series, Vol. 4. Raven Press, New York.

—— Sylvester, R., and Jasmin, C. (1980). Guidelines for the preparation of EORTC cancer clinical trial protocols. *Eur. J. Cancer,* **16,** 871–5.

—— Rozencweig, M., Von Hoff, D., and Muggia, F. (1979). The delta and epsilon errors in the assessment of cancer clinical trials. *Cancer Treat. Rep.* **63,** 1917–21.

—— Sylvester, R., Machin, D., Van Glabbeke, M., De Grauwe, G., Wennerholm, A., Tyrell, J., Renard, G., de Pauw, M., Eeckhoudt, D., Tyrrell, J., and Tagnon, H. (1977). The EORTC Data Center. *Eur. J. Cancer* **13,** 1455–9.

Sylvester, R. J., Machin, D., and Staquet, M. J. (1982). Cancer clinical trial protocols. In *Treatment of cancer* (ed. K. Halnan) p. 861–6. Chapman and Hall, London.

—— Pinedo, H. M., de Pauw, M., Staquet, M., Buyse, M., Renard, G., and Bonadonna, G. (1981). Quality of institution participation in multicenter trials. *New Engl. J. Med.* **305,** 852–5.

TNM Classification of Malignant Tumours (1978). (ed. M. H. Harmer) 3rd edn. International Union Against Cancer, Geneva.

UICC (1978). Controlled therapeutic trials in cancer (ed. R. Flamant and C. Fohanno). *UICC Tech. Rep. Ser.* **32,** Geneva.

US National Institutes of Health (1982). *Compilation of experimental cancer therapy protocol summaries* 6th edn. NIH Publication no 82–1116, US Department of Health and Human Sciences.

Von Hoff, D., Kuhn, J., and Clark, G. (1983). Design and conduct of phase I trials. In *Cancer clinical trials: methods and practice* (eds. M. Buyse, M. Staquet, and R. Sylvester) pp. 210–20. Oxford University Press.

WHO Handbook for reporting results of cancer treatment (1979). WHO Offset Publication no 48. World Health Organization, Geneva.

5 Design of forms for cancer clinical trials

Marleen De Pauw and Marc Buyse

INTRODUCTION

Clinical trials are monitored and their results analysed on the basis of patient data which are collected on forms designed to provide the necessary information. In view of the large number of clinical trials published every year, the design of data report forms represents quite a busy activity, the importance of which is still too often underestimated. Naturally it is generally accepted that 'one of the most decisive and difficult tasks in any inquiry is the construction of an appropriate form of record' (Hill 1971) but unfortunately very little has been contributed to enlighten this task.

Whereas the literature available on the methodology and monitoring of clinical trials unanimously agrees that forms must be clear, unambiguous, short, and simple (Hill 1971; Staquet 1972; Overton 1980), only very few references of some practical assistance are available (Sutherland 1960; Wright and Haybittle, 1979; Gore, 1981; Fox, 1981).

In the field of cancer research, randomized multi-centre clinical trials have become quite common (Staquet, 1978; UICC, 1981) while their complexity has necessitated the establishment of co-ordinating centres. These centres have a central and pivotal role in clinical trials because they are heavily involved in planning and designing a study, and in collecting, editing, storing, monitoring, and analysing the data submitted by the various participants involved. Physicians, nurses, data managers, statisticians, computer scientists, and others are all brought together to collaborate under the leadership of a co-ordinating centre. They will treat patient information received at different stages of a cancer clinical trial usually on the basis of data forms. The design of forms therefore becomes even more important and complex within the framework of a co-ordinating centre.

We will attempt to give some practical guidelines for the design of forms for multi-centre clinical trials in the light of experience acquired through the EORTC Coordinating and Data Center. It goes without saying that it is impossible to outline any stereotyped system for the construction of such forms and that these recommendations will have to be adapted to each particular set of circumstances and environments.

Furthermore, the design of forms to be completed by the patients themselves is beyond the scope of this chapter which will deal only with forms to be completed by investigators or other hospital personnel.

This chapter consists of four parts, the first one dealing with the different sources available for collection of the relevant information to be included on the forms. In the second part the selected information is subdivided according to the different possible types of forms which may be appropriate for a study, while the third part distinguishes between the information necessary only for verification purposes and information which, in addition, must be computerized for inclusion in administrative reports and statistical analyses. Finally, the fourth and last part tackles the design of the form itself.

SOURCES OF INFORMATION TO BE COLLECTED

Standardized methods for reporting cancer clinical trials

One of the main problems in the cancer literature is the difficulty for investigators to compare their results with those of others. These problems originate from inconsistent or incomplete reporting of the patient population under study, the treatment administered, toxicities observed, and the statistical methods employed to assess treatment efficacy. Moreover, there may be important differences from one trial to another as far as the definition of response criteria is concerned.

The development of a 'common language' to describe cancer treatment as well as the use of internationally accepted principles for evaluating data have been the concern of many workers in this field. Chauvergne, Hoerni and Durand (1974) have proposed a common language for the expression of the results of cancer treatment. International classifications such as the *International classification of diseases for oncology* (*ICD–O*) (WHO 1976) and the *Classification of malignant tumours* (*TNM*) (UICC 1978) have been developed by the World Health Organization (WHO) and the International Union Against Cancer (UICC), respectively. Moreover the *WHO Handbook for reporting results of cancer treatment* (WHO 1979) and Miller, Hoogstraten, Staquet, and Winkler (1981) propose a minimum data set which should be reported and provide definitions for criteria such as response, duration of response and duration of survival. In addition a grading system for the reporting of toxicity is provided. As the WHO deals with the reporting of cancer treatment results in general rather than in the specific setting of a clinical trial, Kisner and Sylvester (1980) have proposed a set of guidelines based on the WHO recommendations but adapted specifically to cancer clinical trials. The reporting of results of cancer treatment and the reporting of toxicities are both described in more detail in Part III of this book. The above works should be consulted not only at the time when a trial is being analysed and the results published, but especially when designing protocols since the definitions proposed in these papers should be incorporated in the protocol and data forms at the design stage.

The protocol

The most important document pertaining to any trial is the protocol which provides the scientific basis for the study and describes how the trial is to be carried out. Although the protocol presents the main source of information for items to be included on the data forms, one should carefully select only that information which is relevant to the verification of protocol compliance and to the analysis of the trial objectives.

The study co-ordinator

Since the study co-ordinator is usually the person who writes the protocol or who is at the origin of the clinical trial, he will be aware of possible problem areas which will require careful monitoring. He will also be able to provide guidance as to which data need to be collected for analysis of the trial, for example concerning the potential prognostic factors for the disease under study.

However, as much as it is wise to consult the study co-ordinator about any relevant information to be included on the data forms, one should be conscious of the temptation to record information 'just in case . . .', which usually results in a waste of time and resources. Moreover, collection of marginally useful information may not only detract from the value of the essential data but may also deteriorate the quality of response. Therefore, it is advisable to set up a rule concerning the maximum number of pages allowed per form. In this way the study co-ordinator, the data manager as well as the statistician, will have to proceed even more selectively in choosing only that information which is relevant for the aims of the trial.

The statistician and computer analyst

When collecting the information to be included on the forms, it is wise to check with the statistician and the computer analyst whether all the information required for analysis of the results is included and recorded in a manner which is compatible with the available computer programs.

ORGANIZATION OF THE INFORMATION TO BE COLLECTED

A clinical trial can be subdivided into different stages as follows: the registration or randomization of the patient in a given protocol, his entrance on-study, his treatment and/or follow-up period during the study, the time when he goes off-protocol, the evaluation of the patient's records by the study co-ordinator and, finally, if the patient leaves the protocol alive, the time during which he will be followed for survival and/or progression. Each of these different phases entails the collection of specific information which leads to the design of different types of forms for a given study (Fig. 5.1).

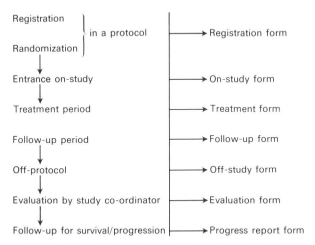

Fig. 5.1. Different phases in a clinical trial requiring different types of forms.

Registration or randomization

Immediately after a patient has been registered or randomized in a given protocol, information pertaining to identification of the patient within the co-ordinating centre, the stratification(s) (if any), and the treatment assigned are coded on a form. This form, usually denoted the *registration form*, becomes the first record in the computer file for that patient, and forms the basis of all future references to this patient by means of his identification number.

Entrance into the protocol

It is of the utmost importance to collect all the necessary information concerning the patient's characteristics at the time he enters a clinical trial. Only in this way can the patient population studied be adequately described in the publication of the results. These data include age, sex, prior anti-tumour therapies, performance status, histopathology, clinical stage, measurability and anatomical extent of the tumour studied.

Moreover, it must be possible to verify whether the patient satisfies the selection criteria stipulated by the protocol and for that purpose additional information such as the presence or absence of chronic diseases, and the results of laboratory and radiological examinations might be required. All well established and potential prognostic factors for the tumour type studied which are not yet included above should also be recorded on this form. For example, prior weight loss, which has been found to be of significant prognostic value for survival in metastatic disease in many tumour types, and for drug response in breast cancer (De Wys, Begg, Lavin, Band, Bennett, Bertino, Cohen, Douglass, Engstrom, Ezdinli, Horton, Johnson, Moertel, Oken, Perlia, Rosenbaum, Silverstein, Skeel, Sponzo, and Tormey, 1980). Finally it is important to be able to *double check* the information supplied at the time of randomization such as the stratifications (if any) and the treatment assigned.

This type of form which gathers information relative to the patient's condition and the status of his cancer before the protocol treatment is started is usually called an *on-study form* or *pre-treatment form*.

The treatment period

Having been entered into a study, the patient will be treated for a certain period of time as defined in the protocol. The sort of information to be recorded during this period, as well as the name to be given to this type of form, depend on the types of treatment under study.

Apart from data pertaining to the treatment administration, such a form usually also includes information regarding the toxicity and response to treatment if applicable. For example, in a clinical trial involving chemotherapy, this form could be denoted as a *chemotherapy form*. It would be completed after each cycle of treatment and record the surface area, the date(s) of administration of the drug(s), the total dose given during the cycle, any delays and/or reduction of the regimen with the reason, haematological and other toxicities, and the response to treatment.

When dealing with trials involving several treatment modalities, a separate form might be necessary only for the principal treatment with the small quantity of information relevant to the other therapies being incorporated in the on-study form. For example, in an adjuvant study in soft tissue sarcoma, patients are randomized after surgery between chemotherapy or no further treatment. The information relevant to the surgery, such as date of surgery, resectability, and surgical procedure could be recorded on the on-study form while a separate chemotherapy form will be designed and filled out after every cycle.

This method should be used with care, however, where it concerns trials involving three or more therapies in that one should avoid combining information pertaining to different treatment disciplines on one form. This is especially true when several investigators complete the data forms. If, for instance, information relative to surgery and radiotherapy is coded on the same form, the time this form will be kept in each department will cause a considerable delay in sending it to the co-ordinating centre, not to mention the problem which will arise if the surgeon does not pass the form on to the radiotherapist or vice versa.

For trials involving simple and well-tolerated oral treatments, a separate treatment form inquiring about the regular intake of the tablets and the eventual side-effects may be unnecessary. Instead, these data may easily be included on the flow sheet or follow-up form described in the following paragraph.

Follow-up in the protocol

Information necessary to follow the progress of a patient during a clinical trial is usually incorporated on a form denoted *flow sheet* or *follow-up form*. This form consists of data relevant to examinations to be repeated at regular intervals and merely serves to monitor the patient's physical condition and disease status. This would involve data on: physical examination including weight and performance status, haematology, biochemistry, X-rays, scans, and any other information pertaining to time to recurrence or progression. This form is usually completed both during and after treatment as long as the patient remains on study.

The time a patient goes off-protocol

Whenever for any reason, the investigator is unable to continue treating a patient or to follow him according to the protocol requirements, the patient is taken off the protocol. The information to be recorded at this stage includes the date and reason for going off-study, the patient's response to treatment, the date and site of progression if applicable, the patient's survival status with the date of death or the date last known to be alive (whichever is applicable), and eventually the cause of death. This form, which is completed when a patient goes off protocol is usually called an *off-study form*.

Evaluation of the patient by the study co-ordinator

Once a patient has been taken off study and his records considered as complete, it is the study co-ordinator's task to review the patient's file in order to make a final decision concerning the evaluability of the patient in the framework of the protocol. This evaluation may be done on the basis of an *evaluation form* which consists of information relative to patient eligibility, major protocol deviations, and completeness of the required patient information.

Progress of the patient off-protocol

Those patients who go off-protocol will usually be followed until progression and/or death. The information to be collected in this case includes: the survival status, the date of death or last known date to be alive, the cause of death, and the date and site of progression if applicable. The form containing this sort of information may be designated as a *progress report form*.

It is essential that each of the forms described above can be easily identified by the co-ordinating centre as well as by the investigator in terms of the patient, the protocol, the institution involved, and the type of form used.

Figure 5.2 shows an example of a one page form designed at the EORTC Data Center. It has been drawn by a plotter connected to a microcomputer and is used in advanced prostatic cancer trials as an off-study form. This form will serve to illustrate several points in the remainder of this chapter. The heading of the form includes: the title of the trial or the name of the co-operative group conducting it, the name or the number of the form, the number of pages it consists of, and the date the form was designed or last modified. Furthermore, the patient's name/number, the name and the address of the participating centre, and the number of the protocol in which the patient is treated must be recorded. To allow incomplete or unclear information to be returned to the investigator, the name of the responsible physician is needed, while the patient's hospital record number (if any) will facilitate the identification of the patient's file within the hospital. However, it is not necessary to repeat these latter two items on each type of form: once, for example on the on-study form, should be sufficient. Finally, one should provide the address of the co-ordinating centre to whom the completed form must be sent with some brief instructions as to when the form should be completed. Forms are usually printed in triplicate so that one copy can be kept at the hospital, another copy can be sent to the study co-ordinator while the top copy can be used by the co-ordinating centre for computerization.

It is evident that the ideas discussed in the above section are based on very elementary principles which may vary depending on the aims of the protocol and the organization of the centre co-ordinating it. Not only may additional forms be necessary, but also the names of the forms will undoubtedly differ among co-ordinating centres, while the decision about the sort of information to be included on each specific form is to a large extent arbitrary. Therefore this paragraph should be considered as an attempt to give an idea of how the design of a set of forms for a clinical trial could eventually be organized, rather than as a set of strict rules to be blindly applied.

COMPUTERIZATION OF THE SELECTED INFORMATION

The information selected for inclusion in data forms can be divided into two categories. The first category consists of information which is essential to perform appropriate computer analyses of the data and which therefore must necessarily be computerized. The other category represents information which allows quality control of the data destined for computerization and is

EORTC GENITO-URINARY TRACT COOPERATIVE GROUP   Form IX   Page 1 of 1
ADVANCED PROSTATE OFF STUDY FORM   March 1982

INSTRUCTIONS: Complete this form WHENEVER A PATIENT IS TAKEN OFF STUDY. Use a
black ballpoint pen and write clearly and firmly. Keep the bottom copy for your
files and send the top two copies to the EORTC DATA CENTER,
1 rue Heger Bordet,
1000 Brussels, Belgium.

Protocol number: _____   Patient's Name: _____

Institution's name and address: _____

1   Patient identification number
                 (DATA CENTER USE ONLY)

22   Date of orchidectomy/start of treatment ⌐
                                              ⊢ (day,month,year)
28   Date of end of treatment (if applicable) ⌐

34   Date off-study (day,month,year)

40   Reason off-study: 1=end of study period
                   2=progression (incl. death due to malignant disease)
                   3=intercurrent death (other than malignant disease)
                   4=excessive toxicity, including toxic death, specify
                   _____
                   5=treatment refused (for reason other than toxicity)
                   6=lost to follow up, specify _____
                   7=protocol violation, specify _____
                   8=other, specify _____
                   9=ineligible, specify _____

41   Response to treatment:
          1=complete remission   5=early death due to malignant disease
          2=partial remission   6=early death due to toxicity
          3=stable disease   7=early death due to other reasons
          4=progression   9=data insufficient to evaluate response

42   Date of progression (day,month,year)

Type of progression   #CODE: 1=no, 2=yes and describe briefly:
                  #
48   Primary prostatic tumour
             #   _____
49   Bone metastases
                 #   _____
50   Visceral metastases
                    #   _____
51   Soft tissue metastases
       #   _____
52   Other, specify _____

53   Patient's survival status: 1=alive, 2=dead, 3=lost to follow up

54   Date of death/last known to be alive (day,month,year)

60   Cause of death, if applicable:
          1=malignant disease   5=other chronic disease
          2=toxicity   8=other, specify
          3=infection   _____
          4=cardiovascular disease   9=unknown

61-80 BLANK

EVALUATION BY THE RESPONSIBLE PHYSICIAN

Was the patient eligible for entry into the study: _____

Are there other reasons for failure for this patient to be fully evaluable:

_____

Date: _____   Signature: _____

Fig. 5.2. Example of a computer-generated form.

therefore supportive in nature. In most instances it will not be necessary to computerize this type of information.

Information requiring computerization

These data comprise all information required for the drafting of administrative and statistical reports based on computer generated analyses. These elementary data can easily be retrieved from the previous paragraphs as follows: data required to adequately describe the patient population studied, all possible prognostic factors, administered treatment doses, reasons for eventual treatment modifications, toxicities reported, response, reason off-protocol, survival, disease-free interval, etc.

Since co-ordinating centers usually monitor multi-centre clinical trials through self-coding forms, the information destined for computer storage is usually coded in boxes numbered from 1 to 80 corresponding to the columns of a computer card (see Fig. 5.2). In this way the forms can be delivered to the keypunch office directly after verification, thus avoiding a manual re-transcription of the original data and an important source of potential error.

Supportive information

Supportive information is fundamental because it documents the computerized data and allows a check on protocol compliance. For example, the overall response to treatment in advanced disease is computerized because it is one of the end-points in the analysis of treatment comparison. It is, however, of paramount importance to be able to check whether the response completed on the forms corresponds with the criteria defined in the protocol. Therefore, it will be necessary to ask for the measurements of all measurable lesions as well as the status of the non-measurable ones before start of treatment and again at regular intervals during treatment. Depending on the tumour type studied, the pre-treatment measurements may be of prognostic value, in which case it will be necessary to computerize them. However, since the person who verifies the forms prior to their entry in the computer file will check the response coded against the measurements given, it is not necessary to store all the subsequent tumour measurements on the computer.

This also holds true for the examinations required to enable an adequate evaluation of the response of the indicator lesion(s), such as the use of lung tomography and/or chest X-rays to evaluate the response of lung metastases. While it is indispensable to be able to check whether the necessary examinations have been performed, there is no further advantage in computerizing these data.

If one suspects that certain aspects of the protocol might be easily overlooked, then it will be most helpful to insert questions which will remind the person who completes the form of the necessity to fulfil certain protocol requirements. For instance, if a histological review of slides is planned, a question asking whether slides have been sent to the referee pathologist(s) will not only remind the investigator of this necessity each time he completes the form, but will also enable the co-ordinating centre to keep track of what is happening. It is clear however that such information need not be computerized.

Whereas information destined for computer storage is usually recorded in numbered boxes, boxes should be avoided when recording supportive information not destined for computerization in order not to confuse the keypuncher (Fig. 5.2).

It should be emphasized however that the situation is not always as clear-cut as described above. Especially where it concerns controversies in the field of cancer, it is advisable to computerize the supportive or raw data instead of, or in addition to, the derived data. In this way possible criticism at the time of publication will be avoided, while analysis of the raw data might possibly lead to interesting findings concerning the controversy itself. For instance, for the staging of testicular cancer at least 10 different classification systems have been proposed (De Wys, Muggia, and Jacobs 1980). Since none of these systems have as yet proved totally satisfactory, it would be advisable to include on the appropriate form a detailed description of the extent of the cancer rather than asking to classify the patient as stage I, II, III, or IV according to an arbitrarily chosen classification system.

Another example pertains to a protocol for the treatment of liver metastases which allows hepatic metastases to be measured by liver scan, echography, or computerized tomography. Although the response to treatment is the end-point of the trial, it is advisable to computerize the supportive information on the methods used to evaluate the response of the metastases in order to permit analysis of, or at least comparisons between, the different methods used.

The idea of distinguishing between information which should or should not be computerized has been put forward to emphasize that even if all the information selected for inclusion on a data form is important for different reasons, only part of the data are essential for computer analysis of the results. Furthermore, reducing the amount of data to be computerized represents a saving of the space needed on both the computer files and output listings, and of time and effort spent in verifying and correcting the information.

DESIGN OF FORMS

Each question must be given the closest thought to see whether it is clear and definite, what the possible answers are; whether the answers can be adequately, if not wholly accurately obtained; how they can be analyzed and put into a statistical table at the end of the inquiry or experiment. If the questions are incomplete, ill conceived or inadequately answered no statistical analysis, however erudite, can compensate for those defects or produce the answers that the worker had hoped to get. The time to remember that is not at the end of an investigation but at its beginning (Hill 1971).

Unfortunately, it is not possible to outline a set of strict rules to be blindly applied in the construction of the questions and their possible answers. However, what can be done is to give some more insight on the basic principles by illustrating the following recommendations with practical examples:

  (i) the questions should be listed in a logical order;
 (ii) questions and answers should be formulated clearly and unambiguously with as little text as possible;
(iii) each question should be self-explanatory and require an answer;
(iv) the codes for the answers should be chosen consistently throughout the forms and reflect the level of measurement for the corresponding questions.

Logical order of requested information

The information requested should be put in a logical order while data on a similar topic should be grouped together. If there is a time element involved, then it is obvious that the order to adopt should be chronological so as to follow as much as possible the order of the information listed in the patient's hospital records.

Example: On-study or pre-treatment form

Patient characteristics:	*birthdate, height, weight, weight loss, sex, performance status, chronic diseases, . . .*
Prior treatment:	*surgery, radiotherapy, chemotherapy, . . .*
Present tumour status:	*stage or category, histology, measurements, . . .*

Treatment assigned by randomization

Clear and unambiguous questions and answers

Formulating clear and unambiguous questions and answers is the most difficult aspect of the design of data forms. Obviously the problem here is how to know which of the questions and answers will be interpreted as fuzzy or confusing by the person who will complete the form. Unfortunately, some of the experience in this field has to be acquired through trial and error, since an ambiguity may arise from those questions for which it is the least expected.

For instance, in a study for papillary carcinoma of the bladder, the size of the largest polyp seen during the cystoscopy performed at entry on-study proved to be of prognostic value. Since these polyps are usually very small it was thought to be a good idea for future studies to ask for the size as precisely as possible, as follows:

☐☐ *Size of largest tumour diameter in centimetres: if greater than 8 cm, code 8.0.*

However, this question was so often coded as │ 1 │   │ that it was deemed necessary to return the forms asking whether this answer meant 1 cm or 1 mm. The replies were mixed and confirmed that the question had been interpreted differently. This ambiguity could have been avoided by formulating the question as follows:

cm mm

☐☐ *Size of largest tumour diameter in centimetres: if greater than 8 cm,*

code │ 8 │ 0 │

e.g. 1 cm = │ 1 │ 0 │ ; *1 mm* = │ 0 │ 1 │.

Another example pertains to the reporting of toxicities in a study including the combination of Cisplatin, Vinblastine, and Bleomycin for disseminated testicular cancer. Since the toxicities inherent to this regimen are well known and were described in detail in the protocol, it was deemed sufficient to record these toxicities on the forms by grouping them as follows: allergic reactions, gastro-intestinal, neuropathy, mucosal and skin toxicity. However, when checking the completed forms it was noted that some centres had classified nausea and vomiting as allergic reactions instead of as gastro-intestinal toxicity. Moreover, constipation which was clearly described in the protocol as being caused by Vinblastine and therefore considered as neurological, was classified as gastro-intestinal toxicity by many investigators. This situation would have been avoided by asking for the actual toxicities which could then be regrouped retrospectively:

☐ *Nausea and vomiting*
☐ *Diarrhoea*
☐ *Paresthesia*
☐ *Loss of tendon reflexes*
☐ *Constipation*
☐ *Abdominal cramps*

etc.

The only way to find out whether all questions are clear and unambiguous is to subject newly designed forms to a trial period, for example by testing them in the first 20 patients entered in the protocol and modifying them if necessary.

Use as little text as possible

As Barnard, Wright and Wilcox (1979) have demonstrated, many people do *not* read or follow instructions when completing a form. Therefore, it is important to formulate questions and answers with as little text as possible. This can be achieved through avoiding repetition of similar answers for different questions by listing the code only once and indicating it, as well as the questions concerned, with an asterisk.

For example:

☐	*Underlying chest wall tumour: 1 = no; 2 = yes; 9 = unknown*
☐	*Skin infiltration: 1 = no; 2 = yes; 9 = unknown*
☐	*Skin ulceration: 1 = no; 2 = yes; 9 = unknown*
☐	*Oedema of the arm: 1 = no; 2 = yes; 9 = unknown*

better:

☐	*Underlying chest wall tumour**	**Code*
☐	*Skin infiltration**	*1 = no*
☐	*Skin ulceration**	*2 = yes*
☐	*Oedema of the arm**	*9 = unknown*

Sometimes it will be possible to combine two or more questions into one single question on the condition that there is only one possible answer among the provided code as shown in the following example.

☐	*Has patient been treated before: 1 = no; 2 = yes*
☐	*If yes, please specify: 1 = chemotherapy*
	2 = radiotherapy
	3 = both chemotherapy and radiotherapy
	8 = other

better:

☐	*Has patient been treated before: 1 = no*
	2 = yes, chemotherapy
	3 = yes, radiotherapy
	4 = yes, both chemotherapy and radiotherapy
	8 = yes, other

Reducing the text whenever possible means less time spent in reading and a quicker completion of the forms.

Self-explanatory questions and answers

As much as one must try to avoid using too much text, one must be careful not to use too little. For instance in asking for dates, instructions regarding the ordering of the day, month, and year are essential because it differs among countries.

Example:

D		M		Y	

Date of mastectomy
(day, month, year)

Moreover, in order to achieve a higher rate of completion, it is advisable to include all the information necessary to answer a question. If one has to consult a separate document to answer a question, the completion of that question will be more readily overlooked, than if the possible answers were at hand. For instance, if one asks for the performance status, the scale should be included on the forms instead of making reference to the protocol.

Every question should require an answer

Whether the person who fills out the form will be able to answer a given question depends as much on the way the question has been formulated as on the codes provided to answer the question. A question which is left unanswered may indicate that the investigator has simply overlooked it or that the answer is unknown. Therefore, every answer must provide enough categories to ensure that all possible situations are covered. In most instances it will be necessary to include special categories providing answers such as 'unknown', 'not applicable', 'examination not done', etc.

For instance if the question

☐ *Liver scan: 1 = normal; 2 = metastases.*

is left blank, then one does not know whether the investigator has forgotten to complete this information or whether it was not completed because a liver scan was not performed. This doubt can be eliminated by adding the category 'not done' as follows:

☐ *Liver scan: 1 = normal; 2 = metastases; 9 = not done.*

However, if the liver scan has been performed but showed abnormalities other than metastases, then this question can still not be answered. Therefore the category 'other' must be included as well:

☐ *Liver scan: 1 = normal; 2 = metastases; 8 = other abnormalities,*
specify: ....
9 = not done

Finally in providing codes to answer a question the code zero (0) may lead to ambiguities when the computer system does not make the distinction between a zero and a blank.

Consistency of codes

The codes adopted must be consistent throughout one specific form, throughout all forms used for a specific trial, and preferably throughout all forms used in a co-operative group. For instance, once the code 1 = no and 2 = yes has been used, all no and yes answers should be recorded as 1 and 2, respectively. Moreover, within co-ordinating centres it seems logical to extend this consistency to forms designed for all clinical trials monitored. This will easily lead to standardization of those codes developed by the co-ordinating centre itself such as: reason off-study, type of progression, survival status, cause of death, evaluability of the patient, etc. (Fig. 5.2).

Example:

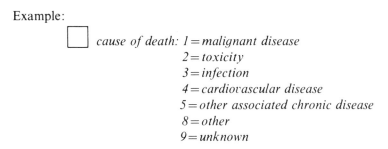

☐ *cause of death: 1 = malignant disease*
2 = toxicity
3 = infection
4 = cardiovascular disease
5 = other associated chronic disease
8 = other
9 = unknown

Such a standardization reduces the errors arising at the coding stage and ensures comparability between different trials.

Level of measurement

Information coded on data report forms will in the end be subjected to some form of statistical analysis, and therefore, as Brigham (1975) has pointed out: 'it cannot be overemphasized that the quantification and statistical analysis of the responses must be considered an integral part of the design of the questionnaire'. In particular, it is important that the codes provided for each variable appropriately reflect the level of measurement of that variable. The intuitive concept of level of measurement was formalized long ago by Stevens (1946) who defined the following scales:

1. Nominal scale (or categorical scale)

This scale consists of numerical codes which are used only as labels. Thus words or letters would serve just as well for the purpose. Typical examples include: reasons off-study, causes of death, sites of disease progression, etc. There is no inherent order in the various categories of this scale. Note that all binary variables are measured on a nominal scale with only two categories which may be called yes/no, present/absent, normal/abnormal, etc.

2. Ordinal scale

The various categories of this scale are ordered but no meaning can be attached to the interval between the successive categories. An example of such a scale is the measurement of the performance status, either on a 0–100 scale (Karnofsky, Abelmann, Craver, and Burchenal 1948) or on a 0–4 scale (Zubrod, Schneiderman, Frei, Brindley, Gold, Schnider, Oviedo, Gorman, Jones, Johnson, Colsky, Chalmers, Ferguson, Dederick, Holland, Selawry, Regelson, Lasagna, and Owens 1960). The 10-point interval between two successive categories on the Karnofsky scale has quite a different meaning whether one drops from 100 to 90 (a minimal loss in ambulatory status) or from 10 to 0 (from moribund to dead).

Ordinal scales are also typically used to report the response to treatment as well as certain toxicities (WHO 1979; Miller, Hoogstraten, Staquet, and Winkler 1981).

If there is an inherent ordering in the categories of a variable, the numerical codes chosen for the categories should reflect it, as in the following example:

☐ *Dukes' grade. Code 1 = No tumour*
       2 = Dukes' A
       3 = Dukes' B
       4 = Dukes' C

3. Interval scale

This scale could be called 'quantitative' as its categories are ordered and equally distant from each other. It is appropriate for measurements such as weight, height, treatment dose, tumour measurements, laboratory data, etc.

The relevance of introducing these various scales here is that the statistical operations which are permitted on a variable depend on the level of measurement at which it is reported. Only frequency counts and the distribution mode and range are applicable to nominal scales. These statistics are also valid for ordinal scales for which one can also calculate the median value and distribution percentiles. Lastly, the widest range of statistics can be calculated for interval scales, i.e. all of the above, plus the mean, standard deviation, etc. The nominal scale is therefore called the lowest scale of measurement and the interval scale the highest. It is advisable, at least in theory, to choose the highest possible level of measurement for each variable. In practice, however, the level selected for some variables will often be a compromise between the ideal situation and the ease of coding.

For instance, in trials where the white blood count has a prognostic influence or in trials aiming at documenting the haematological toxicity of a certain treatment regimen, it is important to know the exact white blood count (interval scale). Otherwise an ordinal scale as proposed by the WHO (1979) will be sufficient, especially if simplicity is sought as illustrated in the following example:

Interval scale:

$\square\square\square\square\square$ *WBC (cells/mm^3)*

Ordinal scale:

$\square$ *WHO code for WBC:*
  0 = ≥4.000 (cells/mm^3)
  1 = 3.000–3.999
  2 = 2.000–2.999
  3 = 1.000–1.999
  4 = <1.000

The choice between ordinal and nominal scales will not always be clear-cut either. Let us consider a trial in which hormonal therapy and chemotherapy are tested simultaneously using a factorial design. There are thus four treatment arms and it is reasonable to assume an ordering of these four arms: from the least aggressive and least toxic arm (no further treatment) to the most aggressive and most toxic arm (the combined modality). Hence the treatment arm could be coded on an ordinal scale. However, two nominal scales (binary scales) could also be used if one wished to emphasize the factorial nature of the trial design.

Ordinal scale:

$\square$ *1 = no further treatment*
  2 = hormonal therapy
  3 = chemotherapy
  4 = both hormonal and chemotherapy

Nominal scale: (multiple binary scale)

$\square$ *Hormonal therapy**   **Code: 1 = no*
$\square$ *Chemotherapy**   *2 = yes*

An instance where multiple binary coding must be used is when the categories of a nominal scale are not mutually exclusive. For instance, the *main* site of distant metastases could be coded on a nominal scale as follows:

☐ *1 = liver ; 2 = lung ; 3 = bone, etc.*

The various categories may be indicated in any order, for example in decreasing order of frequency. However, usually it will be interesting to know not only the *main* metasatic site but the others as well. A multiple binary scale is then appropriate:

☐ *Liver**   **Code : 1 = no*
☐ *Lung**   *2 = yes*
☐ *Bone**

etc.

CONCLUSION

The design of data report forms is one of the first and most decisive steps in the conduct of a clinical trial. Nevertheless, it still represents an often neglected aspect in data collection resulting in detrimental consequences to the outcome of many trials.

In view of the sparce references available in the literature which are of only little practical assistance in the design of data forms, this chapter has been written in the hope to contribute to the enlightenment of this task. Unfortunately, further knowledge will have to be acquired through trial and error.

Modern technology has undoubtedly contributed to a quicker and easier production of data forms (Hanley 1978). At the EORTC Coordinating and Data Center for instance, the typing of forms has been replaced by drawing forms interactively on a plotter connected to a microcomputer. Modern technology will also increasingly enable the transfer of patient data directly from the hospital records into the computer located at the co-ordinating centre (Kronmal, Davis, Fisher, Jones and Gillespie 1978). Even in such a situation some type of data form will be necessary and therefore advances in technology will never dispense with the design of data forms, whether on paper or on videoscreens, as the basis for all further operations in the research process.

REFERENCES

Barnard, P. J., Wright, P., and Wilcox, P. (1979). Effects of response instructions and question style on the ease of completing forms. *J. occupational Psychol.* **52,** 209–26.

Brigham, F. R. (1975). Some quantitative considerations in questionnaire design and analyses. *Appl. Ergonom.* **6.2**, 90–6.

Chauvergne, J., Hoerni, B., and Durand, M. (1974). Langage commun dans l'expression des résultats thérapeutiques en cancérologie. *Bull. Cancer* **61**, no. 2, 235–44.

De Wys, W., Begg, C., Lavin, P., Band, R., Bennett, M., Bertino, R., Cohen, H., Douglass, O., Engstrom, F., Ezdinli, Z., Horton, J., Johnson, J., Moertel, G., Oken, M., Perlia, C., Rosenbaum, C., Silverstein, N., Skeel, T., Sponzo, W., and Tormey, C. (1980). Prognostic effect of weight loss prior to chemotherapy in cancer patients. *Am. J. Med.* **69**, 491–7.

De Wys, W., Muggia, F. M., and Jacobs, E. M. (1980). Staging of testicular cancer: a proposed clinical surgical schema. *Cancer Treat. Rep.* **64**, 669–74.

Fox, J. J. (1981). Design of a record form for a clinical trial. *Clin. Res. Rev.* **1** (2), 157–61.

Gore, S. M. (1981). Assessing clinical trials. Record Sheets. *Br. med. J.* **283**, 296–8.

Hanley, J. A. (1978). A language for computer generation of medical data forms. Biometrics **34**, 288–97.

Hill, B. (1971). *Principles of medical statistics*, 9th edn. The Lancet, London.

Karnofsky, D. A., Abelmann, W. H., Craver, L. F., and Burchenal, J. H. (1948). The use of nitrogen mustards in the palliative treatment of carcinoma. *Cancer* **1**, 634–56.

Kisner, D. L. and Sylvester, R. J. (1980). Guidelines for reporting cancer clinical trials. Colloque INSERM/Direction de la Pharmacie, Evaluation des Médicaments. *INSERM*, Paris **96**, 477–88.

Kronmal, R. A., Davis, K., Fisher, L. K., Jones, R. A., and Gillespie, M. J. (1978). Data management for a larger collaborative clinical trial (CASS: Coronary Artery Surgery Study). *Comput. biomed. Res.* **11**, 553–66.

Miller, A. B., Hoogstraten, B., Staquet, M., and Winkler, A. (1981). Reporting results of cancer treatment. *Cancer* **47**, 207–14.

Overton, H. H. (1980). Perception of the coordinating center. As reviewed by a clinic coordinator. *Control. clin. Trials* **1**, 133–6.

Staquet, M. (1972). Planning and design of multi-institutional trials. In *The design of clinical trials in cancer therapy* (*Symposium, Brussels, 1972*). Editions Scientifiques Européennes, Brussels, and Futura Publishing Co., New York.

—— (ed.) (1978). *Randomized trials in cancer: a critical review by sites*. Raven Press, New York.

Stevens, S. S. (1946). On the theory of scales of measurement. *Science, NY* **103**, 677–80.

Sutherland, I. (1960). The design of records and follow up. In *Controlled clinical trials*, pp. 151–4. Blackwell Scientific Publications, Oxford.

UICC (1978). *TNM, classification of malignant tumours* (ed. M. H. Harmer) 3rd edn. UICC, Geneva.

—— (1981). *Methods and impact of controlled therapeutic trials in cancer*. UICC, Geneva.

WHO (1976). *International classification of diseases for oncology* (*ICD-O*), 1st edn. WHO, Geneva.

—— (1979). *WHO Handbook for reporting results of cancer treatment*, WHO offset publication no. 48. WHO, Geneva.

Zubrod, C. G., Schneiderman, M., Frei, E., III, Brindley, C., Gold, G. L., Schnider, B., Oviedo, R., Gorman, J., Jones, R. Jr, Johnson, U., Colsky, J., Chalmers, T., Ferguson, B., Dederick, M., Holland, J., Selawry, O., Regelson, W., Lasagna, L., and Owens, Jr, A. H. (1960). Appraisal of methods for the study of chemotherapy of cancer in man: comparative therapeutic trial of nitrogen mustard and triethylene thiophosphoramide. *J. chron. Dis.* **11**, 7–33.

6 Computerization of clinical trials

Elisa T. Lee

INTRODUCTION

In the past several decades there has been a sharp increase in the number of cancer clinical trials conducted in pharmaceutical companies, individual hospitals, and, as a co-operative effort, in several hospitals. Advances in microbiology, biochemistry, and pharmacology result in new diagnostic and treatment modalities every day. While these advances have enabled modern medical practice to progress rapidly, they have also created problems. One of the problems is the tremendous amount of history, laboratory, and clinical information accumulated. It can be predicted that the trend will continue and the amount of patient information will no doubt increase even more rapidly in the future. The continual and thorough review of results is a necessary prerequisite for success in clinical trials. An important aspect in a clinical trial is the process of collection and analysis of data. Typically, analysis is considered a statistical task. However, the success of statistical analysis depends heavily on the quality of data collection. Poorly collected and unorganized data will give biased and misleading conclusions. However, the importance of patient information collection and organization for clinical trials has been until recently rather neglected.

WHY COMPUTERIZE?

The traditional patient information collection depends on the medical charts. This method is familiar to physicians, nurses and laboratory scientists. There are no restraints or special requirements on the user. The capacity for accumulation is infinite. However, the advantages are followed by many shortcomings. The shortcomings of the paper record or charts can be summarized as follows.

1. Poor organization: the records may at most be roughly chronological, however, there is no systematic way in organizing the various reports in the chart. This contributes to the difficulty in data retrieval and 'missing data'.

2. Inaccuracy or low reliability: many clinical and laboratory reports are in duplicate. They are often difficult to read. Errors and misinterpretations may be introduced in the process of transcribing information from the chart. This again affects seriously the quality of data.

3. Information not up-to-date: modern medical treatment often requires the co-operation of many specialists, for example a consulting physician, a special laboratory scientist, and a radiation expert. Frequently, their reports may take days or weeks to arrive and be included in the chart. This may delay decisions for treatment.

4. Deficiency in content: basic information about the patient, for example family history of cancer, details about prior treatment, and current status are often incomplete. In addition, staging methods used may not be uniform. All this makes data retrieval extremely difficult. It may require a highly skilled person or even the physician to search for the information needed.

5. Slow access: the charts must be obtained from the records office. They are available for data abstraction only when not being used by the physicians and nurses. Information must be abstracted by searching through the chart. For large and long-term trials, it may take more than one abstractor to collect the needed information for periodic analysis.

6. Slow and inaccurate analysis and reporting: most modern statistical methods require complicated computations, particularly the multivariate techniques. Manual data analysis is extremely time consuming, if not infeasible. In addition, manual computation gives low precision. Slow and inaccurate analysis leads to slow and inaccurate reporting. The ability to quickly respond to a request is very limited. If the clinical trial involves periodic data retrieval and analysis the problem could be very serious.

Revolutionary progress in computer science in the last three decades makes it possible to circumvent many of the shortcomings and difficulties of manual data collection, retrieval, and analysis in clinical investigations. Using computers as a tool for information storage and retrieval as well as statistical analysis becomes a logical step. In general, any clinical trial must go through three steps: (1) trial design, (2) data collection, storage, and retrieval, and (3) data analysis. Because of its incredible speed, large capacity, and high precision, the computer is extremely useful in all three steps, particularly in steps two and three. In the next three sections, the use of computers in these three steps is discussed.

COMPUTERS IN TRIAL DESIGN

Important considerations in trial design include: (1) objectives of the trial, (2) number of patients required, (3) randomization of patients to different treatments, and (4) measures of treatment outcomes (i.e. toxicity, response, remission duration, or survival time). In this step, computer simulation methods can be used in answering these questions, particularly, (2), (3), and (4) for optimizing the design of a clinical trial (for example Knox 1973; Jones 1978; Woodings and Madsen 1978).

Through simulation, the computer can generate an inexhaustible supply of patients with different characteristics and monitor their responses to different treatments throughout the trial. Thus, computerization in this step requires a program which simulates the entry, randomization, and outcome of treatments. Patient characteristics such as age and prognosis may be simulated using different statistical distributions. Assignments of patients to treatments may be done by a computer generated randomization scheme. Measures of treatment outcome may also be generated by assuming a theoretical distribution. For example, the remission duration or survival time may be assumed to follow an exponential or Weibull distribution. If patients can be divided into subgroups according to patient characteristics, different distributions or different parameters may be chosen for each subgroup. The computer then generates random samples from the specified distribution and parameter values as data from a simulated set of patients. The remission or survival data so generated are then compared, for example, by life-table methods. If the simulation procedure is repeated for the same assumptions but different samples (using different random numbers) estimates may be made of the proportion of trials of the type specified in the assumptions which would yield a 'significant' result. This proportion is an estimate of the probability that a trial of this type would detect differences between the treatments for the sample size specified in the assumptions.

The effects of varying the specified assumptions of the trial, that is rate of entry, sample size of each treatment group, distribution of treatment outcomes, etc., may be investigated by repeating the entire simulation procedure with a new set of assumptions. From this an optimum sample size and consequently, an 'optimum' design may be found.

Of course, for a small and simple clinical trial, simulation may not be advantageous. Randomization may be done manually and the sample size for each treatment group estimated by reference to existing tables or graphs. However, if the trial is large and complex, for example if several distinct subgroups of patients are to be entered, the existing tables may not be sufficient and the simulation method may then be useful.

COMPUTERS IN DATA COLLECTION, STORAGE, AND RETRIEVAL

Cancer clinical trials have many facets, most of which relate to the evaluation and comparison of treatments and identification of prognostic factors. Patient characteristics may include personal history, previous treatments, current laboratory test results, and clinical findings. Furthermore, all cancer trials have a long follow-up period after treatment starts, usually from 2 to 5 years. Patients revisit the clinic periodically during this time. Such long active periods of patient observation result in more information accumulation. Periodical review of records is essential to success in cancer clinical trials. The large capacity and high speed of the computer are most desirable in data storage and retrieval.

In the last two decades, major efforts have been devoted to medical data management systems in general. Most of them focus on data collection, storage, and retrieval; only a few have the ability to link to a statistical package. Reviews of the state of the art have been given by, for example, Singer (1969), Ball (1971), and Bekey and Schwartz (1972). A number of the information systems were specifically designed for cancer clinical investigations (Dutreix, Dutreix, and Zummer 1972).

Regardless of the type of clinical trial, computerization of data must go through the following steps:

1. Information must be collected from its source. The source may be the patient, physician, or laboratory.

2. Non-numerical information must be reduced to numerical codes that are readable to the computer.

3. Data must be updated.

4. Data must be retrieved and arranged to the form required by statistical analysis programs.

5. Statistical analysis must be performed and reports generated.

The use of computers in the first four steps is discussed in this section. Computers in statistical data analysis will be discussed next.

In the last two or three decades, medical researchers in clinical trials have used the computer in one way or another. The extent of use or modes of operation depends largely on the computer facilities available in their hospitals. There are, in general, two types of operation available in the computerization of clinical data: in-house service, and outside service or assistance.

In-house service: large and medium size computers

In hospitals with a large- or medium-scale computer, the use of a computer can be grouped into three categories depending on the extent of use:

1. computerized data analysis;

2. batch processing data collection, storage, and retrieval;

3. interactive data collection, storage, and retrieval.

The first category is most common for small clinical studies. It is most frequently used in a one-shot analysis. The second category is often used in large cancer hospitals and co-operative oncology groups. In a batch-processing system, data are first recorded on specially designed forms before entering the computer. Interactive systems usually involve a time-sharing data base. Physicians, nurses, and laboratory technicians record information directly onto the computer from their terminals. Data can also be retrieved from the system by using terminals. In the last two categories, patient data may be retrieved and analysed periodically. The periodic reviews provide updated information on the number of eligible patients, trial progress, opportunities to detect deficiencies and problems, and assistance in deciding whether or not to continue, discontinue, or alter therapy in an active clinical trial. For example, regular reporting of severe toxicity is of vital importance. Therapy may have to be discontinued or revised for patients with severe or life-threatening toxic reactions. Through periodic reviews, patients who failed to return for regular visits can be identified immediately. These patients should not be allowed to disappear from the trial and their reasons for not returning to the hospital should be found out. If they have moved away, their fate should be discovered, if possible, by extensive telephone inquiries, letters, or personal visits. In addition, the computer may be used to register patients and schedule their subsequent visits. This is feasible particularly in an interactive system. Patient data may be entered into the computer as the patient goes through the registration desk, clinics, and laboratories. At the end of the examination, the time for the next visit following the protocol is available on the terminal.

1. Computerized data analysis

Many hospitals have used the computer only for data analysis. Detailed patient information is recorded in traditional charts. At analysis time, the data to be analysed are transcribed onto a computer coding form. These forms are set up with 80 columns that correspond to a keypunched card. Columns are allocated for various variables to be studied. For example, columns 1 to 5 may be for patient number, 6 to 7 for diagnosis, 8 to 10 for age, 11 to 12 for sex, 13 to 14 for prior treatment, 15 to 16 for current treatment, etc. Qualitative variables are assigned different codes, for example for sex, 1 may indicate male and 2 female. Disease stages and classifications may be coded similarly. A sample coding form is given in Fig. 6.1. If 80 columns is not enough for each patient, additional lines or additional coding sheets may be used. For example, one form could contain personal history data, disease category and

Patient no.	Dx (1-AML, 2-ALL)	Age	Sex (1-male, 2-female)	Prior Rx (1-Yes, 0-No)	Rx	WBC	Date of initial Rx	Resp (1-Yes, 0-No)	Relapse date	Surv. status (0-alive, 1-Dead)	Death date
11219	1	25	1	0	2	5450	11075	1		0	9760
12402	1	38	2	1	1	10600	4875	1		10750	
14254	1	50	1	1	1	12100	5750			1	81376
13080	1	65	2	0	2	7980	31575	1	91275	0	
15062	1	49	2	0	1	7145	4875	1	11576	0	
17161	1	70	1	1	2	7000	12975	0	62576	1	72576
17205	1	65	1	0	1	6800	12876	1			
18401	1	79	1	1	2	14700	6875	1	31776	1	32376

Fig. 6.1. Sample coding form.

stage, a second form for prior therapy, a third form for laboratory test results, and a fourth form for response, remission duration and survival time.

Following the coding forms, computer cards are punched and a program to input the data to the computer is written. The data may be stored on a disk or magnetic tape. If the number of cards is not very large, tapes or disks may not be necessary. Or, in some cases, the data may be keyed into the computer directly and stored on a temporary disk.

This method of recording data for analysis is convenient for small trials that involve at most 100 to 200 subjects and do not require periodic reviews of treatment outcomes. It is also the easiest way to record a retrospective study. However, for a large trial or a long-term trial in which periodic reviews are necessary, this method is not efficient. In order to reach maximum data accuracy and completeness, it is important to have a reliable nurse or technician working closely with the investigator to transcribe the data. The coded data must be further checked for possible errors. This can be done manually or by building into the input program an automatic check-list. Unreasonable data entries will be rejected and printed out by the computer.

This method is used in most hospitals where computer facilities and a data processing unit with appropriate statistical software exist. The investigator may need to hire an experienced programmer with a statistical background to work with the statistician. In many hospitals, the investigator may only need to submit the data to the statistician for data entry and analysis.

2. Batch-processing data storage and retrieval

In batch-processing data storage and retrieval, data are first recorded on a specially designed form or forms and then punched on cards for input to the computer or keyed into the computer directly. If the number of items to be recorded is large, the items can be grouped into several categories and recorded on different forms. For example, one form may be designed for pre-study personal and family history, one for prior treatment, one for surgery, one for current treatment and response status, and one for laboratory test results. (Form design is discussed in detail in the previous chapter.) Figure 6.2 gives an example of a pre-study form for a melanoma study. Usually, these forms are kept in the patient's chart and a copy of them is sent to the statistician or computer personnel for input to the computer. The design of these forms is very important. The investigator must consult with the statistician and a computer expert on the kind of information to be collected and the organization of the forms.

A computer program must be written to create a file or files for the data. In most information storage and retrieval systems data are stored in *upright* files. In an upright file, data are arranged as they are collected, that is by patient record. Each patient is a record. Each record is divided into fields that take on one or more data items. The organization or structuring of data items within each record is, in many systems, designated by a 'dictionary'. The dictionary

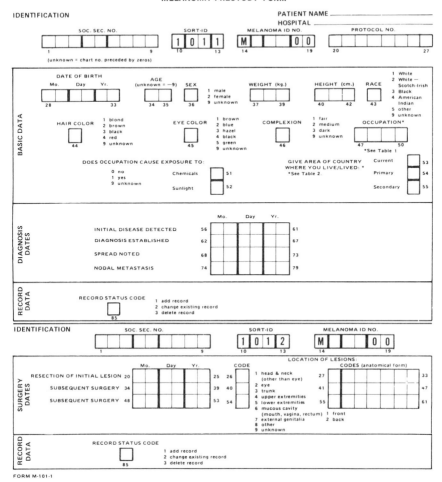

Fig. 6.2. Sample data form.

specifies data item names, type of data, numerical code representations, possible value ranges of all of the data items or fields in a file. For example, field number 6 might be data item name AGE: type of data is numerical, and acceptable values are 1 to 99 and −9 for unknown. Field number 7 might be data item name SEX: type of data is categorical and numerical code representations are 1 for male, 2 for female and 9 for unknown. In every record then, fields 6 and 7 would contain a value for an individual's age and sex.

To specify acceptable values for a field is not only a way to promote quality control of data entry, but also to maintain protocol compliance. There are usually eligibility criteria specified for each clinical trial, for example, diagnostic criteria, age limitations, or criteria based on laboratory test results.

Any entry that does not meet the criteria or specification will be rejected by the computer and an error message printed out.

To retrieve data from an upright file, it is necessary to define the subset of records to be retrieved. For example, in a leukaemia trial, the subset may be all acute myeloblastic leukemias who received no prior therapy. Once the subset of records has been defined, the search criteria are provided. Suppose that AML is coded as 1 in the diagnosis field (DX) and 'no prior therapy' as 0 in the 'prior treatment' field (PT), then the search criteria are $DX = 1$ and $PT = 0$. After search conditions have been specified, they may be combined to make a logical statement using the Boolean AND, OR, and NOT. Records that satisfy the logical statement are then selected. In this example, the logical statement is '$DX = 1$ AND $PT = 0$'.

Data updating is done in a batch mode. Data retrieved from the system may be saved on a disk or tape for statistical analysis, or directly inputed to statistical programs or packages that are available on the same computer.

Most large- and medium-scale computers (for example IBM, CDC, UNIVAC, etc.) have software for file creation. Hospitals with adequate computer facilities may set up their own files to fit their specific needs. There are many batch-processing data systems in the literature, for example, Addison, Coney, Jones, Shields, and Sweeney (1969); Volterrani, Donati, Uslenghi, Sigurta, and Gentenaro (1979), and Mackay (1979).

3. Interactive data storage and retrieval

In the last ten to fifteen years, time-shared systems have been made available by large random-access file storage devices and teleprocessing techniques. Interactive or on-line, real-time data systems have been developed for hospital administration and medical research. The term 'on-line' refers to systems in which terminals at remote locations such as nurse stations, clinics, or laboratories are connected directly to the computer for data input, inquiry, or communication purposes. 'Real time' refers to immediate processing by the computer of information entered through on-line terminals. The completely computerized system may also be connected to statistical analysis programs. Therefore, the researcher may obtain not only patient information but also statistics in minutes or hours. This type of system provides users with convenience and reliability. A number of interactive information storage and retrieval systems have been developed. Among them are MISAR (Karpinski and Bleich 1971), RISS (McLeod and Meldman 1975), CLINFO (Palley and Groner 1974), MEDINFO (Johnson and Barnett 1977), MISAR II (Melski, Geer, and Bleich 1978) and those described by Singer (1969), Fries (1972), Neurath, Bloedorn, Muzenrider and Pedrazzi (1974), Bill, Anderson, O'Fallon, and Silvers (1978), McShan, Haumann, and Glicksman (1979), Glicksman and McShan (1979), Lee (1979), and Wallace and Cooper (1979).

In an interactive data storage and retrieval system, data collection may be done in two modes. The first mode is recording data on paper forms and then entering them onto the computer by a data clerk through a terminal. The computer asks questions on the form and the data clerk responds by typing in the answers. The questions appearing on the terminal may be abbreviated and numbered as on the paper form.

The second mode is direct computer entry without the use of paper forms. As the physician, nurse, or laboratory technician sits at a terminal keyboard inputting information about the patient, the computer responds with questions displayed on the terminal. In general, similar to the batch-processing system, data are coded and the file structure is by record. A 'dictionary' is used to specify fields. However, the data can be maintained in a non-coded manner to allow for easy and flexible input. For example, a pagination system may be designed which would allow the data to be entered as a set of pages or forms. These forms are created by the computer. 'The program allows the user to type a form onto the terminal just as he/she would like to have it appear. The form is then sent to the computer and stored line by line into a random access file' (McShan *et al.* 1979).

Data editing and updating in this case may also be through the terminal or through batch processing. To retrieve data, the user needs to type in the subset criteria and the date items necessary. The computer will search for the subjects, and print out the information specified on the terminal.

An advantage of interactive systems is their immediate feedback. Errors in data entry or lack of protocol compliance can be detected immediately. If the data entered do not satisfy the specifications built into the program, it will be rejected without delay. This advantage allows many transcription errors to be immediately corrected while the data content is still fresh in the minds of the persons dealing with the source information. Another advantage of interactive systems is the minimum requirement on the user. Once the system is working, after a short orientation, physicians, nurses, and technicians can use it without the need of programmers. For a large multi-clinic trail, the interactive, time-sharing system has several advantages. Firstly, the time and trouble of sending forms to the statistical office or computer centre can be saved. Secondly, the average hardware cost to each individual user is considerably reduced. Thirdly, programming cost is also reduced through the sharing of common programs built to serve every clinic. However, an interactive system operation must be staffed with personnel with extensive, up-to-date and detailed knowledge of computers, data file organization, data retrieval techniques, and the clinical trial. The cost of software and hardware (for example terminals) to support the interactive system is high.

For statistical evaluations, two modes of retrieval are used commonly. The first is designed to be interactive. The subset of patients and variables to be analysed are entered into the terminal by name. The user also types in the name of statistical procedures to be used. After the appropriate data are retrieved, statistical analysis will be performed automatically and results appear on the terminal. The second mode is not interactive. It requires data to be extracted and written on a disk or magnetic tape. The data disk or tape may then be used by the statistical software. At this time, not many interactive systems have a complete interactive statistical analysis.

Stand-alone mini or microcomputer system

In the past several years mini and microcomputer development has progressed extremely rapidly. The amounts of central memory and mass storage available to a mini or microcomputer have increased, as has the speed of CPU (Central Processing Unit). Costs of computer hardware, system software development, and communication are enormously reduced. Hospitals have been increasingly looking toward small, inexpensive, locally-owned-and-operated, stand-alone mini or microcomputer systems as an answer to their needs (O'Desky 1977; Wasserman 1977). Examples of mini and microcomputer systems are, respectively, given by Tenenbaum and Weinberger (1979) and Janik, Sharp, Forbush, Wyman, and Jung (1979).

Many of the mini computers today are not really 'mini', for example, Data General's ECLIPSE M/600 has 1500K bytes memory and their MV/8000 is many times larger. Many of the mini computers have a data-base-oriented file management system that allows the user to create, maintain, and use large data bases in multi-terminal, batch, and communication environments. For example, Data General's INFOS software provides the indexed sequential access method and data base access method for data storage and retrieval. It is integrated with Data General's AOS (Advanced Operating System) and executes on a Commercial ECLIPSE C/300 or M/600 mini computer. Mini computers can usually run programs written in BASIC and FORTRAN languages. Statistical programs written in FORTRAN for large computers can easily be run on the mini computer without much difficulty.

Microcomputer technology is still quite young. Though hardware technology continues to advance dramatically, software technology has not. Similar to large computers, microcomputers require that programs for input, editing, updating, retrieval, and statistical analysis be written in the proper language, for example BASIC. For cancer clinical trials, microcomputers suffer from the lack of available sophisticated statistical software. For large and complex trials microcomputers are currently limited by their small central memory (usually less than 64K bytes) and mass storage capacity (usually less than 256K bytes per diskette). However, with on-going technological advances, these limitations will soon be a thing of the past.

Both mini and microcomputers may be linked to a large computer. While a mini or microcomputer is capable of integration into a large computer, it can still be implemented and supported with only limited technical resources. Microcomputers are efficient and convenient for data input and output display when the large computer carries out the analysis. Presently, microcomputers are often used in this capacity.

Outside service or assistance: the service bureau

The application of computerized information systems in hospitals has been most prominent in the business office. In many cases, the computer system for accounting and administrative purposes may not be suitable for clinical and laboratory data. Instead of investing in more computer hardware and personnel, many hospitals look towards outside service. An outside company with a ready information storage and retrieval system may allow hospitals to start with a minimum equipment investment and a minimum of personnel involvement. Usually the hospital is responsible for collecting information by paper forms or terminals and the outside company is responsible for computer data storage, retrieval, and report generating.

There are several large medical information systems available. Among them are PAS (Professional Activity Study), MCAUTO (McDonnel Douglas Automation Company), and SIR (Scientific Information Retrieval).

PAS, a co-operative study conducted by the Commission on Professional and Hospital Activities (CPHA) at Ann Arbor, Michigan, includes centralized collection, processing, and study of data on hospital medical care. It uses a uniform input data form and a uniform disease classification and coding system. It provides an unlimited opportunity to collect and display variable data and generates various reports at a choice of time period (Kaplan and Mendeloff 1975).

MCAUTO, a health service system offered by McDonnel Douglas Automation Company (a division of McDonnel Douglas Corporation) is a large system with multiple subsystems (McDonnel Douglas 1980). One of them, the Patient Care System (PCS), automates patient information associated with drug ordering, scheduling, patient registration, laboratory and radiology results reporting, and history record-keeping. It offers immediate and ready access to a large patient data base. PCS uses multiple, independent in-hospital miniprocessors which allows results to be entered directly into the system by typing on the CRT (Cathode Ray Tube) screen. The Medical Record Information System (MR_{II}) collects, edits, analyses, and reports data from hospital's patient medical records. Data are collected by case abstract forms and processed at MCAUTO's Data Center. All of their data systems are independent of each other, but can be connected and used collectively to produce a composite picture.

Both PAS and MCAUTO use fixed data collection forms. Although they provide the user with numerous reports and statistics, they are mostly summaries or simple tabulations by diagnosis, treatment, etc. No sophisticated statistical analysis of response, remission, or survival is performed by their systems. Therefore, their use in cancer clinical trials is very limited.

SIR, a data base management system, was developed by the Scientific Information Retrieval, Inc. in Evanston, Illinois. This software is available on the following computers and operating systems:

(a) IBM 360/370 running under OS/VS. Interactive processor available with TSO and CMS;

(b) VAX 11/780 running under VMS;

(c) UNIVAC 90 series running under VS/9;

(d) CDC 6000 and CYBER series computers.

In this system, information is grouped into individual cases. Cases consist of records of different types, and records are made up of data items. Users can add, replace, modify, and delete data at any time in both batch mode and interactive mode. Data retrieval may be made from the various record types in the file by sequential search or random access. It provides the user with a set of utility routines for file maintainance. The most attractive feature of SIR is its direct linkage to statistical packages such as SPSS (Statistical Package for the Social Sciences; Nie, Hull, Jenkins, Steinbrenner, and Bent 1975; Hull and Nie 1979), BMDP (Biomedical Computer Programs— P series; Dixon 1977, 1979), and SAS (Statistical Analysis System; SAS 1979). Each of these packages consists of a number of statistical programs, including those for survival data analysis.

Large cancer hospitals with developed computer file management systems, particularly tailored for their own needs, may not find commercially available data base management systems (DBMS) such as SIR useful. However, for hospitals new in the field or small hospitals with limited personnel resources this kind of DBMS may be economical and convenient. Because of its linkage to statistical software, much of the programmer's time can be freed.

The time-sharing service

In this mode, the hospital has access to a large-scale computer, near or remote, through a special communication line. Data are entered by the hospital and reports can be requested. This mode is logical for hospitals that can not afford their own mainframe to pool their needs and share the costs. This mode is ideal for a co-operative group in which participating hospitals are using the same protocols and the hospital that owns the computer functions as the data processing centre. In a time-sharing system, inputs and outputs are usually fixed. Most time-sharing systems operate in a batch update mode. Patient file updating may not be done immediately and requests for specific current information may not be able to be fulfilled at the time of request. In addition, it may also involve high communication costs.

COMPUTERS IN STATISTICAL DATA ANALYSIS

Statistical data analysis is essential in clinical trials. Investigators in cancer clinical trials are usually interested in one or more of the following analyses:

(a) response rates;

(b) distribution of remission durations and survival times;

(c) comparison of response rates, remission durations, and survival times;

(d) identification of prognostic factors related to response, remission duration, and survival time.

All of these analyses except perhaps the response rates require complicated statistical methods and a considerable amount of calculations, particularly the multivariate techniques for the identification of prognostic factors. The computer is indispensable, without it, sophisticated statistical analysis is impossible. Computer programs for many conventional statistical methods are available on many large and small computers. Programs for survival data analysis have been scattered. In general there are three ways to satisfy the need of statistical programs.

1. In-house programming

Hospitals that have a statistical unit, adequate computer facilities, and knowledgeable programmers may develop their own statistical software or implement programs written by others. They may also develop programs for data input to or retrieval from their data system, and arrange them in proper format for the statistical programs. Implementing programs written by others is not usually very difficult, provided that the programs were written for a comparable computer. The size of the programming staff needed depends on the number of ongoing trials. In general, for a small or moderate number of clinical trials, one or two experienced programmers suffice.

2. Subscribing to commercially available statistical packages

Hospitals not wishing to invest in programming may subscribe to one or more of the available program packages. There are a number of statistical packages available, among them, BMDP, SAS, and SPSS provide programs or procedures particularly useful in cancer clinical trials in addition to a number of conventional statistical methods. Each package has its own input language and fixed output, and requires that the data be arranged in a certain manner. The BMDP programs are ready to use on the IBM 360/370. Special arrangements can be made to make them usable on CDC CYBER, Honeywell 600/6000, Univac Series 70, 90 and 1108, and Xerox SIGMA 7. SAS programs run only on IBM 360/370 computers and plug-compatible machines such as Amdahl, Itel, CDC Omega, Magnuson, Ryad, etc. SPSS programs can be run on IBM 360/370, CDC 6000 and CYBER 70, UNIVAC 1100 Series, and Xerox family of computers. BMDP programs can now be accessed through SAS. Suscribing to program packages is convenient if the hospital has the type of computers on which the packages can be run. Programming staff and programming time can be reduced considerably. However, the computers required by these packages are of a large or medium size.

3. A combination of (1) and (2)

Because of the constraints on computers and inflexibility, program packages are not as useful as they should be. Many hospitals are still writing their own programs or searching for available programs to implement. In the following, some of the available programs especially useful in cancer data analysis are given.

Estimation of remission and survival distributions (or curves)

1. The program written by Smith, Putman, and Gehan (1970) in FORTRAN estimates and plots the survival functions (survivorship, density, and hazard) from life-tables.

2. FORTRAN programs PLSURV and LIFETB in Lee (1980) estimate and plot the survival functions based on Kaplan–Meier's product-limit method and Gehan's (1969) life-table method, respectively.

3. Program P1L in BMDP (1979) estimates and plots survival functions based on Kaplan-Meier's product-limit method and Cutler-Ederer's actuarial life-table method.

4. Procedure SURVIVAL in SPSS (1979) estimates and plots survival functions based on life-table analysis.

Comparison of remission and survival distributions

1. The FORTRAN program written by Robertson and Gehan (1970) provides the generalized Wilcoxon two-sample test.

2. The program written by Lee and Desu (1972) in FORTRAN gives a K-sample test for data with right censored observations. The program, named KSAMPLE, is also given in Lee (1980).

3. FORTRAN program TWOST in Lee (1980) provides five two-sample tests: Gehan's generalized Wilcoxon test, the Cox-Mantel test, the logrank test, Cox's F test, and Peto and Peto's generalized Wilcoxon test.

Cox's logistic regression method

This method has been extremely useful in identifying prognostic factors related to response.

1. Program STLOG in FORTRAN by Lee (1974) carries out the procedure in a forward selection fashion.

2. The FORTRAN program written by Morabito and Marubini (1976) allows the user to specify the subset of the independent variables to be fitted.

3. Program PLR in BMDP (1979) allows the variables to be fitted in a stepwise manner.

4. Procedure LOGIST in SAS (1980) provides the user with two choices: a stepwise regression and a backward selection procedure.

Cox's proportional hazard model

This method has been very popular in identifying prognostic factors related to remission duration and survival time.

1. Programs in Kalbfleisch and Prentice (1980) carry out the procedure for the cases of fixed covariates and for time dependent covariates.

2. A FORTRAN subroutine COXMLE by Chang and Pagano (personal communication, 1980).

3. Program P2L in BMPD (Dixon 1979) provides the user with a stepwise option.

4. Procedure PHGLM in SAS (1979) allows the model to be fitted in a stepwise or backward manner.

DISCUSSION AND CONCLUSIONS

The author's intent in reviewing the use of computers in clinical trials has been to provide an overview of the advantages of computerization. In summary, the four modes of operation available in the computerized medical-care field are (1) in-house large or medium computers, (2) in-house small computers, (3) outside service bureau, and (4) outside time-sharing service. In the first mode, the hospital leases or purchases its own large or medium computer, hires competent programming staff, develops their own programs to meet their needs. They may also subscribe to statistical packages as a supplement. In the second mode, the hospital purchases a small computer, that is a mini or microcomputer, hires programmers to develop programs on the specific hardware. The third mode gives the responsibility of data storage, retrieval, and analysis, as well as report generating, to an outside computer service bureau. In the fourth mode, the hospital accesses a remote, large computer through a telephone or leased line. Data are entered by the hospital and analyses done by the large computer, and reports are sent back to the hospital.

A large or medium computer with knowledgeable programmers can certainly provide clinical investigators with a fast and complete service. It would be even more convenient if an on-line system were available. The investigator and/or the originator of the data can interact with the computer directly without going through keypunch operators. Its spontaneous feedback makes it most desirable in quality control, protocol compliance, and report generating. The use of on-line and real-time techniques has been implemented or is at least under consideration. The direction of data systems on large computers is leading towards on-line techniques. However, only large hospitals or cancer centres can afford this mode. Managing a computer centre with competent programmers along with developing and maintaining a data system involves large costs and problems. It is extremely time consuming and costly to develop programs. Commercially available packages may not be flexible enough to meet the specific needs. Thus, an in-house large computer is desirable and may be affordable by large hospitals, but is infeasible to others.

With the recent advances in computer science, mini and microcomputers have become popular. Hardware and software developments for minicomputers have proceeded very rapidly. The amount of memory and storage available as well as the speed of CPU have increased. Computer costs have been reduced considerably. Programs written in FORTRAN for large computers can easily be implemented on mini computers since most of them can run FORTRAN programs. On-line capabilities are available at low cost. A mini computer may be a good solution for a small or medium hospital if the necessary software is available from the computer company or can be written (or implemented) by an in-house programming staff. The microcomputer costs are even lower. However, the microcomputer is not efficient in complicated mathematical computation. Sophisticated statistical programs needed in clinical trials are lacking. An in-house programming staff is still required. At the present, the microcomputer is often interfaced to a larger computer and used as a convenient input and output device.

Many small and medium hospitals use service bureau or time-sharing systems. These two modes require little investment in hardware or personnel on the hospital; they also provide little flexibility. While a service bureau may provide diagnosis and business summaries, its use in cancer clinical trials is very limited. The use of a time-sharing system depends totally on the agreement between the hospital and the institute that owns the computer. If they agreed to provide the needed analyses and reports, this mode is a good solution, otherwise, this mode is of as limited use as a service bureau. Commercially available data base management systems may reduce personnel costs considerably. The problem is that they are available only on certain computers. Hospitals without the right computer will not be able to use the system.

No matter whether the computer is large or small, important phases in the development and installation of a data system are planning and design. No system useful to one hospital is necessarily valid and efficient for any other. It is extremely important to compare various systems before undertaking computerization. It is necessary for the medical director or hospital administrator to be personally committed to computerization. The planning must be based on the total scope of the hospital's activities, for example, the type of clinical trials conducted in the hospital, the need of the users, the range of services provided by the hospital, the philosophy of its management, and the hospital's role in the community.

The system's design should cover the total impact on the hospital of computerization. There are usually five major steps in the design of a data system.

1. The information needed for clinical studies must be identified. This includes patient characteristics to be measured, definitions of disease outcome, and numerical coding schemes for non-numerical characteristics.

2. Methods of recording data used by physicians, nurses and laboratory scientists must be determined. This, of course, is related to the computer system selected. If batch processing is chosen, forms are necessary. However, in an on-line or interactive system, paper forms may not be required. If a form is needed, the goal is to design a single form which could accommodate the patient care requirements and also serve as a source document for data entry into the computer system. The form should provide sufficient flexibility to meet the needs of the physicians and statisticians, and to facilitate computer data entry.

3. The computer hardware configuration must be selected from all that are available. It is indispensible to compare various computers and system software before computerization is undertaken. In the selection process, careful thoughts must be given to the use of various hardware or software. Competent opinions independent of those of the representatives of computer companies should be obtained. If an on-line computer system is preferable, the selection of an appropriate terminal to match the needs of the user may be critical to the success or failure of the data system.

4. Personnel and work flow must be reorganized to match the computer system and to minimize the time necessary to record and retrieve information from the system.

5. Detailed specifications must be prepared for computer programs. These include programs for data entry, editing, retrieval, and statistical analysis. Decisions must be made on the source of programs—in-house programming, commercially available program packages, or a combination of the two.

REFERENCES

Addison, C. H., Coney, M. D., Jones, M. A., Shields, R. W., and Sweeney, J. W. (1969). *General information processing system: application description.* University of Oklahoma, Norman.

Ball, M. J. (1971). An overview of total medical information systems. *Meth. Inf. Med.* **10,** 73–82.

Bekey, G. A. and Schwartz, M. D. (1972). *Hospital information system,* Marcel Dekker, New York.

Bill, J., Anderson, R., O'Fallon, J., and Silvers, A. (1978). Development of a computerised cancer data management system at the Mayo Clinic. *Int. J. bioMedical Comput.* **9,** 477–92.

Dixon, W. J. (1977, 1979). *BMDP—Biomedical Computer Program (P-series),* University of California Press, Berkeley.

Dutreix, J., Dutreix, A., and Zummer, H. (1972). Data recording in radiotherapy. *Comput. Programs Biomed.* **2,** 232–41.

Freis, J. F. (1972). Time-oriented patient records and computer databank. *J. Am. Med. Ass.* **222,** 1536–42.

Gehan, E. (1969). Estimating survival functions from the life table. *J. chron. Dis.* **21,** 626–44.

Glicksman, A. S. and McShan, D. (1979). Interactive computer supported tumor registry in the state of Rhode Island. *Comput. Programs Biomed.* **9,** 274–83.

Hull, C. H. and Nie, N. H. (1979). *SPSS update.* McGraw-Hill, New York.

Janik, D. S., Sharp, E. M., Forbush, L., Wyman, W. L., and Jung, A. L. (1979). Online, realtime, microcomputer clinical data recording, reporting and research. *Proceedings of the 3rd Annual Symposium on Computing Applications in Medical Care,* pp. 319–23.

Johnson, D. C., and Barnett, G. O. (1977). MEDINFO—a medical information system. *Comput. Programs Biomed.* **7,** 191–201.

Jones, D. R. (1978). Computer simulation as a tool for clinical trial design. *Int. J. biomed. Comput.* **10,** 145–50.

Kalbfleisch, J. D. and Prentice, R. C. (1980). *The statistical analysis of failure time data.* Wiley, New York.

Kaplan, B. (1979). Interactive computer patient data entry and analysis system for radiation therapy clinical trials. *Proceedings of the 3rd Annual Symposium on Computing Applications in Medical Care,* pp. 411–16.

Kaplan, S. D. and Mendeloff, A. I. (1975). PAS full coverage areas: a resource for epidemiologic research. *J. chron. Dis.* **28,** 593–9.

Karpinski, R. H. and Bleich, H. L. (1971). MISAR: a miniature information storage and retrieval system. *Comput. biomed. Res.* **4,** 655–60.

Knox, E. G. (1973). A simulation system for screening. In *The future—and present indicatives* (ed. G. McLachlan) pp. 19–55. Oxford University Press for Nuffield Provincial Hospital Trust, Oxford.

Lee, E. T. (1974). A computer program for linear logistic regression analysis. *Comput. Programs Biomed.* **4,** 80–92.

—— (1980). *Statistical methods for survival data analysis.* Lifetime Learning Publications, Belmont, California.

—— Desu, M. M. (1972). A computer program for comparing K samples with right-censored data. *Comput. Programs Biomed.* **2,** 315–21.

Lee, J. Y. (1979). An interactive system for clinical trials. In *Proceedings of the 3rd annual symposium on computing applications in medical care,* pp. 404–5.

Mackey, R. W. (1979). Data management in clinical cancer research: testicular cancer. *Sem. Oncol.* **6,** 1, 130–8.

McDonnel Douglas (1980). *MCAUTO health services overview.* McDonnel Douglas Automation Company, St. Louis, Missouri.

McLeod, D. and Meldman, M. (1975). RISS—a generalized mini-computer relational data base management system. *AFIPS* **44,** 397–402.

McShan, D. Haumann, D., and Glicksman, A. (1979). A new interactive computerized data base and retrieval system. *Comput. Programs Biomed.* **9,** 284–92.

Melski, J. W., Geer, D. E., and Bleich, H. L. (1978). Medical information storage and retrieval using proprocessed variables. *Comput. biomed. Res.* **11,** 613–21.

Morabito, A. and Marubini, E. (1976). A computer program for fitting linear models when the dependent variable is dichotomous, polichotomous or censored survival and non-linear models when the dependent variable is quantitative. *Comput. Programs Biomed.* **5,** 283–95.

Neurath, P. W., Bloedorn, F. G., Munzenrider, J. E., and Pedrazzi, M. G. (1974). A selective patient information system. *Cancer* **33,** 1653–63.

Nie, N. H., Hull, C. H., Jenkins, J. G., Steinbrenner, K., and Bent, D. H. (1975). *SPSS—statistical package for the social sciences.* McGraw-Hill, New York.

O'Desky, R. I. (1977). The impact of microcomputer technology on medical computing. *Proc. Soc. Comput. Med.* **6**, 2, 1.

Palley, N. A. and Groner, G. F. A. (1974). Survey of clinical investigators and their information processing activities. R–1539–NIH. DHEW, Bethesda.

Robertson, C. O. and Gehan, E. A. (1970). A computer sub-program for calculating the generalized Wilcoxon test. *Comput. Programs Biomed.* **1**, 167.

SAS (1979). *SAS user's guide.* SAS Institute Inc., Raleigh, North Carolina.

Singer, J. P. (1969). Computer-based hospital information systems. *Datamation*, **14**, 38–45.

Smith, T. L., Putman, J. E., and Gehan, E. A. (1970). A computer program for estimating survival functions from the life table. *Comput. Programs in Biomed.* **1**, 58–64.

Tenenbaum, A. and Weinberger, G. (1979). A standalone minicomputer system for administration of health care facilities. *Proceedings of the 3rd Annual Symposium on Computing Applications in Medical Care*, 273–5.

Volterrani, F., Donati, G., Uslenghi, C., Sigurta, D., and Gentenaro, G. (1979). A computerized cancer patient information system. *Tumori* **65**, 381–8.

Wallace, J. D. and Cooper, G. A. (1979). Interactive medical questionnaire. In *Proceedings of the 3rd annual symposium onComputer Applications in medical Care*, pp. 406–10.

Wasserman, A. I. (1977). Minicomputers may maximize data processing. *Hospital* **51**, 119.

Woodings, T. L. and Madsen, B. W. (1978). A computer program for experimental design simulation. *Comput. biomed. Res.* **11**, 581–94.

7 Quality control in multi-centre cancer clinical trials

Marc Buyse

The most important component of any clinical investigation is the originality, significance and importance of the idea or the hypothesis being tested, not the methods by which the research is conducted. An even more important principle is that the quality of the research should be judged by the quality of the results (Freireich 1981).

In the last analysis it is always the results that matter. Are the observations well and fairly made? Are they good or bad? If they are bad no tests of significance can compensate—they merely provide a spurious air of respectability to meaningless results (Hill 1971).

INTRODUCTION

This chapter is based on the belief that no statistical technique will ever yield 'good' results from data of dubious quality. Computer scientists repeatedly remind us that a computer cannot convert garbage into fruit salad, and statisticians alike stress that 'no amount of statistical ingenuity can make bad data good' (Gore 1981b). Yet it is not such an uncommon view that the growing sophistication of technology and the refinement of statistical techniques dispense individual investigators from paying careful attention to the data they collect. Perhaps the reverse is true, in that sophisticated technology will increasingly enable one to discover errors in the data that would probably have escaped the scrutiny of the most careful manual checks in the past.

The mere detection of gross errors in the data (a process called data editing) has been thoroughly covered in the literature, but it is only one aspect of quality control in clinical trials. Several authors have stressed that quality control should take place at each step of the research process—in our case, the clinical trial—from the early planning to the final analysis of the data collected (Williams 1979; Friedman, Furberg, and De Mets 1981). This chapter is an attempt to deal not only with the mechanics of data editing (first section), but also with some other aspects of quality control which have received somewhat less attention in the literature so far. The often overlooked impact of missing baseline data and follow-up information will be discussed respectively in the next two sections. Subsequent sections deal with problems pertaining to 'clean' data, that is data that are not missing and have passed the basic edits; there is indeed no guarantee that 'clean' data are 'correct' in an absolute sense. Two sections will outline some indirect ways in which the correctness of data can be verified, namely the presence of systematic outlying observations and the presence of large institutional differences, while the last sections will be devoted respectively to the issues of data consistency and data accuracy.

This chapter deals primarily with multi-centre clinical trials, in which it will be assumed that a central office is responsible for the trial co-ordination and data collection. Quality control will be discussed at the level of the central office, but most of the concepts apply equally well to individual institutions participating in the trial. In this respect, it should be borne in mind that errors should always be detected and corrected at the earliest possible moment in the flow of data from the patient to the publication of the trial results (Falter 1981).

INCORRECT DATA

The importance of proper data management

In multi-centre trials, the data are generally sent by the participating institutions to the central office for computerization, either on paper forms or on some computer readable device (magnetic tapes, cassettes, discs). Kronmal, Davis, Fisher, Jones, and Gillespie (1978) describe an impressive system in which the data are keyed directly into programmable terminals at the various institutions, checked for correctness, and then transmitted over telephone lines to the central office. But their system is likely to be cost effective, at least with today's technology, only for big collaborative studies such as the one they describe. The future will probably see an increasing number of these systems being implemented even for more modest studies, but the apparently old-fashioned method of sending forms to the central office has some advantages on its own. It enables the person in charge of the central data management to check the data *before* the forms are read into the computer, which may be useful to detect gross errors, obvious misunderstandings, illegible data, or high percentages of missing data. In our experience this manual check often uncovers problems which would escape the computer edits, thus preventing data of poor quality to be entered on the computer. The importance of a central data manager, who enjoys an overall view of the study's progress and benefits (in principle) from an aura of impartiality, cannot be overemphasized in the quality control process (O'Fallon, Golenzer, Taylor, Hu, Offord, Bill, and Moertel 1980; Van Glabbeke, Buyse, Renard, and De Pauw 1981). To ensure quality in data collection, appropriately trained personnel should also be appointed within each institution participating in the trial (Evans 1979; Mullin 1981).

Computer edits

Computer edits or checks are performed whenever new data are read in the computer to update the study file. Computer edits can broadly be classified as follows:

(a) Missing value checks

Errors of omission have been identified by Feinstein, Pritchett, and Schimpff (1969) as the major source of imprecision in medical data. Therefore the computer should identify and reject those data sets in which essential information is missing. What is meant by 'essential' is a subjective matter but in practice it will simply be a convenient compromise tending to the ideal situation of requiring all information to be present while keeping the rejection rate reasonably low. In spite of these checks, missing data are so common in any clinical trial that they deserve to be discussed separately in the next section.

(b) Range checks

All data items should be checked to ensure that they fall within a sensible predefined range. For categorical data, the range is simply given by the two extreme codes allowed, while for continuous data, a range must be arbitrarily defined, for example comprising 95 per cent of the population under study. Thus for instance, the haemoglobin concentration of previously untreated patients with solid tumours could be checked against a range, say, of 11–16 g/100 ml; any value outside that range is suspect and worth checking before being inserted in the computer file. Naturally, the edit system must be flexible enough to force the insertion of values outside the range; in our example, a value of 6 g/100 ml should be permitted after checking that the patient is indeed anaemic.

(c) Cross-checks or consistency checks

These are checks which involve two or more data items simultaneously. Examples abound: a body weight of 100 kg is quite plausible for someone 2 m tall but rather unlikely for someone 1·5 m tall, and thus it may be quite useful to cross-check these data before calculating theoretical doses in chemotherapy trials. Other typical examples include the cross-checking of menopausal status with age, of nodal involvement or metastatic extension of the disease with the stage, and so on.

Needless to say, cross-checks are in general much less straightforward to implement than range checks, which can be defined simply by a table indicating the allowed values or range for every data item on file. As a matter of fact, the general description of cross-checks (and their actual computeriz-ation) is as yet a largely unsolved problem. Cross-checks are in most cases performed by tailor-made programs; but this solution is clumsy because it requires a different program to be written for every trial, let alone the communication problems that may arise between the end-users (study co-ordinator, data manager, or statistician) and the computer programmers. This latter problem can be alleviated by having recourse to general file management systems such as SIR (Scientific Information Retrieval; Robinson, Anderson, Cohen, and Gazdzik 1979) which allow the end-users themselves to write whichever cross-checks they need in high level, easy-to-use languages. Again, this approach may not be the most satisfactory as it lacks generality. Fellegi and Holt (1976) have suggested an elegant way of describing certain cross-checks in tabular form, thus enabling the incorpor-ation of these cross-checks in quite a general, table-driven edit system while Karrison (1981) gives a thorough description of an actual system built along these lines.

(d) Sequence checks

These are essentially cross-checks between data items which change over time. An illustrative example is the measurement of height in pediatric studies: a child height at time t must be greater than or equal to the height at time $t-1$. In cancer trials, the most common examples involve the checking of a sequence of dates (for example randomization must be prior to start of treatment, which in turn must be prior to first follow-up exams, etc.). These tests are essential not only because dates are particularly error prone (Friedman *et al.* 1981), but also because the end-points of cancer trials typically involve time periods, that is, differences between various dates.

The implementation of sequence checks is subject to the same difficulties as the other cross-checks discussed above but in addition, they generally require that the entire patient data file be read before they can be performed. Hence these tests suffer from the double handicap of being difficult to define and costly to perform.

(e) Probabilistic checks

All data items which do not pass the computer checks discussed so far are rejected as mistakes. Real life does not always bend itself into this black and white system: some data items can take unusual or rare values without actually being incorrect (see the above example of a low haemoglobin level). It would then be nice to be able to make a distinction between 'fatal errors', which cause data items to be rejected, and 'warnings' which indicate permitted but unusual values, on the basis of a prior probability distribution (hence the term 'probabilistic' checks; Naus 1975). More will be said on unusual values or 'outliers' later in this chapter.

Data correction

A fair percentage of errors detected can be readily corrected at the central office; however, as soon as there is the slightest doubt as to what the correct value should be, it is wise to go back to the local investigator in order to get it. This policy has the additional advantage that it gives feedback to the investigator and sometimes highlights a problem that he was unaware of. On the other hand, going back to the local investigator takes time, money, and energy. Therefore, systems in which the quality control is decentralized and the computer edits performed in each institution (Kronmal *et al.* 1978) undoubtedly have much appeal.

Many authors have presented systems in which the computer itself automatically corrects, whenever possible, the data items found in error (Szameitat and Zindler 1965; Naus, Johnson, and Montalvo 1972; Eichberg, 1980). Such systems of automatic 'imputation' of incorrect data have actually been implemented in large-scale undertakings, where going back to the source of information was either impossible or disproportionately expensive, but there is little room for them, if any at all, in cancer clinical trials.

MISSING DATA

Missing data pose problems no less worrisome than those associated with incorrect data. While the mistakes discovered in incorrect data are often easily explained (for example due to keypunching problems, illegibility, confusion in the units used, etc.), there can, in many cases, be multiple reasons why some pieces of information are missing. Suppose that, in the follow-up examinations of a particular trial, a liver CT-scan is requested and abnormalities on the CT-scan reported. What should be assumed if the information regarding CT-scan is absent for a patient? Probably that the examination was not performed. Yet it is also quite possible that the examination *was* performed, and the result normal, so that the physician did not bother to report it (this is a serious problem in the reporting of treatment toxicities, as will be seen below). Obviously we cannot conclude either way and we shall again have to go back to the local investigator to find out the answer, often at the expense of considerable effort and time lag.

This kind of problem must be avoided at all costs, and trial organizers should therefore resist the temptation to ask for information which is likely to be frequently overlooked by the investigators. Only the follow-up data which are strictly necessary must be requested so that the important data items are not lost in masses of less relevant items. If any data item is then found to be missing, it is really worth making the extra effort to collect it (Peto, Pike, Armitage, Breslow, Cox, Howard, Mantel, McPherson, Peto, and Smith 1977).

The design of data forms is also critical to the amount of missing data (Gore 1981*a*). In particular, explicit codes must be provided on the data forms for 'unknowns', 'not done', 'not applicable', etc. so that all situations can be reported (see Chapter 5 by De Pauw and Buyse on form design in this book).

In spite of these safeguards, there will inevitably be missing data in co-operative trials, and it is therefore of interest to go into some details on the impact of missing data on the trial analysis.

Missing data occurring at random

Let us assume that some fixed percentage of data items are missing and let us further assume, for the sake of simplicity, that missing data occur at random, that is, the probability that a data item be missing is uniform among all data items and among all patients. These hypotheses are admittedly simplistic, but the point is to show how detrimental missing data can be and not to carry out fancy calculations. Table 7.1 indicates the proportion of patients for whom there will be *no* missing data under these hypotheses. It shows how strikingly low that proportion can be. For example, assuming that overall as a few as 1 per cent of data items are missing, and that there are 100 items per patient, then only 37 per cent of the patients have all their data items completed, or conversely 63 per cent of the patients have at least one missing data item somewhere!

This situation may create a problem, for example, if we wish to fit a multi-variate model to our data. A patient has to be excluded from the model as soon as one data item is missing for that patient (there are ways around this problem, but we will not consider them here). Naturally, we shall never have to use the 100 data items (or variates) in the model, but even if we limit ourselves to the 10 most interesting variates, Table 7.1 indicates that we still might loose as many as 10 per cent of the patients—always under the assumption of only 1 per cent of missing data overall. It is fair to say that the above hypotheses are not very realistic: missing data rarely occur at random among all data items but rather in direct proportion to the difficulty of obtaining them. Thus the figures of Table 7.1 may be overly pessimistic. But on the other hand, the overall percentage of missing data was assumed to be very low: 1 per cent is unfortunately an underestimation for many real life situations, so that after all the figures given may not be too far from reality.

Table 7.1. *Proportion of patients in whom no data are missing, assuming various overall percentages of missing data items (columns) and various numbers of data items per patient (rows). Missing data are assumed to occur at random.*

Number of data items per patient	Overall percentage of missing data items			
	0.1%	0.5%	1%	5%
5	99	98	95	77
10	99	95	90	60
50	95	78	60	8
100	90	61	37	1

Missing data not occurring at random

In practice, some data items, viewed as less important by the investigators, will tend to be missed out more often than the essential ones. Although this attitude may be intuitively correct, it can lead to serious problems, if the neglected data item is one which turns out later on to be of great prognostic importance. A good example of this occurred in an EORTC melanoma trial, started in 1974, in which both the tumour level of invasion according to Clark (1967) and the tumour thickness according to Breslow (1970) were requested. Clark's level, at that time the most widely accepted technique for assessing tumour depth, was reported on all cases, while the tumour thickness was often missing or grossly rounded off. Hence some patients had to be excluded from a multivariate analysis in which Breslow's thickness was one of the most important variables (Cochran, Buyse, Lejeune, Macher, Revuz, and Rumke 1981). Should this study be run today, now that the Breslow's thickness has been demonstrated to be of superior prognostic value to the Clark's level, in addition to its being a more reliable measurement (EORTC Melanoma Pathologists' Group 1980), there would probably be no missing values for thickness at all. Thus missing values can create a vicious circle in the search for new or better prognostic factors.

Missing values can create even more serious problems when they depend on some characteristic of the patient, or worse still, on the treatment. A case in point in this respect is when a treatment is compared to a 'no treatment' control group. There is then considerable potential for bias in the evaluation of results if the follow-up of treated patients is more rigorous than that of control patients (Brown 1982). The presence of more missing data in the control group than in the treated group would certainly constitute a warning that such a bias might indeed be present. If, for example, in a digestive tract cancer trial, the carcinoembryonic antigen levels were missing more frequently in one arm than in the other, tumour recurrences might be suspected earlier in the latter arm, prompting earlier confirmatory examinations of such possible recurrences and also their earlier treatment.

Leaving aside this rather extreme situation, several checks can usefully be carried out on missing data. First, their frequency for all variables under investigation can point to difficulties in obtaining or coding some of these variables. A high frequency of missing values for a variable will cast doubt on any analysis involving that variable; Wermuth and Cochran (1979) discuss a converse example in which the complete *absence* of missing values for a variable led them to suspect the way in which this variable had been coded! (this variable was coded 'yes' if the patient had had nephritis during a particular time period, and 'no' otherwise). Secondly, a comparison of the percentage of missing values between the institutions is often a direct (if only partial) reflection of the quality of the data gathered from them. Thirdly, it is well worth checking if the subgroup of patients with a missing value for one particular variable is comparable with the other patients in the trial. In a paper comparing data bases and randomized clinical trials, Byar (1980) rightly states that, 'in general, we should not expect patients with missing data to resemble those for whom data are available.' Whenever a variable of potential prognostic importance is analysed with respect to the study end-points, the group of patients with a missing value for that variable should automatically be compared with the other groups to detect any bias in the analysis. The necessity of such a comparison was strikingly apparent in a recent EORTC trial on the adjuvant treatment of patients operated for a malignant brain glioma by radiation therapy, combined or not with a radiosensitizer (misonidazole). Only patients in whom steroid administration could be discontinued after surgery were eligible for the study; however, occasional administration of steroids was allowed during radiotherapy. When examining the impact on disease-free interval of whether or not patients had received steroids during radiotherapy, it appeared that patients not receiving steroids had a better prognosis ($p = 0.01$), but it was also clear that patients for whom this information was missing formed a very different group from both others ($p < 0.001$, Fig. 7.1a). This striking difference was readily explained by the fact that the information on steroid administration was in most cases provided only at the time of disease recurrence, and was thus missing precisely for those patients who were enjoying the longest disease-free intervals. Now it is obvious that the comparison between patients receiving steroids and the others can be drastically affected by the group with missing information: taking the extreme (but not foolish) assumption that all patients with missing information did receive steroids, the difference between the two groups vanishes (Fig. 7.1b). In reality, the converse happened to be true in that only a small porportion (three out of 17) of these patients had in fact received steroids, and thus the difference between the two groups became even more significant ($p = 0.002$, Fig. 7.1c).

PROBLEMS RELATED TO FOLLOW UP DATA

Delayed follow-up

Delayed reporting of follow-up data can seriously affect or even bias the statistical analysis. Chlebowski, Weiner, Ryden, and Bateman (1981) mention it as one of the reasons why the significant treatment difference that they had detected in an interim analysis, became non-significant at the end of a phase III trial (the interim analysis had already been published long ago, though!). A precaution that can partially safeguard against hasty conclusions is to look at the delays of reporting and average follow-up time in each treatment arm. But this gives only partial protection, as illustrated by the fact that Chlebowski *et al.* (1981) could find no difference in the pattern of reporting between their two treatment arms. Thus excessive delays in reporting are potentially misleading

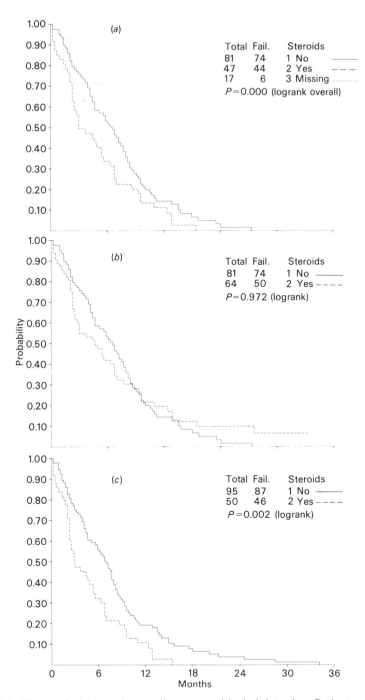

Fig. 7.1. Disease-free interval according to steroid administration. Patients with a missing value for steroid administration are either shown separately (a), grouped with patients receiving steroids (b), or classified in the group they were found later to belong to (c).

even if they are not grossly imbalanced between the treatment arms. In phase II studies, too, they can deceive the investigators in situations where 'good news travels first', and may perhaps explain the remarkable downward time trend in the response rate to many new chemotherapeutic regimens.

Reporting delays can certainly be shortened by regulary requesting follow-up information according to the protocol schedule. At the EORTC Data Center, several computer-printed documents are used for this purpose:

(a) an 'administrative' report, summarizing the forms received and patient status for all institutions participating in a particular study;

(b) a 'request of forms' report, which is a complementary document indicating for each patient what forms are overdue and for how long (prospective reminders would probably be more effective, as argued by McDonald (1976));

(c) an 'activity' report, which reflects the quality of participation from each institution by giving the proportion of patients with missing baseline information, with missing follow-up information or who violate the inclusion criteria defined in the study protocol.

What helps even more than these documents are the sanctions that can be imposed on the institutions with a poor quality of participation record, especially if these sanctions go as far as excluding some institutions from the publication of the study results.

A more lenient and more positive attitude is to organize, whenever possible, on-site visits to the institutions where troubleshooting appears necessary. McFadden (1980) reports that in the ECOG such visits revealed the same problems were experienced by all the institutions in difficulties. Thus some visits are probably warranted to identify these problems and suggest remedies. Mowery and Williams (1979) further suggest that 'ideally, each clinical center should be visited twice a year'. Whether this is feasible depends on the financial resources available and the number of institutions involved. But whether this is desirable and cost-effective for institutions entering only a few patients in the study, is very doubtful. Unfortunately, in our experience at the EORTC, it is in those institutions entering only a few patients that the administrative problems tend to occur the most frequently. Sylvester, Pinedo, De Pauw, Staquet, Buyse, Renard, and Bonadonna (1981) have shown that an institution's degree of participation in a multi-centre trial tends to correlate with the quality of its participation, in terms of both protocol compliance and promptness to send the relevant information to the central office. However, this experience is not shared by all co-operative groups (*New England Journal of Medicine* 1982).

Losses to follow-up, withdrawals, and exclusions

In most trials lasting longer than a few weeks, some patients are inevitably lost to follow-up, and any information on these patients is therefore almost impossible to recover. In contrast, it is perfectly possible and highly desirable to collect all data on patients who withdraw from a clinical trial or who are excluded from it retrospectively, that is at any time after randomization (Gore 1981*b*). These patients must be followed as carefully as the others because, while it was stated previously that there was no reason to expect patients with missing data to resemble the others, we now have all reasons to believe that patients who withdraw do *not* resemble the others.

The statistical problems related to losses to follow-up, withdrawals and retrospective exclusions are beyond the scope of this chapter: they are fully discussed, for example by Peto, Pike, Armitage, Breslow, Cox, Howard, Mantel, McPherson, Peto, and Smith (1976), Sackett and Gent (1979), and in the next chapter by Brown (1983). Schwartz and Lellouch (1967) have attempted to classify the reasons why patients withdraw and the impact of the various withdrawal reasons on the analysis of a binary outcome variable (such as response to treatment). In any case, the proportion of patients who are not properly followed-up for any reason must be kept to an absolute minimum (Evans 1979) and is a partial but crucial indicator of a trial's overall quality.

OUTLIERS

The detection of outliers, that is the identification of unusual or extreme observations in the distribution of some variables, is a useful way of uncovering errors. 'Unusual' observations are here taken as those values that fall within acceptable limits but are expected to occur only rarely. A large amount of work has been devoted in the statistical literature to the identification of outliers: the interested reader could usefully refer to the paper of Anscombe (1960) or to the landmark survey of Barnett and Lewis (1978). Much of the work deals with the identification of outliers when the distribution of the underlying variable is assumed to be normal, or roughly normal. Unfortunately, data collected in clinical trials may rarely be assumed to fulfill this condition of normality, and other parametric or non-parametric approaches would then be warranted. In practice however, the naive approach of taking a look at the distribution of all variables under investigation will probably be deemed sufficient to detect the most obvious outliers (Wermuth and Cochran 1979). Similarly, looking at two-way (or three-way, etc.) distributions is a practical method of discovering multi-variate outlyers, that is combinations of values which are unusual even if these values, taken individually, seem quite well behaved. Here again, more sophisticated methods have been proposed to detect these kinds of outliers; multivariate techniques such as principal component or discriminant analysis may prove valuable (Gnanadesikan and Kettenring 1972).

Whether outliers should be rejected from or incorporated in the analysis is another much debated question which will not be discussed here: when an outlier is identified, every effort should be made to check its correctness by going back to the local investigators. This process will either disclose an error made in the measurement or coding of the variable, or confirm the questioned value as being a genuine outlier. In this latter case, one should not worry too much as long as the statistical techniques used to analyse the data are relatively insensitive to the presence of outliers. For example, when assessing the prognostic influence of Breslow's thickness on survival in a melanoma study, one may form groups of increasing thickness: say under 1·5 mm, from 1·5 mm to 3·0 mm, and over 3·0 mm. A truly outlying thickness of, say, 10 mm is thus simply included in the third group above and the analysis is completely insensitive to the fact that this tumour is in fact exceptionally thick. On the other hand, if one incorporates tumour thickness as a continuous variable in some statistical model, it will be wise to assess the sensitivity of the model to the presence of this unusually large value.

The detection of outliers has been extended by Canner, Huang, and Meinert (1981) to monitor institutional performance in multi-centre clinical trials. They propose to compare the institutions with respect to the incidence of various events (for example operative mortality, patient adherence to the treatment regimen, etc.) and they derive a test statistic to identify outlier institutions at some predetermined significance level. Naturally, their tests 'should not be used in and of themselves to provide a ranking of clinics on how well they are doing', but rather as a tool for quantifying large institutional differences.

INSTITUTIONAL DIFFERENCES

In fact, differences among institutions are probably a common feature of most multi-centre trials. While this is not a problem *per se*, it does call for care in analysing the data and reporting the trial results. Examining institutional differences can be used as a way of assessing data quality and revealing problem areas.

Differences in reporting

Consider Fig. 7.2. It shows the proportion of patients for whom side-effects or toxicities to a new chemotherapeutic agent were reported in a multi-centre phase II study involving 15 European institutions. The degree of the toxicity (coded 'mild', 'moderate', 'severe', etc.) and its time of onset are not considered here, but merely whether or not a toxicity was reported at any time during the trial period. Figure 7.2 clearly emphasizes that in institution A there are systematically less cases reported with toxicity than in all the others, and this, surprisingly, is true of both haematologic and non-haematologic toxicities. Conversely, in institution B, there is an obvious and systematic over-reporting of cases with toxicity as compared with the average. Note that institutions A and B entered respectively 28 and 31 patients in the study (out of

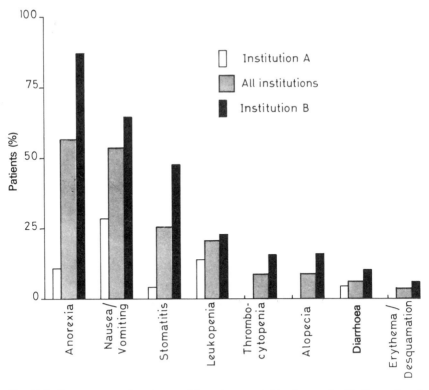

Fig. 7.2. Percentages of patients with various toxicities in two institutions, A and B, compared to all institutions participating in a multi-centre trial (111 patients).

a total of 111 patients) and were in fact the two major participants, hence the wide differences in percentages depicted on Fig. 7.2 are not just due to small denominators.

Multivariate analyses performed on these toxicity data showed that the differences were not attributable to apparent variations in the patient population (age, extent of disease, etc.) or in the treatment administration: total dose, number of cycles, etc. It seems therefore unlikely that the differences that appear on Fig. 7.2. actually reflect true underlying differences in toxicity; it is much more probable that differing attitudes on the part of the investigators led them to report toxicities differently from one institution to the next. It was clear that some investigators tended to report unexpected toxicities in preference to those which had already been documented in earlier publications on the drug. Also, the most frequent toxicities to this drug were essentially digestive, and the definition of such toxicities lacks precision. As Feinstein (1967) pointed out in his excellent discussion on the acquisition of clinical data, symptomatic designations are often ambiguous and imprecise, even the most widely accepted ones: as to digestive toxicities, 'does diarrhea refer to loose stools, many stools, or both—and constipation to hard stools, few stools, or both? Does anorexia signify lack of desire for food, lack of appealing food, or unwillingness to eat lest the intake of food be followed by discomfort?' Moreover, the assessment of the degree of these toxicities is rather subjective and therefore liable to considerable measurement error (Herson 1980).

As could be expected, the wide differences of Fig. 7.2 were not found in the reporting of haematological toxicities to other more myelosuppressive chemotherapies, although this is probably not so much because haematological toxicities can be objectively and precisely measured as because bone marrow depression is dose-limiting for these myelotoxic drugs. Recommendations such as those made by the World Health Organization, which attempt at defining precise categories for each toxicity, constitute a definite improvement over the vague degrees used in the past ('mild', 'moderate', severe', etc.) (WHO 1979; Miller, Hoogstraten, Staquet, and Winkler 1981). But these recommendations will only lead to a more effective reporting of toxicities if a precise assessment of toxicities is deemed sufficiently important to be emphasized as an end-point of the trial.

In all fairness to the example discussed above, it should be mentioned that the lack of drug activity was soon divulged, which prompted the investigators to let things slide and contributed to poor data quality. The point remains, though, that under-reporting of non-critical events may (and therefore will) occur in clinical trials.

Differences in patient management

In some instances, the institutional differences that emerge when analysing the data reflect a genuine variation in patient management—and it may then be important to identify the cause for this variation.

This was the case in an EORTC multi-centre phase III trial of immunotherapy combined with post-operative chemotherapy and radio-therapy in patients with primary breast cancer presenting with positive axillary nodes. The post-operative chemotherapy adopted in both treatment arms was the classical CMF schema. Figure 7.3 displays the distribution of patients who received less than 50 per cent, from 50 to 75 per cent, and over 75 per cent of the theoretical dose of methotrexate for the four major participants in this trial (denoted A, B, C, and D). The four institutions have been ordered so that A is closest to the protocol (no patients received less than 50 per cent of their theoretical dose of methotrexate) while D is the furthest (nearly half the patients received less than 50 per cent of their theoretical dose of methotrexate). A similar pattern was also apparent in the two other drugs, 5-fluorouracil and cyclophosphamide.

The co-operative group running this trial made some enlightening discoveries in trying to explain these wide institutional variations in treatment

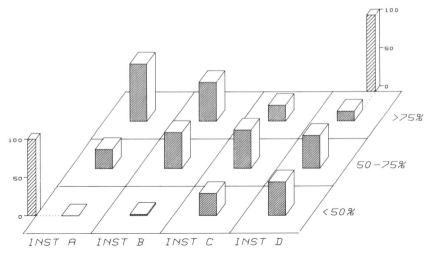

Fig. 7.3. Percentages of patients receiving less than 50 per cent, from 50 per cent to 75 per cent, or over 75 per cent of the theoretical dose of methotrexate, in four institutions: A, B, C, and D (199 patients).

administration, particularly as regards the timing of radiotherapy and chemotherapy. A more detailed discussion would obviously be beyond the scope of this chapter, but these findings certainly call for caution, especially in performing any analysis involving the doses of chemotherapy received, or in comparing treatment results in different institutions.

This rather extreme example highlights the need for a close and continuous monitoring of the essential variables across the institutions participating in a clinical trial. At the minimum, this could be done by the study co-ordinator, but it is preferable that a group be appointed to continuously assure quality data collection and adherence to protocol (Knatterud 1981). Glicksman, Reinstein, Brotman, and McShan (1980) describe an impressive system used to ensure protocol adherence in chemotherapy trials: the drug doses are calculated interactively using a central computer on the basis of data such as the patient's weight and height, performance status, and haematologic condition on the day of treatment.

INCONSISTENT DATA

In their paper, Glicksman and colleagues (1980) also stress the need to carry out a retrospective review of all therapeutic and pathological data in order to assess their consistency. Data are said to be consistent if they are the same when the observation is repeated by the same observer (repeatability) or when they are reported by other investigators (reproducibility). Some authors use the term 'reliability' rather than 'consistency'.

Review panels

A systematic review of pathological data is common practice in many co-operative groups. This generally entails sending pathological materials (slides) to a central review panel which reassesses them blindly and independently of the local investigators. Problems arise when there is a discrepancy or inconsistency between the review panel and the local pathologist, particularly when the protocol excludes certain histological types or when treatment depends upon histology.

In case of an inconsistency, the opinion of the review panel must be given priority, both to ensure standardization across institutions and because this opinion is (or should be) the result of several independent reviews of the material. However, it is interesting to keep track of the local pathologist's opinion in order to detect systematic differences between this pathologist and the panel. It may also be of interest, as pointed out by Tilley, Forthofer, and Harrist (1981), to test the hypothesis that the level of agreement between a local pathologist and the review panel meets a predetermined standard.

Inter-observer agreement

Although review panels are widely accepted for assessing the consistency of data pertaining to pathology or response to treatment, much less attention is usually paid to other data which may nevertheless show considerable inter-observer variability, such as symptom descriptions (Koran 1975), diagnostic examinations (Kahn 1979), or the assessment of performance status (Hutchinson, Boyd, and Feinstein 1979). All these papers tend to indicate that data consistency can rarely be taken for granted. Even such crucial data as tumour measurements have been shown to be rather inconsistent when assessed either by clinical methods (Moertel and Hanley 1976) or from X-rays (Henderson, Martin and Zacharski 1981). It is clearly out of the question to appoint specialist panels to review all trial data, however replicate examinations as well as inter-observer studies can be set up to check on the consistency of the most important data items.

This may be particularly relevant for the critical events under investigation in clinical trials, because agreement regarding abnormalities (which are associated with the critical events) is usually lower than agreement regarding normality (Koran 1975). For instance, the inter-observer agreement when assessing performance status decreases as the patient's performance status decreases, at least until total dependence is reached (Jette and Deniston 1978). This being said as a word of caution, one should not overestimate the importance of *some* inter-observer variability. For instance, in spite of its relatively poor reproducibility, the Karnofsky performance status scale has been shown, for example by Yates, Chalmer, and McKegney (1980), to have considerable validity (a notion which will be defined in the next section).

But in recognition of the inevitable presence of inter-observer variability, one must beware of potentially biasing treatment comparisons in phase III trials. In the trial schema depicted in Fig. 7.4, for instance, one might fear that a difference of opinion between two observers (the surgeon and the chemotherapist) would systematically affect treatment comparisons based on end-points less reliable than survival.

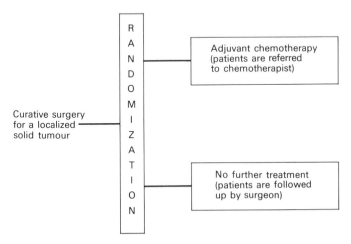

Fig. 7.4. A trial schema where systematic inter-observer differences may bias treatment comparisons.

Another point which trial organizers should always keep in mind is that when explicit criteria are defined for the assessment of clinical events, the inter-observer agreement is substantially higher than when the observers do not use criteria (Boyd, Pater, Ginsburg, and Myers 1979). Hence the need to define explicit criteria and to attempt to standardize the information collected in clinical trials.

This chapter is not the place to discuss the various measures used to quantify inter-observer agreement; in addition to the papers cited above, the interested reader could consult the historical reference of Cohen (1969), in which he introduced a coefficient of agreement called 'kappa', which has been extended by Light (1971) and is now in wide use. Kramer and Feinstein (1981) provide an excellent review of the different statistics of concordance.

INACCURATE DATA

According to Feinstein, Pritchett, and Schimpff (1969), 'the most basic scientific questions about any type of data deal with the issues of precision, accuracy and consistency'. Data precision and consistency have already been discussed above, so we should finally turn to the issue of accuracy (or validity) of the data. Data are said to be accurate (or valid) if they measure what they purport to measure. For example, as was mentioned above, the Karnofsky scale is a valid indicator of the patients' functional status, because it correlates well with several other variables relating to physical function, and because it is in many instances an excellent predictor of survival duration or response to treatment.

Unfortunately, there are all too frequent examples of invalid measurements in clinical trials, even for data which at first sight would be considered of prime importance by most investigators. This was illustrated in a trial on hormonal treatment of patients with advanced prostatic cancer. The required pre-treatment studies included a determination of the histopathological grading according to the *TNM classification of malignant tumours* (Harmer 1978) which is based on the worst degree of tumour differentiation that can be identified (G0 = no evidence of anaplasia, G1 = high degree of differentiation, G2 = medium degree of differentiation, G3 = low degree of differentiation or undifferentiated). The biopsy technique was not standardized; the techniques most frequently used in the 248 randomized patients were needle biopsy and/or transurethral resection (TUR, which for our purposes will be regarded as a biopsy technique, leaving aside its therapeutic intent). The data on histopathological grading presented some disturbing characteristics (Sylvester, Suciu, and De Pauw 1983). First, the degree of differentiation could not be assessed in some 7 per cent of the patients (in whom the tumour was probably missed by the biopsy). Secondly, the G grade was correlated with the biopsy technique employed: the average G grade was significantly worse in the patients who had undergone both TUR and needle biopsy than in the others, pointing to a probable understaging of these latter patients. This correlation persisted after adjustment for all other patient characteristics and hence was not spuriously due to the fact that patient characteristics influence the choice of the biopsy technique. Instead, the choice of the technique varied considerably across institutions, reflecting different attitudes on the part of the physicians involved. Thirdly, a significant correlation between the response to treatment and the initial G grade was found only in those patients with both TUR and needle biopsy. It was clear from these analyses that the histopathological data provided by some of the biopsy techniques were grossly inaccurate.

In general, grossly inaccurate data will yield meaningless or even potentially misleading results. To prove with a statistical analysis that data are indeed inaccurate will in most cases be much more difficult than in the example above, if not impossible. Therefore, data which are thought *a priori* to bear a high risk of being inaccurate should not be requested at all in clinical trials. If they are of great importance in the trial interpretation, one should worry about their possible inaccuracy; if not, they will probably add an unnecessary workload on the investigators.

CONCLUSION

One may wonder why quality control, a somewhat boring issue, has recently attracted so much attention, to the point of becoming one of the most fashionable topics in conferences and periodicals devoted to clinical trials. Perhaps this fashion is explained, at least partly, by the very disappointing reproducibility of cancer trial results. The literature is fraught with false positive results, which lead disenchanted investigators to repeat published trials for themselves before investing too many hopes in the achievements claimed by others.

Several different mechanisms may be accused of concurring to produce this large number of false positives. Improper methodology, including inadequate statistical techniques, has long been recognized as one of the major contributing mechanisms (Altman 1981). Preconceived ideas, self-fulfilling prophecies, the 'hot stuff' effect, and various other sources of bias have been identified (Sackett 1979) which may play a role too. Maybe many of the positive trials which are published belong to those 5 per cent which inevitably yield significant results just by chance. But there is also at least a possibility that some of the wrong conclusions were actually drawn from shaky data.

This may be the reason why data quality assurance has become an important issue in clinical trials. As Falter (1981) put it, 'quality must be consciously built into the scientific process'. Contrary to false results, it will not happen by chance.

ACKNOWLEDGEMENTS

I am grateful to several colleagues who have provided me with the examples quoted in this chapter, and to the EORTC co-operative groups for permission to use their data.

This work is supported by grant number 2 UIO CA 11488–13, awarded by the National Cancer Institute, Department of Health, Education, and Welfare.

REFERENCES

Altman, D. G. (1981). Statistics and ethics in medical research—improving the quality of statistics in medical journals. *Br. med. J.* **282,** 44–6.

Anscombe, F. J. (1960). Rejection of outliers. *Technometrics* **2,** 123–47.

Barnett, V. and Lewis, T. (1978). Outliers in statistical data. Wiley, New York.

Boyd, N. F., Pater, J. L., Ginsburg, A. D., and Myers, R. E. (1979). Observer variation in the classification of information from medical records. *J. chron. Dis.* **32,** 327–32.

Breslow, A. (1970). Thickness, cross-sectional areas and depth of invasion in the prognosis of cutaneous melanoma. *Ann. Surg.* **172,** 902–8.

Brown, B. (1983). Statistical problems related to protocol non-adherence. In *Cancer clinical trials: methods and practice.* (eds. M. Buyse, M. Staquet, and R. Sylvester) pp. 124–36. Oxford University Press.

Byar, D. P. (1980). Why data bases should not replace randomized clinical trials. *Biometrics* **36**, 337–42.

Canner, P. L., Huang, Y. B., and Meinert, C. L. (1981). On the detection of outlier clinics in medical and surgical trials. I. Practical considerations; II. Theoretical Considerations. *Cont. clin. Trials* **2**, 231–52.

Chlebowski, R. T., Weiner, J. M., Ryden, V. M. J., and Bateman, J. R. (1981). Factors influencing the interim interpretation of a breast cancer trial: danger of achieving the 'expected' result. *Cont. clin. Trials* **2**, 123–32.

Clark, W. H. Jr (1967). A classification of malignant melanoma in man correlated with histogenesis and biologic behaviour. In *Advances in biology of the skin* (eds. W. Mongagna and Hu. Funan) Vol. 8. Pergamon, London.

Cochran, A. J., Buyse, M. E., Lejeune, F. J., Macher, E. Revuz, J., and Rumke, P. (1981). Adjuvant reactivity predicts survival in patients with 'high-risk' primary malignant melanoma treated with systemic BCG. *Int. J. Cancer* **28**, 543–50.

Cohen, J. (1960). A coefficient of agreement for nominal scales. *Educ. psychol. Measure*. **20**, 37–46.

De Pauw, M. and Buyse, M. (1983). Design of forms for cancer clinical trials. In *Cancer clinical trials: methods and practice* (eds. M. Buyse, M. Staquet, and R. Sylvester) pp. 64–82. Oxford University Press.

Eichberg, J. (1980). *Getting the data plausible*, pp. 102–07. COMPSTAT 80, Physica-Verlag for the International Association for Statistical Computing.

EORTC Melanoma Pathologists' Group Writing Committee: Prade, M., Sancho-Garnier, H., Cesarini, J. P., Cochran, A. J. (1980). Difficulties encountered in the application of Clark classification and the Breslow. *Int. J. Cancer* **26**, 159–63.

Evans, J. T. (1979). Internal monitoring: patient and study management at the clinic. *Clin. Pharmacol. Ther.* **25**, 712–16.

Falter, K. H. (1981). Data quality assurance. In *Statistics in the pharmaceutical industry* (eds. C. R. Buncher and Jia-Yeong Tsay), pp. 301–26. Marcel Dekker, New York.

Feinstein, A. (1967). *Clinical judgment*. Williams and Wilkins, Baltimore.

Feinstein, A. R., Pritchett, J. A., and Schimpff, C. R. (1969). The epidemiology of cancer therapy. III. The management of imperfect data. *Archs intern. Med.* **123**, 448–61.

Fellegi, I. P. and Holt, D. (1976). A systematic approach to automatic edit and imputation. *J. Am. statist. Ass.* **71**, 17–35.

Freireich, E. J. (1981). Presidential address to the American Society of Clinical Oncology (ASCO), 23 June. Unpublished.

Friedman, L. M., Furberg, C. D., and De Mets, D. L. (1981). Fundamentals of clinical trials, pp. 112–21. John Wright, PSG Inc., Boston.

Glicksman, A. S., Reinstein, L. E., Brotman, R., and McShan, D. (1980). Quality assurance programs in clinical trials. *Cancer Treat. Rep.* **64**, 425–33.

Gnanadesikan, R. and Kettenring, J. R. (1972). Robust estimates, residuals, and outlier detection with multiresponse data. *Biometrics* **28**, 81–124.

Gore, S. M. (1981*a*). Assessing clinical trials—record sheets. *Br. med. J.* **283**, 296–8.

—— (1981*b*). Assessing clinical trials—rash adventures. *Br. med. J.* **283**, 426–8.

Harmer, M. H. (ed.) (1978). *TNM classification of malignant tumours*, 3rd edn. International Union Against Cancer, Geneva.

Henderson, W. G., Martin, J. F., and Zacharski, L. R. (1981). Comparison of local versus central tumor measurements in a multicenter cancer trial. *Cont. clin. Trials* **2**, 70 (abstract).

Herson, J. (1980). Evaluation of toxicity: statistical considerations. *Cancer Treat. Rep.* **64**, 463–8.

Hill, B. A. (1971). *Principles of medical statistics*, 9th edn. The Lancet, London.

Hutchinson, T. A., Boyd, N. F., and Feinstein, A. R. (1979). Scientific problems in clinical scales, as demonstrated in the Karnofsky index of performance status. *J. chron. Dis.* **31**, 573–80.

Jette, A. M. and Deniston, O. L. (1978). Inter-observer reliability of a functional status assessment instrument. *J. chron. Dis.* **31**, 573–80.

Kahn, H. A. (1979). Diagnostic standardization. *Clin. Pharmac. Ther.* **25**, 704–11.

Karrison, T. (1981). Data editing in a clinical trial. *Control. clin. Trials* **2**, 15–29.

Knatterud, G. L. (1981). Methods of quality control and of continuous audit procedures for controlled clinical trials. *Control. Clin. Trials* **1**, 327–32.

Koran, L. M. (1975). The reliability of clinical methods, data and judgments (in two parts). *New Engl. J. Med.* **293**, 642–6; 695–701.

Kramer, M. S. and Feinstein, A. R. (1981). The biostatistics of concordance. *Clin. Pharmac. Ther.* **29**, 111–23.

Kronmal, R. A., Davis, K., Fisher, L. D., Jones, R. A., and Gillespie, M. J. (1978). Data management for a large collaborative clinical trial (Cass: Coronary Artery Surgery Study). *Comput. biomed. Res.* **11**, 553–66.

Light, R. J. (1971). Measures of response agreement for qualitative data: some generalizations and alternatives. *Psychol. Bull.* **76**, 365–77.

McDonald, C. J. (1976). Protocol based computer reminders, the quality of care and the non-prefectability of man. *New Engl. J. Med.* **295**, 1351–5.

McFadden, E. (1980). Basic guidelines for institution data management in multicenter clinical trials. *Cont. clin. Trials* **1**, 172 (abstract).

Miller, A. B., Hoogstraten, B., Staquet, M., and Winkler, A. (1981). Reporting results of cancer treatment. *Cancer* **47**, 207–14.

Moertel, C. G. and Hanley, J. A. (1976). The effect of measuring error on the results of therapeutic trials in advanced cancer. *Cancer* **38**, 388–94.

Mowery, R. L. and Williams, O. D. (1979). Aspects of clinic monitoring in large-scale multiclinic trials. *Clin. Pharmac. Ther.* **25**, 717–19.

Mullin, S. M. (1981). How valid are the data collected in a complex multicenter clinical trial? *Cont. clin. Trials* **2**, 69–70 (abstract).

Naus, J. I. (1975). *Data quality control and editing*. Marcel Dekker, New York.

——, Johnson, T. G., and Montalvo, R. (1972). A probabilistic model for identifying errors in data editing. *J. Am. statist. Ass.* **67**, 943–50.

New England Journal of Medicine (1982). Quality of institutional participation in multicenter trials. *New Engl. J. Med.* **306**, 813–14.

O'Fallon, J. R., Golenzer, H. J., Taylor, W. F., Hu, T., Offord, J. R., Bill, J., and Moertel, C. G. (1980). Data quality control for a data management system for multiple clinical trials, *ASA Proceedings of the Statistical Computing Section, Washington*, pp. 66–75. American Statistical Association, Washington, DC.

Peto, R., Pike, M. C., Armitage, P., Breslow, N. E., Cox, D. R., Howard, S. V., Mantel, N., McPherson, K., Peto, J., and Smith, P. G. (1976). Design and analysis of randomised clinical trials requiring prolonged observation of each patient. I. Introduction and Design. *Br. J. Cancer* **34**, 585–612.

—— —— —— —— —— —— —— —— —— —— (1977). Design and analysis of randomised clinical trials requiring prolonged observation of each patient. II. Analysis and examples. *Br. J. Cancer* **35**, 1–39.

Robinson, B. N., Anderson, G. D., Cohen, E., and Gazdzik, W. F. (1979). *S.I.R. scientific information retrieval. User's manual*. SIR, Evanston.

Sackett, D. L. (1979). Bias in analytic research. *J. chron. Dis.* **32**, 51–63.

—— and Gent, M. (1979). Controversy in counting and attributing events in clinical trials. *New Engl. J. Med.* **301**, 1410–12.

Schwartz, D. and Lellouch, J. (1967). Les manquants dans l'essai thérapeutique. *Biometrics* **32**, 145–52.

Sylvester, R. J., Pinedo, H. M., De Pauw, M., Staquet, M. J., Buyse, M. E., Renard, J., and Bonadonna, G. (1981). Quality of institutional participation in multicenter clinical trials. *New Engl. J. Med.* **305**, 852–5.

Sylvester, R., Suciu, S., and De Pauw, M. (1983). The correlation between grading and clinical response. In *Cancer of the prostate and kidney* (eds. P. H. Smith, M. Pavone-Macaluso) pp. 459–66. Plenum, New York.

Szameitat, K. and Zindler, H. J. (1965). The reduction of errors in statistics by automatic corrections. *Bull ISI, Proceedings of 35th Session, Belgrade* **41**, 395–417.

Tilley, B., Forthofer, R., and Harrist, R. (1981). Analysis of quality control data: using Fleiss' extension of Cohen's kappa to test that observer agreement achieves a predetermined standard. *Cont. Clin. Trials* **2**, 70 (abstract).

Van Glabbeke, M., Buyse, M., Renard, J., and De Pauw, M. (1981). Computer-aided data management and data quality control in multicenter clinical cancer trials. *Control. Clin. Trials* **2**, 87 (abstract).

Wermuth, N. and Cochran, W. G. (1979). Detecting systematic errors in multi-clinic observational data. *Biometrics* **35**, 683–6.

WHO (1979). *WHO handbook for reporting results of cancer treatment*. WHO Offset Publication no. 48. WHO, Geneva.

Williams, O. D. (1979). A framework for the quality assurance of clinical data. *Clin. Pharma. Ther.* **25**, 700–02.

Yates, J. W., Chalmer, B., and McKegney, F. P. (1980). Evaluation of patients with advanced cancer using the Karnofsky performance status. *Cancer* **45**, 2220–4.

8 Problems related to protocol non-adherence

Byron W. Brown, Jr.

INTRODUCTION

The importance of the written protocol has been emphasized elsewhere in this book. The purpose of this chapter is to discuss the kinds of difficulties that can arise if the protocol is not followed closely. Deviations from protocol can affect the results of a clinical trial in various ways. Some deviations can dilute the power of the trial, that is, the chance of detecting a real difference in efficacy among the treatments under test. Other deviations can lead to biases in the results, causing differences between treatments that are not reflective of true differences in efficacy.

In the following sections, deviations from protocol are categorized and discussed under the headings of deviations from prescribed procedures for random treatment assignment, methods of measurement, treatment regimens, follow-up, data management, and statistical analysis. In each section the importance of proper procedure is emphasized. Common deviations from such procedures are noted, along with steps for avoidance of deviations from protocol, and accommodations that might be made in case of protocol deviation. Specific references are not given in the individual sections, but useful general references are listed at the end of the chapter.

RANDOMIZATION

The protocol for the randomized clinical trial will contain a detailed prescription of how the random assignment of treatments to patients is to be carried out. The method should ensure that the decision to admit the patient to the trial is made without knowledge of which treatment the patient will get if admitted. Ideally the treatment identity will be unknown to the medical team *during* treatment, but such *masking* or blindfolding is rarely possible in cancer trials, where different modes of therapy are compared, and different drugs have distinctive side-effects. The randomization will usually be designed to ensure that the treatment groups are balanced on important characteristics, such as the numbers of patients assigned to the groups, times of admission, institution treating the patient (if the trial is multi-institutional), severity of disease, age, and sex.

For example, in a Northern California Oncology Group randomized chemotherapy comparison for oat-cell lung cancer, each patient is registered by telephoning the statistical centre. After checking all the eligibility criteria, the statistical centre co-ordinator enters the patient's identification and characteristics into the computer, and the computer randomly assigns the patient to a treatment group. The assignment is selected randomly but with a probability biased ($p = 3/4$) towards the assignment that will better balance the treatment groups simultaneously on a predetermined set of baseline measurements. A method of random assignment that balances the treatment groups on the basis of previous assignments is called an *adaptive procedure*. Of course, other non-adaptive methods of randomization are more common, but even the simple envelope system, or prearranged and numbered series of treatment packages, or bottles involves a decision to admit and then the selection of the next appropriate treatment group assignment.

Deviations from a protocol procedure for randomization can create serious problems in the evaluation of clinical trial results. One common deviation from a valid randomization procedure is to allow the persons who decide on patient eligibility for the study to know prior to entry what treatment the patient would get if the patient were admitted to the study. This knowledge may be available to the admitter through a flaw in the procedure, through misunderstanding on the part of the admitter, or even through deliberate violation of the protocol. A typical flaw is to assign treatment by birth date, hospital chart number, or last digit in the social security number—all of which would be available to the person examining the patient for admission to the study. Use of a series of sealed envelopes, each containing a treatment assignment for an admitted patient, might be a better system, but the naïve admitter may open the envelope first and thus know the next treatment before the next patient candidate arrives. The non-naïve admitter may try to discover the envelope contents through more devious methods.

The bias that can be brought about by knowing the treatment assignment before deciding on patient admission comes through *failing to admit* certain patients who would otherwise be assigned a particular one of the several treatments. Such bias in a study is difficult to prevent since it can be eliminated only through a foolproof, cheat-proof protocol. The bias itself is even more difficult to detect in the data when the study is complete. However, some steps can be taken. Of course, the best insurance against admission bias is the masked trial, where the admitter is unaware of the next treatment to be assigned prior to the patient's actual entry on study *and also after entry*. If the treatments are identical to the senses and arranged in random order, in numbered containers (bottles, phials, tubes), the admitter can easily be kept in ignorance of the identity of the treatment next up for the next patient admitted. If this ideal situation is not realizable, then the next best method would require the admitter to decide on admission and then register the candidate by name and other characteristics, and only then be instructed by the registration centre as to which treatment the patient is to receive.

After the trial is completed, the patients in the several treatment groups can be compared with regard to their average characteristics at baseline—age, severity of disease, history of disease, and so forth. Statistically significant differences among the groups (taking the multivariate nature of the comparison into account) would seriously compromise the credibility of the study, perhaps beyond repair. But such comparisons are *not* sensitive to admission bias and may fail to detect important biases. Preventive measures in the protocol are the best approach.

Patients are sometimes admitted to a study, randomly assigned to a treatment group, and then found to fail one or more of the eligibility criteria. For example, after admission and commencement of treatment, it may be found that the patient did not fall in the required age range, or that the patient did not have the specified diagnosis (gram-negative instead of gram-positive infection, or non-oat-cell instead of oat-cell lung cancer). This problem can be minimized to some extent by clearly specifying the criteria and by forcing the person admitting the patient to specify on a check-off form a 'yes' or 'no' for each criterion. The method is even more effective if the admitter goes over the list with a registration centre, as described above. Problems arise when data on eligibility are to be reviewed later by other 'experts', for example a panel of pathologists, reviewing slides for a cancer diagnosis. Honest disagreements can arise, and the patient may ultimately be judged ineligible. The problem can be even more acute if the decision for admission to the study must be made quickly, before all of the data on eligibility are available. For example, disease stage in a lymphoma trial may determine the protocol and thus the possible treatment assignments, yet the physician is eager to get treatment started, without waiting for the final staging conference. In these cases, some questions arise as to how to conduct the randomization and how to analyse the results containing data on patients inadvertently started on the 'wrong' protocol or treatment.

One is tempted to terminate ineligible patients from the study or protocol as soon as they are discovered to be ineligible and to ignore them in the analysis. This practice is most common in cancer clinical trials. In practice, one can easily find studies in which one of the eligibility criteria is that the patient must live long enough to complete a full cycle of therapy, lasting for several weeks after random assignment. One can even find examples in which a patient is deleted from analysis due to findings at autopsy that suggest misdiagnosis.

These examples clearly reveal the dangers of bias in the practice of deleting patients from the study or the analysis, based on events, review of data and/or judgements occurring after the admission of the patient to the study and the random treatment assignment. Biases can arise in the review of patients for eligibility, especially if the reviewers know which treatment the patient received; the danger is even more acute if the reviewers know the course of disease for the patient after admission. Biases can also arise if the treatment itself can affect the chance of deletion, as would be the case if the treatment failed or caused life-threatening toxicity, thus preventing completion of the application of the full treatment cycle, or if the treatment caused death and thus made careful autopsy review possible in these special cases. Differential drop-out due to toxicity could easily happen in a trial comparing adjuvant chemotherapy with placebo or no treatment.

Cardiovascular trials often employ a view quite different from that in cancer, in regard to errors in eligibility; they require retention of every patient in the group originally assigned, and a primary statistical comparison, based on this grouping. This approach has the advantage of providing an unbiased and statistically sound comparison of the treatment groups as defined by the randomization. It has the disadvantage of comparing groups whose definitions are blurred by the various violations of clear-cut criteria, some violations avoidable perhaps and other violations unavoidable except through *post hoc* review. It would seem foolish to include in the evaluation of a study of therapy for post-myocardial patients, substantial numbers of patients known on retrospective review to have not had a myocardial infarction (MI), even though this retrospective judgement might be subject to some bias.

Some steps can be taken in design and in analysis to meet the problems here. First, it is clear that masking or blindfolding can be a big help. If review and *post hoc* judgements are made without knowledge of treatment assignment and course of disease following admission to the study, but based only on data dealing with the patient to the time of admission, most bias will be eliminated. Furthermore, the statistical analysis should compare the patients judged eligible with those judged ineligible in any reviews, separately for each treatment group. This is *not* a sensitive test for the existence of bias, unless both those eligible and those ineligible are numerous, but if this tabulation does reveal bias, the trial validity would certainly be suspect.

Deletion of patients based on events or data generated *after admission*, such as whether the treatment cycle is completed or not, or histology findings at autopsy, should be avoided. The causal linkages can be such as to threaten any inference about differences among treatments. Of course, in all questions about statistical analysis, if several approaches (for example, eligibles only as compared with an analysis involving all patients) lead to the same conclusions, the reader is thus assured that the results do not differ materially according to the policy chosen.

If the results *do* depend materially on how the question of ineligible patients is handled, *and* the question of bias has been minimized through masking, then the several conflicting results must be reconciled. Such discrepancies are unusual. However, if such a discrepancy occurs, the 'pure' analysis (that is, omitting ineligible patients and patients incompletely treated) may suggest a treatment difference, while the more conservative approach based on all patients will suggest a smaller, statistically insignificant difference. For example, one might find little difference between two chemotherapy regimens for metastatic breast cancer, but then find that there is a marked difference among the subset of patients treated most aggressively, as determined by the nadir of the white blood cell count. One of several possible interpretations is that, although the regimens do not differ much in efficacy over all eligible patients, there is a difference in a small subgroup who can tolerate aggressive therapy.

The distinction between the treatment effects in groups of patients defined by the data at hand when treatment was initiated and the effects among subgroups defined retrospectively is clear. The former deals with questions directly relevant to patient management, the latter to basic questions of treatment mechanism and effect. The distinction is clear in cancer trials where patients are declared ineligible for treatment evaluation if they do not survive long enough or cannot otherwise tolerate the treatment. Even though *post hoc* editing of the data may be fraught with physician bias, and bias due to short-term treatment toxicity, the clinical scientist wants to discover whether the treatments differ *when applied to the right patients and when the treatments have had a chance to have effect*, a question of basic importance in evaluating the possibility of ultimate therapeutic utility. The stance regarding misassignment and incomplete treatment must be decided by the question asked and the possible role of bias in the results. In adjuvant studies, it seems most appropriate to compare treatment groups as formed at the point of randomization, including patients who drop out as well as those who faithfully adhere to the protocol. However, in the treatment of advanced disease, an argument might be made for comparing responses or survival on those subgroups receiving at least minimal therapy.

Some deviations from protocol in random assignment can be minimized through anticipation and planning. Others are unavoidable, due to unavailability of data at admission and necessary retrospective review. If substantial numbers of patients ultimately fail the eligibility criteria, the validity and credibility of the study will be threatened. The protocol should carefully describe how the problem will be handled in execution and in analysis, and what conclusions can be drawn when the results of the various approaches to analysis are in conflict.

MEASUREMENT PROCEDURES

A protocol will be written in such a way that the measurements taken, especially with regard to the end-points used for evaluation and comparison of the treatments for toxicity and efficacy, will not be biased in favour of one or another of the treatments. Biases which affect all treatments equally are common and acceptable, even desirable in certain situations though this is often misunderstood. For example, in studies of drugs, toxicity data of higher reliability and greater statistical power will be obtained if each patient is queried specifically as to the occurrence of various possible side-effects, for example nausea, dizziness, and headaches. This will result in higher rates of side-effects reported in the study, but will affect all treatment groups equally in this regard. The study will be a more powerful study for detecting differences in rates among the treatments, but pharmaceutical firms are sometimes reluctant to use the technique because the deliberate upward bias may not be clearly appreciated by other persons reading the study reports.

Differential treatment bias in the observations is the more serious problem. Of course, the main source of such bias arises through unmasking of the persons making the observations. If the investigator in a randomized clinical comparison of two therapeutic regimens for liver cancer knows which therapy the patient is on, it is clear that such knowledge can bias his/her observations as to the course of the disease in the patient. Optimism can cause him/her to see improvements among patients receiving the new therapy, but not among those receiving the standard therapy. Conservatism might result in an opposite bias. The less objective the measurement or observation, the more the danger of bias. Interpretation of liver scans and measurements of tumour mass are inherently unreliable and subject to bias. Length of disease-free interval is less so, and interval from study admission or date of randomization to death would seem least subject to measurement bias.

Some sources of measurement bias that can differentially affect treatment groups are not so widely appreciated. A common bias comes from more frequent or more intensive observation in one of the treatment groups. The protocol should be written with enough care, detail, and cautionary remarks to obviate this problem, but that is difficult to do. If one of the treatments is suspected of possibly causing kidney damage, and monitoring is thought to be necessary, then *all* patients should be monitored. Monitoring of any group of people, especially people who are under treatment for some disease, *will* uncover unsuspected problems, such as minor, maybe even significant, kidney damage. Without the benefit of like monitoring of the other treatment groups, the results for the one suspect group may be difficult to interpret. Comparison will be especially suspect if different observers monitor the several treatment groups, for example, radiotherapists following the radiotherapy group and chemotherapists the chemotherapy group.

Different intensities or frequency of monitoring can lead to accidental biases not related to the reason for the monitoring. Further, the differential monitoring itself may be accidental, at least with regard to the investigator. For example, one of the therapies may cause a minor side-effect, say nausea, that brings many of the patients into the office for attention. This increase in office visits will itself increase medical surveillance, measurement of temperature, pulse, blood pressure, routine blood parameters, and so forth, thus increasing the probability of detecting real or chance aberrations, to be attributed to the single treatment that causes nausea, itself perhaps an unimportant side-effect.

Of course, the main methods of avoiding biases that unfairly favour one or another treatment are to write the protocol carefully, in awareness of the possibility of bias, to include masking of evaluators where possible to make sure the same evaluators are monitoring all groups, and then to make sure that the protocol is followed. Where the clinician administering treatment cannot be masked, it is sometimes possible to use evaluators different from the clinicians, for example in reading scans. In any case, objective measures should be used where masking is not possible, for example measures such as laboratory parameters and survival times.

TREATMENT

The treatments themselves are the focus of the therapeutic trial. They usually receive the most thorough and detailed attention in the planning of the study and are described most completely in the protocol. However, less attention is given to the management of the patient with regard to ancillary treatment during the protocol treatment period, to the management of the patient in the event that the assigned treatment is not effective, and to treatment following the protocol-prescribed treatment. It is clear that ancillary treatment in any of these three categories, effectively administered, can distort the difference between two treatment groups, either causing an apparent difference in efficacy not actually there, or hiding a real difference in efficacy. Again the best remedy lies in masking the identity of the treatment group, but this is rarely possible in cancer trials. Further remedy is always the tightly written protocol that specifies which ancillary treatments can be used and when, with the specifications to be applied equally to the several treatment groups. The study forms must provide space for well-defined documentation of all ancillary therapy, including documentation that no such therapy has been given or received.

Difficulties arise in situations where the treatments under study are such that the ancillary therapy, if necessary, cannot be the same for the several treatment groups. For example, in a trial comparing simple mastectomy with tumorectomy, the treatments of local failure will differ, and interpretation of the results will depend on the approaches used. Another example is the question of follow-up treatment of failures in a comparative trial of orchidectomy with hormonal therapy for advanced prostate cancer. In either of the above examples, a difference in efficacy can be obscured by the approach to ancillary or follow-up treatment, the choice of end-points, and the handling of the data.

The problem can be handled in several ways:

1. The protocol can specify in detail what constitutes treatment failure, and the groups can be compared on time to treatment failure. Treatment

subsequent to failure of the assigned treatment will be at the physician's discretion, and outside the purview of the study design *and analysis*.

2. The above solution is somewhat unsatisfactory if it is at all imaginable, or likely, that treatment failures in one group are better off than those in the other group, *given that they have failed*. In the breast cancer example cited above, local failures are certainly not comparable in the two groups with regard to prognosis and prospects for further treatment. The point is even clearer in the case of failure in advanced prostate cancer. Equal failure rates following orchidectomy and hormonal therapy certainly would not assure equal prognosis in the two groups, since the options for further treatment are quite different.

The examples demonstrate the need for a protocol that standardizes all treatment of the patients during the study period, that is to the specified end-points of the study. This is especially important in adjuvant studies where survival is the end-point.

Clearly, one might follow all patients through successive, well-defined courses of therapy, contingent on the individual courses of disease. The analysis would compare the treatment groups as defined by the original randomization, though the random assignments really constitute assignment to treatment regimens, dependent in part on response to therapy. If the protocol is followed, this is all quite logical and valid, and clear-cut inferences can be drawn. The temptation, however, is to regroup patients according to the treatments they actually receive through the study. For example, in an adjuvant trial comparing adjuvant chemotherapy with no further treatment, one is tempted to regroup any adjuvant patients who receive little or no adjuvant therapy with the no-treatment or control group. The bias in such an analysis is obvious, since the reasons for non-adherence, for example toxicity, may well be associated with the defined end-point.

Equally obvious, *deletion* of the patients in question from the analysis will also yield a biased evaluation. In other examples, where deletion or regrouping is done based on subsequent treatment, the biases may not be so obvious, but in all cases the practice is dangerous. In short, to avoid bias, the analysis should be based on the original random treatment group assignment, though additional analyses can be done, using regroupings and subgroupings of the patients.

FOLLOW-UP

Clinical trials in chronic disease are particularly prone to deviations from protocol with regard to follow-up observation, because such trials usually call for follow-up of long duration for each patient in the trial. For example, in studies comparing treatments for early stages of Hodgkin's disease, patients will be followed from diagnosis to death, and substantial numbers of such patients will survive more than 10 years.

In such trials there are several common violations of protocol that threaten the proper interpretation, credibility, or even the validity of the study. The most obvious problem is the loss of the subject to continued follow-up. If patients move away or refuse to continue participation in the study, their therapeutic outcomes will not be available for analysis. Analysis of the remaining patients will not be entirely satisfactory, since it may be easy to imagine that the lost data, if available, might seriously change the total complexion of the result. For example, it might well be that patients who dropped out of one of the two treatment groups did so because of some serious problem associated with the treatment, a problem presaging treatment failure, perhaps, or a problem of toxic reaction to the treatment.

What can be done about follow-up problems? A number of preventive and adaptive measures can be recommended:

1. First, anticipate the problem in the design stage so as to hold dropouts to a minimum. Include, in the eligibility requirements, criteria that exclude persons unlikely to stick by the study, for example persons who live hundreds of miles from the treatment centre, persons on temporary assignment to the area, and so forth. Also, be sure that the subject is fully informed as to the commitment he/she is making, in terms of time, clinic visits, expense, and so forth.

2. Secondly, make it as easy as possible for the subject to particpate in the trial. Without serious compromise of the basic aims of the study, require as few clinic visits as possible; hold the time per visit to a minimum; use a minimum of painful, tedious, and otherwise bothersome procedures. Other steps that can be helpful are to furnish transportation to and from the clinic, make home visits, obtain information by phone, and so forth. Also, frequent communication with the subject, free information, and small rewards for continued participation can be used.

3. Despite the best of efforts, however, there will be drop-outs, some due to moving and some due to refusal to continue participation. Several steps can be taken. When a subject moves, it is sometimes possible to see that the subject continues to receive therapy and/or follow-up attention in his/her new area, through the co-operation of local physicians. If a subject refuses further collaboration, the reasons should be ascertained through a tested procedure, and the information should be recorded and checked in the same way that all other data in the trial are handled. This information should be used to adjust the study protocol, where possible, to avoid future similar losses. Furthermore, the information can be used in the evaluation of results to estimate the possible magnitude of bias due to the drop-out problem.

4. For all drop-outs, continued effort should be made to obtain at least minimal information on the course or outcome for the subject. The survival status of each subject can usually be ascertained, even if the subject moves to another city or state. Often the subject who drops out will consent to a minimal, final evaluation, at the planned termination of his/her follow-up

period, even though intervening treatment and/or follow-up is not acceptable. Again this information can be very valuable in bounding possible bias due to drop-out.

5. In the analysis of data for a clinical trial in which there have been drop-outs, there are several widely accepted principles. First, statistical analyses should be presented on the question as to whether the drop-outs have occurred with roughly equal frequency, and to subjects of the same baseline characteristics, across the several treatment groups. If drop-outs from one of the groups are more numerous, or distinctly different (for example more severely ill at admission to the study) the study results present serious problems in evaluation. If all treatments seem equally subject to drop-out, the question of bias due to drop-out becomes less acute. However, in any case, the preferred procedure is to include the drop-outs in the main analyses where this is possible. For example, in a comparison of standard maintenance therapy with a very aggressive multi-drug regimen, in leukaemia patients, there may well be more drop-outs from the specified regimen in the experimental group. However, the principal analysis should focus on all patients initially assigned to each group. Weight loss and smoking cessation experiments are studies that commonly experience large drop-out rates. Subjects who do not lose weight at the beginning of the experiment will drop out in discouragement. Their data should be used, through an analysis that takes into account the series of weight measurements for each subject, and the length of each series. In smoking cessation experiments it is important to include all subjects in the analysis, perhaps assuming that drop-outs resume their baseline habits.

DATA MANAGEMENT AND STATISTICAL ANALYSIS

The protocol should include a careful description of the methods of data management and the statistical analyses that are to be carried out. The results of a study can be biased in the editing of the data as the data are received in the statistical office. This can happen if the editor knows the treatments the patients have received and has leeway or options in interpretation of the data, exercises closer scrutiny for errors and error correction for selected patients, and has some freedom for decisions on the classification or deletion of patients in the analysis. Again the ideal would demand a masking of the data editors, but this is not done in very many studies. Minimization of editorial bias can be achieved through (i) design of forms that require little editing and subjective review and coding, and (ii) a detailed protocol for editing, including specific directions as to which forms are acceptable and which require further information.

Biases can also occur through purposive selection of time points for analysis, choice of end-points, choice of the method of statistical analysis and decision for stopping the study. These areas should be covered in the protocol, and the statistical plan for analysis ahould be followed if at all reasonable.

Deviation from the protocol for statistical analysis should be mentioned in any report, together with the reasons for the deviation. Such deviation will almost certainly affect the credibility of the study, whereas the planned study, followed to the anticipated conclusion, gains much in inferential force.

MONITORING THE CLINICAL TRIAL

The preceding sections have dealt with the common sorts of protocol violations, methods for minimizing such violations and problems in dealing with such violations in the evaluation of the results of the trial. Here we deal with the question of measuring the degree of adherence to the protocol. In studies of fairly long duration, prompt measurement can even reveal trouble spots during the trial, and lead to a certain amount of quality *control* or *adjustment*.

Some of the methods of monitoring have been suggested in the preceding sections, but will be mentioned again along with others.

1. The best monitor for admission and randomization is to require that the admitter register the potential candidate with the statistical office, go over the eligibility requirements while making out a check form, and then either receive the treatment assignment (if unmasked) or go to the next sequential treatment package. If this method cannot be used, the check-off eligibility form is still strongly advised, and should be forwarded immediately to the statistical office along with the treatment assignment, so eligibility criteria and treatment assignment can be checked and registered.

2. The administration of treatment assigned, plus ancillary treatments, should be recorded on study forms, and sent regularly to the statistical office for editing and verification of protocol adherence.

3. Where possible, actual adherence of the patient to the protocol should be monitored. In drug studies, tracers in urine or serum can be monitored on a periodic or random basis. Pill counts are not as satisfactory but are often used. The data should be made available to the statistical office on a regular basis.

4. End-points must be measured, recorded, and made available to the statistical office on a regular basis. Regular quality checks on measurement reliability and validity should be conducted. For laboratory tests, this means the submission of blind specimens to the laboratory(s) making the study determinations. For EKGs, X-rays and the like, similar control procedures can be initiated. Extramural review of pathology slides, radiation therapy films, organ and bone scans, by central reviewers, can lead to more uniform data and enhanced credibility. For measurements and observations made in the clinic or at the bedside, for example blood pressure, or tumour size, observers should be trained, tested, and then retested at intervals. This may require visits of measurement specialists, or reports to the various observers in the study. It should be added here that it is possible, perhaps even too common, to initiate control procedures that are *too stringent*, without thought

to the quality and control necessary to assure validity and credibility sufficient to the goals of the study. Careful evaluation is necessary here, or great amounts of money can be wasted in attempting to achieve *far greater control than is necessary*. It should always be borne in mind that anything more than that necessary for the treatment of the patient in the study, can only be justified by the scientific ends of the trial itself, and the scientific ends of a clinical trial are largely focused on group averages, not individual values.

5. It is important to facilitate and monitor follow-up. This is best done by frequently generating lists of patients due for follow-up visits or contacts, and lists of those overdue. Losses to follow-up must be identified promptly so that remedial measures can be taken, before the patient is lost completely or essential information is beyond retrieval.

6. The quality of the data, whether on the eligibility forms, admission forms, or treatment and follow-up forms, must be monitored as the forms come into the statistical office. Each form must be checked for errors, for completeness, for consistency with previous data. Inadequacies must be corrected promptly. The quality of the data should be measured and monitored, so that trouble spots can be identified, trends can be gauged, and remedial action taken. The remedial action will usually be the clarification of the protocol, an improvement in the forms, or further training of the study personnel.

7. Checking of the study data to determine whether they have been validly recorded, in the clinic or at the bedside, is a point of growing concern. Short of looking over the shoulder of the observer as each observation is made and recorded, there seems no perfect way of doing this. However, some steps have been taken in this direction in recent studies. The United States National Cancer Institute is currently developing requirements for each co-operative clinical cancer group to initiate visits from the statistical centre to each clinic and hospital, to compare, entry by entry, study patient data with data in the patient's records in the clinic or hospital. This would be done for a randomly selected set of patients at each facility. Pharmaceutical firms are also developing similar monitoring plans for the physicians participating in their clinical trial programmes, with a certain degree of encouragement from the regulatory agencies. Such efforts are yet to be evaluated with regard to need, effectiveness, and cost. However, it does seem reasonable to expect that regular visits to the facilities will spruce up the quality of each to some extent.

SUMMARY

The importance of the protocol for a clinical trial cannot be overemphasized. The protocol itself should anticipate the occurrence of deviations from prescribed procedure and should include measures for holding such deviations to a minimum and accommodating to those that occur. Adjustment to deviations from protocol are made in the implementation, for example the decision to follow up or not to follow up a patient who drops out, and in the statistical analysis, for example in the decision to include or exclude certain ineligible patients in the analysis. In every accommodation the first thought must be to the goal of the study and the validity of the results in regard to this goal. Secondly, the credibility of the study in the view of the target audience must be borne in mind. The third consideration will be reliability, cost efficiency, and simplicity.

BIBLIOGRAPHY

The following references constitute a good starting point for reading on the methodology of clinical trials. Each deals in part or *in toto* with problems of protocol adherence. The more recent references provide a good starting point for a comprehensive study of the subject. The book by Friedman, Furberg, and DeMets (1981) is especially recommended.

REFERENCES

Armitage, P. (1979). The design of clinical trials. *Aust. J. Stat.* **21,** 266–81.

Friedman, L. M., Furberg, C. D., and DeMets, D. L. (1981). *Fundamentals of clinical trials.* John Wright, PSG Inc., Boston.

Mosteller, F. (1979). Problems of omission in communications, *Clin. Pharmac. Ther.* **25,** 761–4.

Peto, R., Pike, M. C., Armitage, P., Breslow, N. E., Cox, D. R., Howard, S. V., Mantel, N., McPherson, K., Peto, J., and Smith, P. G. (1976). Design and analysis of randomized clinical trials requiring prolonged observation of each patient. I. Introduction and design. *Br. J. Cancer* **34,** 585–612.

—— —— —— —— —— —— —— —— —— —— (1977). Design and analysis of randomized clinical trials requiring prolonged observation of each patient. II. Analysis and examples. *Br. J. Cancer* **35,** 1–39.

Sackett, D. L. and Gent, M. (1979). Controversy in counting and attributing events in clinical trials. *New Eng. J. Med.* **301,** 1410–12.

—— and Haynes, R. B. (1976). *Compliance with therapeutic regimens.* Johns Hopkins University Press, Baltimore.

Schwartz, D. and Lellouch, J. (1967). Explanatory and pragmatic attitudes in therapeutic trials. *J. chron. Dis.* **20,** 637–48.

Simon, R. (1979). Restricted randomization designs in clinical trials. *Biometrics* **35,** 503–12.

Temple, R. and Pledger, G. W. (1980). The FDA's critique of the Anturane Reinfarction Trial. *New Eng. J. Med.* **303,** 1488–92.

Tukey, J. W. (1977). Some thoughts on clinical trials, especially problems of multiplicity. *Science* **19,** 679–84.

Part III
Reporting

9 Reporting treatment results in solid tumours

Barth Hoogstraten

In evaluating the results of cancer therapy the response rate is of limited importance, response duration is of greater value and survival is the most important criteria of success.

INTRODUCTION

The reporting of treatment results proceeds along a path laden with problems, errors, abuses and failures in following accepted guidelines. Much of this results from lack of knowledge or from having a little knowledge. Unfortunately in part it is due to an effort to improve treatment results. Before proceeding with describing the 'rules' for reporting treatment results in solid tumours the most common pitfalls will be discussed. Much of this presentation was the subject of two meetings on the standardization of reporting results of cancer treatment. These meetings were organized by the World Health Organization with representatives of the European Organization for Research on Treatment of Cancer (EORTC), the National Cancer Institute of the USA, the International Union against Cancer (UICC), and the Council for Mutual Economic Assistance (CMEA), as well as with members of several other organizations.

The combined efforts of 37 investigators from 18 countries were reported in the *WHO Handbook for Reporting Results of Cancer Treatment* (1979). The conclusions and recommendations have recently been reported by Miller, Hoogstraten, Staquet, and Winkler (1981).

MATURATION OF DATA

'There is no substitute for maturation of data.' The value of this statement can be exemplified by two studies of the treatment of adult acute leukaemia conducted by the Southwest Oncology Group. One study, called 10-day OAP, opened on 9 July 1973 and was closed on 1 January 1975. This study served as the 'historical control' for the subsequent protocol, called CIAL, which was activated on 6 March 1975 and closed on 1 January 1977. Table 9.1 gives the median survival times for the two studies on seven dates of analysis. While the median for the 10-day OAP study remains at 18 weeks, the median for CIAL was still decreasing as of July 1979. The levels of significance for the differences in survival with time changes from a statistically significant $p < 0.01$ to a p value of 0.07.

Table 9.1. *Median duration of survival in two successive studies of acute leukaemia: effect of the maturation of data*

Date	CIAL			10-day OAP			
	Patients (n)	Deaths (%)	Median (weeks)	Patients (n)	Deaths (%)	Median (weeks)	p value
9/76	184	40	—	174	56	26	<0.01
12/76	397	41	81	179	72	18	<0.01
4/77	470	50	48	179	79	18	0.01
9/77	518	54	43	179	81	18	0.02
1/78	522	62	44	178	81	18	0.03
10/78	543	71	42	177	82	18	0.06
7/79	543	80	38	179	87	18	0.07

Figure 9.1 shows the survival curves at a three-year interval. The curves for the two studies both changed considerably with time. However, while in 1976 the 10-day OAP study was at least partially mature as far as its data are concerned, the CIAL data were still very immature. With time the difference in survival between the two studies decreased markedly and the percentages surviving at two and three years are very similar.

The comparison between the two studies was reported only in abstract form by McCredie, Hewlett, Gehan, and Freireich in 1977 when the median survival times for the two studies were 67 + weeks with CIAL and 24 weeks with 10-day OAP; the 'p value' was still <0.01. The authors concluded that CIAL prolongs the survival of patients when compared with the previous regimens.

The analyses of these two studies serve to stress three points:

1. The use of historical controls remains a dubious practice.

2. Statistically significant differences are subject to considerable change in the course of time.

3. Maturation of data or lack thereof should be given more attention by both investigators and statisticians.

THE 'p' VALUE

The contributions made by the biostatisticians have without the slightest doubt been beneficial for the conduct of clinical trials in cancer. Their positive input far outweighs the negative influence when some statisticians occasionally step beyond the boundaries of their understandably limited clinical knowledge and arrive at faulty or questionable conclusions. The real danger of

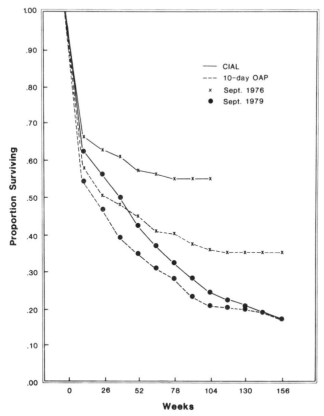

Fig. 9.1. Survival curves at a three-year interval for 10-day OAP, CIAL trials.

statistics in medicine lies with clinical investigators, who become unduly impressed by the results of their findings and 'hide behind a *p* value' to justify their conclusions—a *p* value which at times should not have been calculated. All too often one hears a presentation at national and international meetings in which the presentor arrives at far-reaching conclusions without sufficient justification. An example can be drawn from the abstracts of the American Society of Clinical Oncology in 1980. Of the hundreds of abstracts a review was made of five successive abstracts of clinical trials in which *p* values were used (Table 9.2).

In Abstract A the authors condemn one treatment modality even though that modality was used in the three successive treatment plans. The conclusion was based on a comparison with 'results in the literature'. The conclusion from Abstract B, although quite logical, makes little sense. In Abstract C the authors fail to mention the considerable imbalance in prognostically important factors between the treatment arms. Only in Abstract D were the authors somewhat cautious in their conclusion. In Abstract E the third

Table 9.2. *Review of five successive ASCO abstracts in which* p *values were used*

Patients (n)	Randomization	p value	Conclusion by authors
A. 36	No—three sequential groups of 7, 11 and 18 cases	≤0.006	One treatment modality makes contribution
B. 75	two way	<0.01	Inferior arm offers no advantage over the superior arm
C. 151	three way	0.02 and 0.03	One arm gives superior survival
D. 94	two way, two stratifications	0.10	In subsets of 18 and 19 survival appears to be improved
E. 146	Partially, three treatments	<0.01	Superior disease-free survival for one treatment
F. 228	two way	<0.03	One arm gives superior CR rate
		0.2	Superior survival for same arm

treatment plan was instituted after the previous two randomized arms were closed. The duration of follow-up for this treatment arm is considerably shorter than that of the other arms and yet the authors claim its superiority over the two 'historical control' arms. Abstract F is not successive and was chosen because the authors arrived at a correct conclusion as far as the CR rate is concerned, but are clearly overly optimistic about the survival. These six abstracts give rise to several questions:

Were the calculations made by a statistician?

If yes:

A. Did the statistician have a good working knowledge of the medical area under investigation?

B. Did the statistician help in the design of the study?

C. Did the statistician have access to all data?

D. Did the statistician approve the final conclusions?

If not:

A. Did the investigator understand the limitations of the statistical evaluations?

B. Did the investigator know which correct calculations to use?

C. Did an unbiased investigator review the study design, the data and the abstract?

D. Did the investigator consult with a statistician?

The poor reporting of treatment results is not confined to meetings and abstracts. It is nearly impossible to read an issue of leading clinical cancer journals without giving rise to serious questions about study design, data collection, definitions of response, determination of results, and the reporting of results.

NUMERATOR AND DENOMINATOR

The numerator is the number of patients in whom events occur during a given period of observation. Bias can play an important role in arriving at a numerator. Even when a standard method for calculating tumour size is used, human error in tumour measurement can play a significant role as was so clearly shown by Moertel and Hanley (1976). Their study was designed to simulate the conditions which the physician encounters in oncological practice when measuring tumours in the abdomen, lymph nodes, and subcutaneous metastases. Sixteen experienced oncologists each measured 12 simulated tumour masses. Twelve solid spheres were selected, measuring from 1.8 to 14.5 cm in diameter, the total diameter being 66.8 cm. The oncologists deviated in their measurements with a range of 3.1 to 22.5 cm, which is 4.6 to 33.6 per cent. Two sets of 'tumours' had the same diameter which allowed an estimation of the reproducibility of each physician's measurements.

Moertel and Hanley also determined the error rates if the same size tumour is measured by two different investigators (Table 9.3). In that situation there were a total of 1920 configurations. If a tumour regression of at least 25 per cent were required the percentage of false-positives would be 24.9 per cent, while if at least 50 per cent shrinkage was stipulated, the error rate would fall to 6.8 per cent. Conversely in reporting tumour growth the false-negative rates were 31.5 per cent and 17.8 per cent respectively, for ≥ 25 per cent and ≥ 50 per cent growth.

Table 9.3. *Erroneously declared objective responses and progressions when two investigators measure a tumour which has remained the same size*[*]

	Objective response	
	$\geq 25\%$ Shrinkage	$\geq 50\%$ Shrinkage
False-positive	24.9%	6.8%
	Objective progression	
	$\geq 25\%$ Growth	$\geq 50\%$ Growth
False-negative	31.5%	17.8%

[*] After Moertel and Hanley (1976).

Their study was conducted under ideal conditions and one can anticipate larger error rates when the oncologist measures irregular masses through the abdominal wall of uncomfortable patients. Based on this study the importance of at least 50 per cent reduction of the product of the longest perpendicular diameters of a clearly measurable tumour mass was again emphasized. And even then an erroneous recording of objective response must be anticipated for between 5 and 10 per cent of patients treated.

With the introduction of newer diagnostic techniques an important new factor in determining the numerator is being added: the non-oncologist, the non-participating investigator. This is especially true for the following techniques: computerized axial transverse (CAT) scans; radio-isotopic scans; and ultrasonography. These highly specialized studies require interpretation by experts and the oncologist thus becomes dependent on others for the evaluation of tumour size. And of necessity the quality of these interpretations will vary with the quality of the radiologist and his interest in accuracy.

It is human nature for investigators to choose on the positive side when the question arises whether a patient has attained a remission or not. This is especially the case when several tumour masses are being measured in a single patient and when measurability cannot easily be defined. Not infrequently the study chairman will bend the data even a little further, so that all-in-all the numerator of the responses inadvertently becomes biased positively—larger than a more critical observer may allow.

Recently this was emphasized by Sears and Olson (1980) who performed an extramural review of 385 clinical responses of advanced breast cancer. These cases were contributed by investigators from seven institutions. Sears and Olson agreed with the investigators' interpretation in only 79 per cent, disagreed in 5 per cent and found the documentation of 60 patients (16 per cent) insufficient to permit evaluation of the result of therapy.

The denominator is the total number of patients at risk during a given period of observation. Rarely are the results of cancer treatment reported in a fashion where the denominator has not been tampered with in one or several ways. Often a single denominator is used from which many patients of the original population have been declared ineligible or non-evaluable for a variety of reasons. The extent to which this occurs is not known, but some indication can be obtained from a report by Hoogstraten and Fabian (1979) who determined the efficacy of single drugs in the treatment of advanced breast cancer. A literature search of articles written in English resulted in 4948 patients treated with 35 different drugs. Articles which used an objective response defined as a reduction in tumour mass of less than 50 per cent, and articles which excluded the non-evaluable patients from the denominator, comprised a total of 1933 cases. Thus at least 39 per cent of the patients studied were of questionable value.

The 'eligibility' of patients should be determined either at the time of patient registration or very soon thereafter, but definitely before the investigator and study co-ordinator know the outcome of the treatment. Declaring a patient 'ineligible' prospectively is an acceptable practice, while doing so after the results are known may lead to tampering of the data.

The reasons most often used for declaring a patient non-evaluable are shown in Table 9.4.

Table 9.4. *Reasons most often given to reduce the denominator: non-evaluable patients*

1. Early death
2. Lost to follow-up
3. Failure to complete therapy due to toxicity
4. Refused further therapy
5. Inadequate data
6. Major protocol violation
7. Other reasons

'Early death' usually comprises the largest portion. Rarely is this defined in the protocol and the study co-ordinator all too often selects an arbitrary time limit after the study has been completed. That time limit supposedly is chosen to give the treatment a fair chance, but one only needs to remember the dramatic improvement which can take place within a few days of therapy in children with acute leukaemia or adults with small cell cancer of the lung to realize that most early deaths really are treatment failures.

The next three categories 'lost to follow-up', 'failure to complete therapy due to toxicity' and 'refused further therapy' consist of patients who failed to have a satisfactory response, patients who have a good response and see no need for further therapy, or those who could not cope with the toxicity. Again in most instances it is the treatment which is at fault. 'Inadequate data' is really the judgement of the study chairman who can be too lenient or too strict. In actual practice it is rare for a study chairman to exclude a good responding patient because of 'inadequate data', whereas he is more apt to do it with the non-responder.

When Sears and Olson (1980) reviewed the 385 patients with breast cancer these had already been declared evaluable by the investigators and they had rendered their opinion as to the result of therapy. Sears and Olson could not make an evaluation in 16 per cent of these evaluable patients. Their extramural review changes both numerator and denominator for an overall change of 21 per cent in interpretation.

A variety of 'other reasons' have been used and frequently the author of a manuscript does not bother to delineate these reasons. Probably the only valid cause to reduce the denominator should be major violations in the treatment programme, since these are usually spelled out in the protocol.

The combination of the inflated numerator and the reduced denominator leads to spuriously high response rates. The practice of manipulating clinical data is widespread and it behooves the readership of medical journals to carefully evaluate the 'Materials and Methods' section of a manuscript before accepting response rates at face value. There is, of course, no harm when investigators attempt to report the efficacy of a new therapy in adequately treated patients, provided that at least one other denominator is also used. The WHO conference recommends that at least two of three denominators be used for reporting results:

(a) registered and eligible;

(b) registered, eligible, and treated: this includes all patients who were registered, were eligible, and were given therapy regardless of how little or how much therapy was given;

(c) registered, eligible, and adequately treated.

When other denominators are used, they should be clearly defined.

EVALUATION OF DATA

Accurate and mature data do not necessarily guarantee the completeness of data evaluation. But they do allow a more in-depth study of the data when this becomes necessary. A recent example of the virtue of detailed analysis can be found in the well-known area of adjuvant treatment of breast cancer with cyclic combination chemotherapy consisting of cyclophosphamide, methotrexate and fluorouracil (CMF). The investigators, Bonadonna, Brusamolino, Valagussa, Rossi, Brugnatelli, Brambilla, DeLina, Tancini, Bajetta, Musumeci, and Veronesi (1976), are all experienced and most reliable. Only five of 391 patients entered into the study were excluded from analysis. In an updated analysis (Bonadonna, Rossi, Valagussa, Banfi, and Veronesi 1977), the authors concluded that the advantage of giving CMF is apparently limited to pre-menopausal women. In another large study conducted by the Southwest Oncology Group L-PAM was compared with CMF to which prednisone and vincristine were added, CMFVP. The important finding in this study is that CMFVP is effective equally well in post-menopausal women.

One expects that the menopausal status would not influence the outcome of adjuvant chemotherapy, as age has no bearing on the efficacy of combination chemotherapy in advanced disease as shown by Hoogstraten, George, Samal, Rivkin, Costanzi, Bonnet, Thigpen, and Braine (1976). Bonadonna subsequently went back to his original data and in careful re-analysis of the actual drug doses given to the patients, he demonstrated that post-menopausal women who received the higher doses benefitted as much as the younger women (Bonadonna *et al.* 1981). This retrospective and more complete analysis, which led the authors to radically revise their conclusions, is a credit to the investigators and the reliability of their data.

With good data it is best to do a very detailed analysis. Reviewers and editors can always ask that a portion of the analysis be deleted, they cannot add to the manuscript.

RELEVANT TUMOUR DATA

The data relevant to the tumour can be divided into two parts.

Subjective tumour data

Performance status

The classification of the performance status is the most helpful and most often used aid in determining the subjective effect of cancer treatment. The recommended classification uses five grades and is especially useful since it encompasses the Karnofsky scale as well (Karnofsky, Abelman, Craver, and Burchenal 1948):

Grade	Scale
0	Fully active, able to carry on all predisease performance without restriction (Karnofsky 90–100)
1	Restricted in physically strenuous activity but ambulatory and able to carry out work of a light or sedentary nature, e.g. light housework, office work (Karnofsky 70–80)
2	Ambulatory and capable of all self-care, but unable to carry out any work activities. Up and about more than 50 per cent of waking hours (Karnofsky 50–60)
3	Capable of only limited self-care, confined to bed or chair more than 50 per cent of waking hours (Karnofsky 30–40)
4	Completely disabled. Cannot carry on any self-care. Totally confined to bed or chair (Karnofsky 10–20)

Weight

The second most useful subjective parameter for the evaluation of the impact of the tumour or of the treatment is the weight of the patient. Weight loss almost certainly indicates advancing disease, unless of course excess body fluid has been eliminated. On the other hand, when the patient is gaining 'healthy' weight this can be considered a good sign, and objective improvement is likely to follow.

It is unfortunate that the definition of subjective response is so difficult or nearly impossible. Unlike the clinical investigator, the vast majority of patients are not much interested in an objective decrease in tumour size, unless they can personally observe this. Objective data are the main tool of the oncologist, while the patients are more interested in how they feel. And how they feel has direct bearing on treatment, especially in drug therapy. A patient who feels good will tolerate more chemotherapy, and thus has a greater chance of response to that treatment.

Objective tumour data

A minimum set of information is desirable.

1. Site of the primary tumour

The ICD–O classification is recommended for topography coding (WHO 1976).

2. Histopathology

The ICD–O morphology codes (WHO 1976) are most often used for delineating the histopathology, tumour type, grade, and stage of the tumour. The surgico-pathological stage should also be recorded when surgery has been used to complete the staging of the disease.

3. Tumour measurability

All measurements should be recorded in metric notations (centimetres), using a rule or calipers. Direct measurement along two axes remains the most reliable method for determining tumour size (Hayward, Carbone, Heuson, Kumaoka, Segaloff, and Rubens 1976). Difficulty arises when several tumour sites are involved, and when more than one tumour mass is measured. The Combination Chemotherapy Subcommitee of the Breast Cancer Task Force of the National Cancer Institute, USA (see Hoogstraten *et al.* 1977) has proposed rather elaborate charts to determine the overall response, but their usefulness or lack thereof has not yet been adequately tested.

Four categories of tumour measurability are useful:

(a) Measurable, bidimensional—the surface area of the tumour is approximated by multiplying its longest diameter with its greatest perpendicular diameter.

(b) Measurable, unidimensional—malignant disease measurable in only one dimension. For the evaluation of treatment efficacy this is a much less reliable category than the previous one. Examples are:

Abdominal mass—the accuracy is tempered by the findings of Moertel and Hanley (1976) which indicate the limited value of measuring intra-abdominal tumours by palpation alone.

Mediastinal and hilar masses—these can be measured accurately when a pre-involvement chest X-ray is available, by subtracting the normal mediastinal or hilar width from the width containing malignant disease. When a pre-involvement X-ray is not available only clinical judgement can be used and it becomes virtually impossible to declare complete resolution of the tumour.

Hepatomegaly—the sum of three linear measurements to the liver edge is used most often: from the xiphoid notch and from the costal margins 10 cm bilateral from the xiphoid notch. The value of this measurement is limited since not all hepatomegaly constitutes a tumour.

(c) Non-measurable, evaluable—malignant disease which is not measurable by rule or caliper, but its progress is readily evaluable. Response or increasing disease can only be estimated. Examples include: ill-defined pelvic or abdominal masses; lymphangitic lung metastases; malignant ascites or pleural effusions uninfluenced by diuretics; ill-defined skin metastases; bone metastases. This category is of special importance for gynaecological malignancies and cancer of the gastrointestinal tract. The determination of treatment response can be highly biased, and considerable caution is advised before results are accepted at face value.

(d) Biological markers, chemical values—unless specifically stipulated in treatment protocols these markers and laboratory results are not used to evaluate response. However, some markers are so tumour-specific that they can be more important for following the disease than the actual tumour measurements. A good example are the gonadotrophins for the trophoblastic tumours, which can detect active disease long before or after the tumour can be measured in centimetres.

4. Number of tumours to be measured

Investigators should always attempt to measure several tumours when possible. It is well known that malignancies, especially melanoma, can show marked regression in some masses while others remain the same in size or even grow. The term 'mixed response' is sometimes used to describe this phenomenon, but this should be avoided. Whenever one of the masses continues to grow this constitutes progressive disease, which resists the treatment and therefore the patient cannot be considered as a responder.

5. Methods of tumour measurement

Physical examination and radiographs have always been the most important modes of tumour measurement. But lately other highly sensitive studies have become available and others can be expected in the future. Investigators should always remain receptive to new methodology, and include those methods which can increase the accuracy of tumour measurement.

Physical examination—superficial and palpable lesions can often be measured with great accuracy, and physical examination remains a valuable method of tumour measurement. Care should be taken that the same observer performs the measurements in a given patient, since considerable difference can exist between two or more observers.

Radiographs—the usefulness of X-rays is especially obvious for lung tumours and bone metastases. They can also be used in special situations, such as deviation or obstruction of ureters.

Photographs—in patients with breast cancer there is no better way for following skin involvement than the colour photograph. Photographs are indispensable for intraoral cancer, and in special circumstances, such as laparoscopy.

Computerized Axial Transverse (CAT) scan—probably no other new method has had as large an impact on following tumour masses as the CAT scan. This techique has introduced a refinement that made several other methods obsolete, and constitutes a strong argument against the use of the 'historical control'. The CAT scan is invaluable for brain tumours and intra-abdominal tumours.

It is still too early to determine its full impact, but already questions can and are being raised, whether the CAT scan has outmoded the radio-isotope scan of brain and liver, ultrasonogram, or lymphangiography. Currently its drawback is the degree of sophistication necessary for the interpretation of the scans, and close co-operation with the expert radiographer is advisable.

Lymphangiography—this may be used as an indicator of anti-neoplastic response, provided abnormalities clearly represent malignant disease. The criteria for measurable or non-measurable, evaluable disease must be met. Nodes of patients with solid tumours containing only small peripheral defects cannot be used as either measurable or non-measurable, evaluable disease. Lymphangiography should be repeated as necessary to adequately evaluate response.

Laboratory studies—these include the usual blood counts and blood chemistries all of which can aid in the evaluation of the patient. Bone marrow biopsy, tumour markers, and disease-specific excretory products can be useful.

Bone scan—these continue to be of great value for the evaluation of bone metastases. However, not all 'hot spots' on a bone scan represent malignant disease and X-ray should be taken of all positive or suspicious areas. Occasionally a biopsy may be indicated.

RESPONSE

The guidelines proposed by the Breast Cancer Task Force in the USA (Hoogstraten, Irwin, Ahmann, Band, Fink, Greenspan, Sears, Sedransk, Smalley, Talley, Tormey, Carter 1977), those outlined by the UICC project (Hayward *et al.* 1977), the report by Miller *et al.* (1981), and the WHO guidelines (WHO 1979) form the basis for the criteria of response used in this chapter.

In the past some investigators have used decreases of less than 50 per cent as responses, but Moertel and Hanley (1976) have demonstrated the fallacy of this practice. On the other hand a 25 per cent increase in tumour size is most widely used and recommended to designate progressive disease and that may not be enough for the palpable tumours.

Most oncologists use four weeks measured from the onset of response as the minimum duration of tumour regression before calling it a response. Some investigators are more conservative in using 3 months as the minimum duration in which case it is often measured from the first day of therapy. A shorter duration may sometimes be useful when a new drug is being tested.

Definitions

Complete response (CR)

(a) Clinical—complete disappearance of all clinically-detectable malignant disease for at least four weeks.

Bone metastases: (i) patients with radiographic evidence of bony metastases prior to therapy must have normalization of radiographs or complete sclerotic healing of lytic metastases in association with a normal bone scan; (ii) patients with an abnormal bone scan and normal radiographs prior to therapy must have normalization of the bone scan, provided that the abnormalities represent malignant disease as proven by biopsy.

(b) Pathological—pathological proof of a clinically complete response after rebiopsying areas of known malignant disease.

Partial response (PR)

A greater than, or equal to, 50 per cent decrease in tumour size for at least 4 weeks, without an increase in the size of any area of known malignant disease of greater than 25 per cent or appearance of new areas of malignant disease.

(a) Measurable, bidimensional—a greater than, or equal to, 50 per cent decrease in tumour area of an organ site, or in the sum of the products of perpendicular diameters of multiple lesions in the same organ site for at least four weeks.

(i) Mediastinal and hilar width response can sometimes be accurately determined by the following formula:

A = on-study width
B = normal width (pre-involvement X-ray)
C = width after treatment

$$\text{PR if } \frac{(A-B)-(C-B)}{(A-B)} \geq 0.3.$$

Unfortunately there is only infrequently a pre-involvement X-ray available.

(ii) Palpable masses that can be measured in only one dimension are evaluated for response by using the formula:

A = on-study measurement
B = measurement after treatment

$$\text{PR if } \frac{A-B}{A} \geq 0.3.$$

(iii) Liver sizes—A partial response of malignant hepatomegaly has occurred if the liver measurements below the costal margin(s) in the midclavicular lines (or other consistently used points) and the tip of the xyphoid decrease by greater than, or equal to, 30 per cent.

(b) Non-measurable, evaluable—a definite improvement in evaluable malignant disease estimated to be in excess of 50 per cent and lasting for at least four weeks and agreed upon by two independent investigators.

(i) Serial evaluations of chest X-rays (i.e. confluent multi-nodular and lymphangitic metastases, malignant pleural effusions) and physical measurements (i.e. abdominal girth) should be documented in records and by photograph when practical.

(ii) A partial response of bony metastases occurs if there is a partial decrease in the size of lesions, partial sclerotic transformation of lytic lesions, or decreased density of blastic lesions, lasting for at least four weeks.

No change (NC)

No significant change in measurable or evaluable disease for at least four weeks (greater than, or equal to, twelve weeks for bony metastases).

(a) No increase in size of any known malignant disease.

(b) No appearance of new areas of malignant disease.

(c) This designation includes decrease in malignant disease of less than 50 per cent, or decrease in unidimensional measurable disease of less than 30 per cent, or increase in malignant disease of less than 25 per cent in any site.

Progression (P)

Significant increase in size of lesions present at the start of therapy or appearance of new metastatic lesions known not to be present at the start of therapy.

(a) Measurable, bidimensional, and unidimensional:

(i) Greater than, or equal to, 25 per cent increase in the area of any malignant lesions greater than 2 cm, or in the sum of the products of the individual lesions in a given organ site (comparison of products of the longest diameter by the greatest perpendicular diameter).

(ii) Greater than, or equal to, 50 per cent increase in the size of the product of diameters if only one lesion is available for measurement and was less than 2 cm in size at the initiation of therapy.

(iii) Greater than, or equal to, 25 per cent increase in the sum of the liver measurements below the costal margins and xyphoid.

(iv) Appearance of new malignant lesions.

(b) Non-measurable, evaluable:

(i) definite increase in the area of malignant lesions estimated to be greater than 25 per cent;

(ii) appearance of new malignant lesions;

(iii) increase in size or number of bony metastases (pathological fractures do not represent progression unless there is a documented increase in bony disease);

(iv) adjuvant—definite clinical evidence of recurrent or metastatic malignant disease. Biopsy-proven evidence of recurrence should be obtained when feasible.

No evidence of disease (NED)

A lack of clinically identifiable malignant disease in non-measurable, non-evaluable, or adjuvant patients.

Recurrence

(a) appearance of new lesion(s) in a patient with no evidence of disease (NED);

(b) reappearance of lesions in a patient who has had a complete response (CR);

(c) a 25 per cent increase in size of lesions or appearance of new metastatic lesions in patients with a partial response (PR).

Response by organ site

The evaluation of the effect of therapy on an involved organ site is influenced by several factors, that is, number of measurable lesions, methods of measurement, and degree of measurability. Because of this it becomes necessary to establish some rules to be used in the evaluation of an individual organ site.

(a) Record responses as complete (CR), partial (PR), no change (NC), progression (P), or NED under appropriate methods of evaluation.

(b) If more than one type of evaluation method exists for a given organ site, each must be recorded separately.

(c) An organ site PR occurs if there is a greater than 50 per cent decrease in the sum of the products of the perpendicular diameters of all measurable lesions in that organ site.

(d) In patients with measurable disease, the worst response prevails in determining response by organ site.

(e) Stabilization of evaluable disease does not detract from a PR of measurable disease by organ site but reduces a CR to a PR.

(f) Progression in any classification of measurability or evaluability in an organ site prevails as the response for that organ site.

Total patient response

In determining the overall (total) objective response the following rules apply:

(a) if both measurable and unmeasurable disease is present in a given patient, the result of each should be recorded separately;

(b) in patients with measurable disease, the poorest response designation prevails;

(c) 'no change' in unmeasurable lesions does not detract from a partial response in measurable lesions, but reduces a complete response in measurable lesions to partial response overall;

(d) if in the totals of responses by organ site there are equal or greater numbers of complete plus partial responses than of 'no change' designations, then the overall response will be partial;

(e) if progressive disease exists in any lesions or when a new lesion appears, then the overall result is 'progressive disease'.

Duration of response

The responding patient may undergo a period of continuing improvement and eventually reach a complete response. It may be desirable to separate the duration spent in complete response from the overall duration. Duration is defined by a beginning and an end-point. While there is no controversy regarding the end-point of a response, there is a difference of opinion about the onset of response.

One school of thought claims that in the responding patient the overall response began on the first day of treatment and lasted to the date of first observation of progressive disease. Very often it is difficult to determine when a partial response has actually occurred or when a partial response is so good that one can speak of a complete response. This is especially true for the intra-abdominal tumours and skeletal metastases.

A second school is more puritan and insists on a sharp delineation of the onset of response. The proponents of this school are faced with the obvious problem that in patients with solid tumours they may have to choose a date arbitrarily.

The difficulty has been approached by the various task forces in different ways. The Breast Cancer Task Force (Hoogstraten *et al.* 1977) gives the duration of response as being from onset of response until relapse, and states that the onset of response is that time when the criteria for a particular response are first met (i.e. ≥ 50 per cent decrease for PR and complete disappearance for CR).

The UICC Task Force (Hayward *et al.* 1977) used the start of therapy as the onset of objective regression and thus carefully avoided the 'onset' of response. This task force found it essential to categorize a patient as having a regression at a stated time. It is not quite clear what is meant by this.

The WHO Task Force (WHO 1979) compromised and called the onset of complete response as the date when it was first recorded, but used the first day of treatment as the onset for partial response.

The entire problem can be minimized as long as the investigators clearly define the onset of response in their protocol and in their report. The duration of response is the period between onset of response and the date thereafter on which progressive disease is first noted. In patients who first spend some time in a partial response and subsequently a period in complete response, one should calculate the period of overall response.

SURVIVAL

The definitions of survival are simple:

1. disease-free survival is the period during which there is no evidence of disease activity;

2. survival covers the period from the date of an event to the date of death. The event can be the diagnosis, the start of therapy, or any other clearly defined happening.

CONCLUSION

At the beginning of this chapter this author stated his personal philosophy regarding the evaluation of cancer therapy. The problems are many, and it is doubtful that full agreement regarding criteria for response and the evaluation of response will be reached in the near future. And even when there is such agreement, the investigators are likely to differ in their interpretations.

Duo cum faciunt idem, non est idem. This Latin proverb by Terence says it so well: 'If two people do the same thing, it is not exactly the same.'

Nevertheless the reporting of results can be greatly improved if the authors adhere to five self-imposed guidelines:

● Let the data mature,
● Make use of an informed statistician,
● Do not tamper with the numerator and denominator,
● Remain strictly objective ('honest'),
● Stay with the facts and do not make the pitfall of overinterpretation.

REFERENCES

Bonadonna, G., Brusamolino, E., Valagussa, P., Rossi, A., Brugnatelli, L., Brambilla, C., DeLina, M., Tancini, G., Bajetta, E., Musumeci, R., and Veronesi, U. (1976). Combination chemotherapy as an adjuvant treatment in operable breast cancer. *New Engl. J. Med.* **294**, 405–10.

——Rossi, A., Valagussa, P., Banfi, A., and Veronesi, U. (1977). The CMF program for operable breast cancer with positive axillary nodes. *Cancer* **39**, 2904 – 15.

——Valagussa, P., Rossi, A., Tancini, G., Brambilla, C., Marchina, S., and Veronesi, U. (1981). Multimodal therapy with CMF in resectable breast cancer with positive axillary nodes—the Milan Institute experience. In *Adjuvant therapy of cancer III* (ed. S. E. Jones and S. E. Salmon). Grune and Stratton, New York.

Hayward, J. L., Carbone, P. P., Heuson, J. C., Kumaoka, S., Segaloff, A., and Rubens, R. D. (1979). Assessment of response to therapy in advanced breast cancer. *Cancer* **39**, 1289–93.

Hoogstraten, B. and Fabian, C. (1979). A reappraisal of single drugs in advanced breast cancer. *Cancer clin. Trials* **2**, 101–9.

—— George, S. L., Samal, B., Rivkin, S. E., Costanzi, J. J., Bonnet, J. D., Thigpen, T., and Braine, H. (1976). Combination chemotherapy and adriamycin in patients with advanced breast cancer. A Southwest Oncology Group Study. *Cancer* **38**, 13–20.

—— Irwin, L., Ahmann, D., Band, P., Fink, D. J., Greenspan, E., Sears, M. E., Sedransk, N., Smalley, R., Talley, R., Tormey, D. C., and Carter, S. (1977). *Breast cancer: suggested protocol guidelines for combination chemotherapy trials.* DHEW Publication No. (NIH) 77–1192. Bethesda, Maryland.

Karnofsky, D. A., Abelman, W. H., Craver, L. F., and Burchenal, J. H. (1948). The use of nitrogen mustards in the palliative treatment of carcinoma. *Cancer* **1**, 634–56.

McCredie, K. B., Hewlett, J. S., Gehan, G. A., and Freireich, E. J. (1977). Chemoimmunotherapy of adult acute leukaemia (CIAL). *Proc. Am. Ass. cancer Res.* **18**, 127.

Miller, A. B., Hoogstraten, B., Staquet, M., and Winkler, A. (1981). Reporting results of cancer treatment. *Cancer* **47**, 207–14.

Moertel, C. G., and Hanley, J. A. (1976). The effect of measuring error on the results of therapeutic trials in advanced cancer. *Cancer* **38**, 388–94.

Sears, M. E., and Olson, K. B. (1980). Extramural review of clinical response of breast cancer to cytotoxic chemotherapy. *Cancer* **46**, 2928–9.

WHO (1976). *International classification of disease for oncology* (ICD–O) 1st edn. World Health Organization, Geneva.

—— (1979). *WHO handbook for reporting results of cancer treatment*, WHO Offset Publication No. 48, WHO, Geneva.

10 Reporting treatment results in non-solid tumours

Robert Zittoun and Harvey D. Preisler

INTRODUCTION

While there has been substantial improvement in the therapy of non-solid tumours, the ability to collect and interpret information has lagged behind the profusion of new therapeutic strategies. The results of clinical trials are usually reported in terms of percentage complete remission, duration of remission, and survival, with final statistical analysis being performed on these end-points. This approach leads to the underutilization of information which is readily available for broader usages and hence leads to the design of successor protocols which are not based on a complete and logical interpretation of the previous studies. Moreover, many reported trials do not utilize appropriate methodology (George 1978; Peto, Pike, Armitage, Breslow, Cox, Howard, Mantel, McPherson, Peto, and Smith 1977), nor do they show evidence of originality. The same pitfalls as those exposed in the previous chapter about solid tumours apply to haematological malignancies; some pertinent results need longer follow-up, especially those describing a 'plateau'. Historical controls cannot substitute for a fully comparable series. The p value, the numerators and denominators are submitted to the same biases which reduce the value of many results and prevent a proper comparison between therapeutic trials.

Initial parameters

There is generally agreement on the *initial parameters necessary* for a valid analysis. The most important are:

Parameters which allow the selection of a homogeneous population and exclude other diseases with similar features but different prognoses and treatments. For instance, hairy cell leukaemia must be excluded from a study of chronic lymphocytic leukaemia (CLL), and angio-immunoblastic lymphadenopathy from a study of Hodgkin's Disease (HD). Therefore, pathological material should be reviewed by referees. This review must be done prior to randomization whenever there is an appreciable risk of including patients whose disease does not correspond to the group being studied.

The parameters having known or potential prognostic value, such as age, performance status, clinical staging, and blood counts. Age distribution as well as performance status should be carefully analysed, since variations in these parameters undoubtedly explain many differences in reported results (Keating, Smith, Gehan, McCredie, Bodey, Spitzer, Hersh, Gutterman, and Freireich 1980; Wiernik and Serpick 1970). Secondary diseases—such as acute leukaemia following a pre-leukaemic state, or occuring in patients treated for another cancer—have a poor prognosis (Preisler and Lyman 1977) and should be studied separately.

The moment for a patient to be considered on-study and to start the treatment must be carefully defined and previous treatments recorded. Even in diseases such as leukaemia, variations in the time lag between the first signs, the diagnosis, and the start of the induction treatment can lead to heterogeneity of results.

Measurability of non-solid tumours

In most haematological malignancies, *the entire initial tumour mass* can only be roughly estimated. Assessment has been made possible in multiple myeloma, by measuring the rate of synthesis of the total circulating M component as well as the *in vitro* synthesis per myeloma cell (Salmon and Durie 1975). The tumour mass has been shown to fluctuate around 10^{12} cells, a number close to those previously estimated in widespread haematological malignancies. Correlations of the measured tumour mass with current parameters have given a scientific basis to the clinical staging (Durie and Salmon 1975). Such staging must be defined according to criteria which have already received wide acceptance or those which have been proposed more recently in various diseases, such as chronic lymphocytic leukaemia (Rai, Sawitsky, Cronkite, Chanana, Levy, and Pasternack 1975), chronic myelocytic leukaemia (Tura, Baccarani, Corbelli, and the Italian Cooperative Study Group on Chronic Myeloid Leukaemia 1981), multiple myeloma (Durie, Salmon and Moon 1980) and Hodgkin's Disease (Carbone and Kaplan 1971). In Hodgkin's Disease and non-Hodgkin's lymphoma, clinical staging must be made according to the Ann Arbor classification. However, the number of involved areas and the volume of tumours should also be taken into account (Sweet and Golomb 1980).

Variations of the tumour mass during treatment are difficult to assess. In acute leukaemia, the leukaemic cells decrease to less than 10^{10} during complete remission, but their exact level cannot be determined. The time to relapse depends (in addition to the effect of subsequent treatments) on this residual tumour mass (Frei and Canellos 1980), and its proliferative capacity, but neither are currently measurable. The study of biological markers has led to some disappointment: for example it has been shown that some cells labelled with the common acute lymphocytic leukaemia (ALL) antigen may correspond to normal regenerating cells (Janossy, Bollum, Bradstock, McMichael, Rapson, and Greaves 1979). Other biological assays such as the thymidine-labelling index (Stryckmans, Debusscher, Ronge-Collard, Socquet, and Zittoun 1980) and *in vitro* growth on agar (Vincent, Sutherland, Bradley, Lind, and Gunz 1977) cannot be currently applied to large multi-center trials and are still questionable. Nevertheless, the precision attainable in acute leukaemia by carrying out blood and bone marrow examinations, gives a clear-cut definition of complete remission.

In chronic leukaemias, the white blood cell count is related to tumour mass, but its partial or complete normalization during treatment does not generally correspond to a true complete remission. In chronic myelocytic leukaemia (CML) the bone marrow cells are still Ph^1 positive, and in CLL, lymph node and spleen enlargements frequently persist. In CML, other biological parameters have been utilized for monitoring the reduction of tumour mass, such as vitamin B_{12} binding capacity (Hyman and Reiquam 1975), or level of Ph^1 positive cells.

In multiple myeloma, frequent follow-up of M-component data is currently used to determine the time to maximum regression as well as remission duration (Durie *et al.* 1980).

In Hodgkin's Disease and non-Hodgkin's lymphoma (NHL) enlarged lymph nodes can be measured in the same way as in solid tumours. Once the treatment is started, response is generally comparable in the various localizations. Persisting enlarged lymph nodes or spleen are usually considered to be evidence of therapeutic failure, but histological studies remain necessary to assess recurrences.

The treatment protocol

Precise formulation of the treatment protocol is needed, including doses and schedules. Apparently, small variations can modify the results to a large extent. Duration of the induction treatment and the number of courses required to attain remission must be reported, since they can be of prognostic importance for the duration of remission. The time, or number of courses, to complete remission or maximum regression seems to correlate negatively with the duration of response or survival in acute leukaemia (Keating *et al.* 1980), but it correlates positively in multiple meyloma (Durie *et al.* 1980), and shows no correlation in nodular lymphoma (Portlock, Rosenberg, Glatstein, and Kaplan 1976).

A minimum of two cycles is usually necessary to judge the effect of the treatment in highly proliferative diseases, such as acute leukaemia, HD and large-cell-diffuse NHL (DeVita, Serpick, and Carbone 1970). Complete absence of anti-tumoral effect after the first (or the first two) cycle(s) makes the later induction of a complete remission unlikely. On the contrary, slowly proliferative NHL may need many months of treatment before achieving a complete remission (Portlock *et al.* 1976).

Response and relapse

At least three definite events must be adopted as end-points: the occurrence of a response, the time to relapse, and the time to death, with a completely separate analysis of the entire trial for each of these end-points (Peto *et al.* 1977). For example, in acute myeloid leukaemia (AML), age has been proven to be of prognostic value in many studies with respect to remission induction, but not for time to relapse once a complete remission is achieved (Gale and Cline 1977).

Acute myeloid leukaemia will be used as a model to discuss the problem of response and relapse, but the points apply equally as well to other haematological malignancies.

Remission induction therapy for AML must be viewed from three perspectives:

1. *The clinical efficacy of the regimen:* the number of patients who enter remission versus the number of patients who do not. For this analysis, every patient who is treated according to the protocol under study must be counted regardless of whether or not the patient was removed from the study and whatever the reason for removal. Studies which report the results of 'adequate trials of therapy' are misleading, since the clinical efficacy of the regimen is by definition the overall effects of the regimen on all patients and not simply its effects on patients who can survive the complications of either the disease or the treatment. The clinical efficacy is the net effect of points 2 and 3 below.

2. *The anti-leukaemic effects of the regimen:* the ability of the regimen to destroy leukaemic cells. Naturally the induction of a complete remission is proof that the regimen is effective, but significant anti-leukaemic effects may be produced even if the patient does not enter remission because of death due to intercurrent disease, to the side-effects of the regimen, etc. Hence, the anti-leukaemic effects of a regimen may not be correctly evaluated if only the outcome of remission induction therapy is recorded.

3. *The toxicity produced by the regimen:* evaluation of this component is important, since the production of little or no toxicity can indicate that the intensity of a regimen can be increased. Conversely a high death rate, due to side-effects, mandates that the intensity of a regimen be decreased and such a decrease may result in an increase in clinical efficacy.

The section on AML which follows describes a system for classifying remission induction failures (Preisler 1978). This system permits an assessment of the anti-leukaemic effects of an induction regimen, as well as an estimation of the proportion of patients who may be remission induction failures because of excessive toxicity of the regimen or inadequate control of leukaemia-related problems. By providing data as to the cause of treatment failure one can carefully assess its anti-leukaemic efficacy, the ability of the regimen to prevent death due to leukaemia, and the toxicity of the regimen. Clearly if one is comparing two regimens, each of which produces a 50 per cent remission rate, one would need to know the reasons for induction failure in order to compare the regimens properly. If one found that all the remission failures associated with one regimen were due to persistent leukaemia, while all the failures of the second regimen were hypoplastic toxic deaths, then it would be apparent that the regimens were not equivalent and that the intensity of the former regimen should be increased while the intensity of the latter decreased, and the effects of the regimens re-evaluated.

Other problems regarding the interpretation of reports of remission induction protocols relate to the nature of the institutions in which the studies were performed and the comparability of patients. Institutions vary in the number of patients they see and hence in their experience in treating AML. Furthermore, the availability of platelet and granulocyte transfusions, the policies regarding their use, as well as the use of antibiotics, are all factors in determining the outcome of remission induction therapy. These factors determine the ability of physicians, nurses, and house staff to recognize and treat the problems unique to remission induction therapy. When treatment results are reported an effort must be made to describe these aspects of supportive care.

Given the paucity of information provided in the literature it is practically impossible to compare different consolidation/maintenance regimens, except for the overall duration of complete remission associated with administration of the regimen and the drugs administered. A more complete reporting of essential data would correct this problem and a reasonable starting-point would be the collection of data on the depth and duration of pancytopenia produced, how often it was produced, and the overall duration of therapy. At least in this way one could compare the intensity of different therapies using haematologic toxicity as a point of comparison.

Uniform criteria for defining leukaemic relapse do not exist nor are there specific intervals for obtaining bone marrow specimens to monitor remission. Given the fact that early relapse in the marrow may not effect peripheral blood counts for several months, care must be given when reporting and comparing remission durations.

Finally it is often assumed that relapse indicates resistance to prior therapy and that response to subsequent therapy is an indication of a lack of cross-resistance between drugs and regimens. This assumption is frequently incorrect. If the patient has not received the agents used to induce remission within 3 to 4 months of having relapsed, if he received the drugs but not by the same route, at the same dose level, or duration of administration as employed during remission induction therapy, then relapse does not necessarily indicate the presence of drug-resistant disease. The situation is further complicated by the fact that an equivalent dose of a drug like adriamycin produces lower plasma levels in some patients who have been treated previously with the drug (Gessner, Robert, Bolanowska, Hoerni, Durand, Preisler, and Rustum 1981). Unless plasma drug levels during therapy are quantified, even failure to achieve complete remission is not necessarily an indication of leukaemic cell resistance to the drugs in question. A precise definition of resistance is necessary when conducting and interpreting the results of any clinical study.

Other required clinical evaluations

Haematological toxicity

Haematological toxicity is more difficult to assess in acute leukaemia than in solid tumours, since these diseases *per se* produce a bone marrow failure. The nadir of polymorphonuclears and the duration of this aplastic phase (currently 2 to 3 weeks) must be reported. The nadir of the platelet count is more difficult to define, due to the use of prophylactic platelet transfusions.

Once CR is achieved, haematological toxicity can be easily assessed during consolidation and maintenance treatment according to the WHO criteria (WHO 1979). Progressive cytopenia may be due to impending relapse rather than drug toxicity. A few circulating immature cells and/or an increase (>5 per cent) in bone marrow blast cells are sometimes observed during the recovery from the toxicity produced by the therapy. One should remember that in acute leukaemia, relapses are almost always of the same cytological type (Zittoun, Cadiou, and Smadja 1969). When a definite conclusion cannot be reached, a second bone marrow examination should be carried out 1 to 2 weeks after stopping treatment.

Haematological toxicity is more easily recognized in the other non-solid tumours. It is related to the drug dose and toxicity *per se*. Bone marrow involvement may increase the toxicity of chemotherapy. It usually leads to reduced doses, preferentially according to precise and prefixed rules. The overall results, as emphasized above, are superior when the total doses are not very different from the theoretical, or optimal ones, whereas the chance of response and cure decreases when toxicity, or other factors such as age, leads to decreased doses (Frei and Canellos 1980) and/or an increase in the time between courses of therapy.

Long-term toxicity

Non-solid tumours are frequently treated by polychemotherapy, including alkylating agents, in association with radiotherapy. Growth in children and fertility should be evaluated regularly.

The occurrence of a second malignancy should be carefully watched for. A reduction in the frequency of leukaemia and other secondary cancers should be a major goal of future therapeutic trials in Hodgkin's Disease.

Evaluation of quality of life

This evaluation is still neglected in most reported results, as oncologists seem to give their attention only to duration, and not to the 'quality of life' during induction, remission, and even after cure. It is obviously difficult to quantify objectively the 'quality of life'. However one should indicate, along with the duration of disease-free interval and survival, the time spent at the hospital (Brennan and Lewis 1980) and, periodically, the performance status. Methods for evaluation of 'quality of life' with questionnaires and subjective scales (Priestman and Baum 1976) have been recently developed and should be included in new trials, mainly in those with toxic regimens and a poor prognosis. The number of null results can be reduced if the search for a possible improvement in the methods of eliminating disease and extending life is complemented by an attempt to reduce the disruptive and painful effects of disease and treatment and to improve the socio-economic efficiency (Ciampi and Till 1980).

ACUTE LEUKAEMIA STUDIES

Eligibility and stratification

To be eligible for the study, the diagnosis of leukaemia should have been made on the basis of the cytological features and the blood and bone marrow smears. Myeloid and lymphoid types must be carefully separated. The criteria described by the French–American–British proposals for classification of leukaemia are at present widely used (Bennet *et al.* 1976). Prior to the initiation of study treatment and to the randomization (if a randomized study is contemplated), attempts should be made to control any immediate medical problems such as bleeding, infection, and metabolic abnormalities. Patients who die after randomization, even if they do so before the initiation of therapy, should be reported when the overall results of the study are published since they also represent a failure of therapy.

Studies comparing two or more approaches to therapy should be both prospective and randomized with stratifications being carried out to ensure a balance of prognostic factors in the different treatment arms. Age is an important prognostic factor, with increasing age being associated with an increasingly poor prognosis (Gehan, Smith and Freireich 1976). Individuals, 15 years of age or less, should be considered to be eligible for paediatric studies given the important prognostic effect of age; stratification of patients as ≤ 15, 16 to 60, >60 years should be considered. Other potential criteria for prognosis include a history of prior radiation therapy or chemotherapy (Preisler and Lyman 1977), or of having experienced a pre-leukaemic syndrome since both are significant adverse prognostic factors. Consideration should also be given to the important influence of infection at the time of diagnosis on the outcome of therapy (Gehan *et al.* 1976). For studies of ALL, stratification is recommended with regard to white blood cell count. The presence of extramedullary disease, surface marker characteristics (Sallan, Ritz, Pesando, Gelber, O'Brien, Hitchcock, Coral, and Schlossman 1980), cytogenetic abnormalities (Golomb, Vardman, Rowley 1978; Preisler, Reese,

Marinello 1983), and FAB type (L_1, L_2, or L_3) represent significant prognostic factors. In ALL and AML, cytogenetic studies using recently described banding techniques should be performed with a special search for Ph[1] chromosome in ALL or translocations and aneuploidy in AML; these are findings of proven or potential prognostic value (Rowley 1981).

Evaluation of response to therapy

Complete remission should be defined as the disappearance of all manifestations of leukaemia (Hyman and Reiquam 1975). The bone marrow should be normocellular, and should contain a maximum of 5 per cent blast cells (and no leukaemic cells); cells of the granulocytic, erythrocytic, and megakaryocytic series should be morphologically normal and should be present in the normal range except for drug-related abnormalities, with haemoglobin ≥ 10 g/100 ml, neutrophils $\geq 1000/\mu l$ and platelets $\geq 100\,000/\mu l$. The bone marrow and peripheral blood should remain normal for at least 1 month before a complete remission can be said to have been induced (WHO 1979). Leukaemic cell infiltrations of the skin or other sites should not be present. If appropriate, organ biopsy may be necessary to rule out the presence of residual disease. Other potential measures of the 'completeness' of remission are cytogenetic studies and cell surface marker studies for patients whose leukaemic cell lines were marked in this fashion. At the present time, however, while these ancillary studies are not uniformly available, efforts should be made to employ them when remission status is being evaluated.

Partial remission is usually characterized by bone marrow containing 5.1–25 per cent blast cells, or 10.1–30 per cent blast cells plus promyelocytes. In addition, peripheral blood must contain ≥ 9 g/100 ml haemoglobin, $\geq 1000/\mu l$ neutrophils, $\geq 50\,000/\mu l$ platelets and no more than 5 per cent blast cells. (Ohnuma, Rosner, Levy, Cuttner, Moon, Silver, Blom, Falkson, Burningham, Glidewell, and Holland 1971). These conditions must be met after a fixed number of courses of induction treatment (usually one or two) since patients in partial remission after one (or two) induction course(s) can achieve complete remission thereafter.

The outcome of induction treatment should be reported as either complete remission, partial remission or remission induction failure. Remission induction failure should be further defined in terms of the type of failure (Preisler 1978). Table 10.1 provides a system for classifying remission induction failures. Failure type for each course of remission induction therapy should be reported.

Remission duration and criteria of relapse

Defining the duration of complete remission presents many problems. The problem of the starting-point can be eliminated by calculating the disease-free interval and remission duration from registration or randomization.

Table 10.1.

Failure type	Different types of failure of the induction treatment in acute leukaemia
I	'Significant drug resistance': administration of a course of remission induction therapy fails to produce significant marrow hypoplasia in a patient who survives for 7 or more days after the completion of drug administration.
II	'Relative drug resistance': (a) a course of chemotherapy produces severe marrow hypoplasia but leukaemic cells repopulate the marrow within 40 days of completion of the course of therapy; (b) partial remission (see text).
III	Regeneration failure: chemotherapy renders the marrow severely hypoplastic and it remains so for more than 40 days after the end of the course of chemotherapy.
IV	Hypoplastic death: patient expires during a period of severe marrow hypoplasia. If this death occurs more than 40 days after the end of a course of therapy the patient is considered to be a type III failure.
V	Inadequate trial: patient expires less than 7 days after the end of a course of chemotherapy with a cellular bone marrow.
VI	Patient achieves complete haematologic remission but leukaemic cells persist in extramedullary sites (i.e. central nervous system, liver, spleen, etc.).

Relapse should be defined by overt circulating blast cells (≥ 100/ml) or by careful analysis of the bone marrow smears.

A small increase in the proportion of myeloblasts in the bone marrow of a patient with AML in remission is difficult to assess unless Auer rods are present. Because of this, relapse of AML should be defined as an increase in the percentage of myeloblasts to > 10 per cent or the sum of myeloblasts + promyelocytes to > 20 per cent found on two occasions separated by 2 weeks. The presence of other abnormal appearing cells (such as megaloblastoid erythroid abnormalities in patients with FAB type M6, or monocytoid cells in patients with FAB type M4 or M5) in patients receiving chemotherapy is difficult to interpret unless the abnormal erythroid cells are PAS positive or the monocytoid cells are identical in appearance to, and have the same histochemical characteristics of, the leukaemic monocytoid cells present at the time of initial diagnosis. Cytogenetic studies at this time may permit a distinction to be made between leukaemic relapse and drug effect. For the sake of consistency these clearly abnormal cells should also constitute 10 per cent of the marrow cells in order for a diagnosis of relapse to be made. Also for reasons of consistency the presence of Auer rods should be recorded, but should not by themselves be sufficient to remove a patient from study if the above criteria for relapse have not been fulfilled. The same is true when cytogenetic abnormalities are detected in a patient who otherwise would be classified as being in complete remission.

Leukaemic relapse can occur either in the bone marrow or in an extramedullary site. A diagnosis of extramedullary relapse should be based on a tissue diagnosis and not simply on the basis of organomegaly.

Monitoring of patients during complete remission

Peripheral blood counts should be obtained at least once every 2 weeks and bone marrow examinations obtained at least every 8 weeks (at shorter intervals in case of unexpected cytopenia). For patients with ALL, particular attention should be paid to the testes, ovaries, and central nervous system since these are frequent sites of extramedullary relapse. These may become problem areas in AML as greater numbers of patients experience prolonged survival.

Serial cell surface marker studies, using monoclonal antibodies, measurements of the proportions of Tdt (terminal-deoxynucleotidyl-transferase) positive cells, and serial studies of marrow cytogenetics may prove useful in the future for assessing the proportion of residual leukaemic cells present in remission patients and for monitoring fluctuations in the numbers of leukaemic cells during therapy.

Comparison of treatment regimens

The reporting of treatment results for acute leukaemia should include complete remission rate, median duration of remission, and survival curves for all patients and also for just those patients who enter complete remission.

Data should also be provided for patients who were not entered on study but who were seen at the institution during the time the study was carried out, and the reasons for not being entered in the study.

With respect to the remission induction component of the study the time to complete remission (CR), the number of courses to CR, and the failure type for patients who did not enter CR, together with the number of courses, and time to treatment failure should be reported. Non-haematological toxicity should also be reported according to the WHO criteria (WHO 1979). In addition the duration of time spent at the various levels of toxicity should be recorded. If several institutions are involved in a study a breakdown of the data by institution should be provided so that inter-institutional differences can be evaluated.

The therapeutic efficacy of a maintenance regimen is always evaluated in terms of remission duration and survival; however, the reporting of maintenance regimens should also include information about the frequency and doses of drugs administered, when courses were given, the number of days per course, the *level and duration* of therapy-induced pancytopenia, and the total number of courses administered until therapy was discontinued. Data regarding reductions in intensity, frequency, and/or the duration of courses of therapy should also be reported. Needless to say, other toxicities should be reported as well.

Studies of relapsed disease

As defined above, relapsed disease is not synonymous with disease that is resistant to the agents with which the patient has been treated. Resistance to previously administered agents can be assumed to be present only for patients who fail to enter remission after administration of the identical agents, administered at the same dose levels and at the same schedule that previously produced a CR. Functional resistance probably can be assumed to be present if patients relapse within 3 months of receiving an aggressive course of chemotherapy with the agents in question. It should be remembered, however, that therapeutic resistance is not synonymous with leukaemic cell resistance to the drugs employed, since therapeutic resistance can result from the absence of therapeutically-active plasma drug levels due to the matabolism of the drugs by the patient (Gessner *et al.* 1981).

Special considerations in childhood

There are several aspects of paediatric leukaemia which present special problems. Paediatric AML is more frequently responsive to prednisone/vincristine therapy than is AML in adults (Land, Sutow, and Dument 1976), and unlike adult AML appears to involve the central nervous system as frequently as does ALL (Choi and Simone 1976). These facts must be taken into account in the design of protocols and in the comparison of the results of treatment regimens used to treat children and adults with AML.

Given the special situation of children when therapeutic regimens are being evaluated, data should be provided regarding the effects of the regimens on physical growth, psychological development, the development of consequent neoplasms, and other long term effects of therapy.

CHRONIC MYELOCYTIC LEUKAEMIA

Given the distinctively different phases of the disease and of the therapeutic goals for each phase, the following discussion will be divided into a chronic phase and a blastic phase disease.

Chronic phase disease

Diagnostic criteria and prognostic factors

The diagnosis of CML is usually suspected when there is persistent leucocytosis without apparent cause. For a diagnosis of chronic myelocytic leukaemia to be made the presence of the Philadelphia chromosome must be confirmed, and recent cytogenetic studies have demonstrated that chromosomal banding should be part of the initial study since the Ph^1 chromosome may be 'masked' (Marinello, Morita, and Sandberg 1981). In addition, the clinical significance of unusual translocations are presently unknown and should be evaluated. The myeloproliferative syndrome known as Philadelphia negative CML has a different clinical course than Ph[1] positive CML and hence Ph[1] negative patients should be stratified separately if they are studied along with Ph[1] positive patients.

Patients who are thought to be in early blastic crisis or to have Ph[1] positive acute leukaemia should not be included in studies of conventional CML. Patients in these categories include those who present with: (1) marrow blasts greater than 20 per cent; (2) peripheral blood blasts greater than 10 per cent; (3) peripheral blood blasts + promyelocytes greater than 20 per cent; (4) evidence of extramedullary disease such as involvement of the bones, lymph nodes, central nervous system, etc. The biology of this disease and the response to therapy differs from that of chronic phase or blastic CML and hence these patients should be studied separately.

Prior to initiation of study treatment, patients should be evaluated for the stage of the disease. Tura and co-workers have demonstrated that there are substantial differences in time to death for patients who had various combinations of adverse prognostic factors at the time of therapy. These include hepatomegaly, splenomegaly, hyperleucocytosis, thrombocytopenia or thrombocytosis, > 1 per cent peripheral blood blast cells, and > 20 per cent peripheral blood granulated precursors (Tura *et al.* 1981). The grouping of patients into early disease (zero or one adverse factor), intermediate disease (two or three adverse factors) or later disease (four to six adverse factors) led to highly significant differences in the time to death. Therefore, assessment of the stage at diagnosis and at the initiation of therapy will lead to the appropriate stratification of patients, and permit assessment of the comparability of patients participating in various studies.

It has been proposed that the cytogenetic constitution of Ph[1] patients is of prognostic significance and can be used to 'stage' patients. Patients in whom chromosomal abnormalities are found in addition to the Ph[1] chromosome, have a poorer prognosis than patients in whom only the Ph[1] chromosome is detected (Sakurai *et al.* 1976). The significance of persistent normal metaphases has recently been called into question (Sokal 1980), and the fact that many metaphases have to be characterized to include or exclude significant levels of genetic mosaicism (25 identical metaphases must be characterized to exclude the possibility that a second clone is present at a level of 12 per cent), reduces the utility of this approach for most studies (Hook 1977).

Evaluation of therapy

The goals of therapy of the chronic phase of the disease are to control and reduce white cell counts, relieve symptoms, and delay or prevent the onset of blastic transformation. More recently, attempts have also been made to affect a cytogenetic reversion to normal. The criteria for clinical control of the disease are reduction of the white cell counts to normal or near normal levels (WBC $< 15\ 000/\mu l$), maintenance of the counts at these levels, disappearance of (or prevention of the development of) hepatosplenomegaly, and control of constitutional symptoms such as fever, fatigue, and weight loss. Reporting of treatment effects should include these aspects of the illness and attention should be paid to the platelet count since thrombocytosis is often a problem. Patients should be monitored and data recorded at least every 3 to 4 months. Needless to say the side-effects of therapy should be reported. The WHO or the Cancer and Acute Leukaemia Group B toxicity schemas are appropriate but as described earlier, provision should be made for reporting the duration of side-effects as well.

The most critical measurement of the efficacy of any therapeutic approach to the chronic phase of the disease is the delay of the onset of blastic crisis. That is not to suggest that deaths due to other causes (bleeding, thrombosis, etc.) should not be recorded but rather that blastic crisis is undoubtedly the most common cause of death. The criteria for diagnosing blastic crisis or accelerated disease are provided in Table 10.2. Despite reports that the appearance of cytogenetic abnormalities in addition to the Ph[1] chromosome is an indication of impending blastic transformation, the reproducibility of these observations is unknown and hence evaluation of the effects of chronic phase therapy on the course of the illness (even therapy directed at suppressing newly emerging clones) should be based upon measurements of the time to the clinical onset of blastic crisis.

Attempts to produce cytogenetic reversion of Ph[1] patients to normal or to suppress newly emerging clones during the latter stages of the chronic phase of the disease are extremely difficult to evaluate. As noted above, many metaphases have to be characterized if one wants to exclude or recognize levels of mosaicism which are quite substantial.

Table 10.2. *Criteria for accelerated disease and blastic crisis of CML*

A. Accelerated disease
(1) Myeloblasts in bone marrow or peripheral blood ≥ 10 per cent, but < 20 per cent or myeloblasts + promyelocytes ≥ 20 per cent, but < 30 per cent.
(2) Appearance of extramedullary tumours
(3) Doubling time of immature cells (myeloblasts + promyelocytes + myelocytes) in the peripheral blood of ≤ 5 days
B. Blastic crisis
(1) ≥ 20 per cent myeloblasts or ≥ 30 per cent meyloblasts + promyelocytes in peripheral blood or bone marrow

---

These criteria do not include other phenomena suggestive of, or associated with, accelerated/blastic phase disease such as fever unrelated to infection, persistent anaemia not ascribable to chemotherapy, eosinophilia, basophilia, marrow fibrosis, and appearance of new cytogenetic abnormalities; these do not provide definitive evidence of metamorphosis of the chronic phase.

Blastic crisis

The criteria for diagnosing a blastic crisis are listed in Table 10.2. The criteria for accelerated disease are also provided since it represents a stage in the evolution to blastic crisis and can be used as an indication of the end of the chronic phase. The criteria for evaluating response to therapy and toxicity of the regimen under trial are identical to those described for the acute leukaemias. These should be adhered to since a review of the current literature demonstrates that one cannot determine the proportion of blastic crisis patients who fail therapy because of drug resistant failure or who die during a period of marrow hypoplasia. This information is essential for evaluating the effects of therapy on the disease and for comparing the effects of different therapeutic approaches.

The type of blastic crisis (myeloid, lymphoid, or mixed) should be defined when different regimens are being compared since their response rate differs considerably. Needless to say stratification should be made on this basis as well. Changes in subtype of blastic crisis as a result of therapy should also be recorded. While morphological and histochemical criteria can be used to recognize some cases of lymphoid crisis, the most reliable means for recognition are methods capable of recognizing lymphoid surface markers and Tdt (Marks, Baltimore, and McCaffrey 1978). Pre-therapy cytogenetic constitution should also be recorded.

For patients who enter remission, it should be specified whether the remission was characterized by reversion to the chronic phase of the disease or to a state of normal haematopoiesis. Repeat cytogenetic studies are useful in this regards.

Pediatric CML

Pediatric disease represents a special case since the Ph^1 chromosome is not detectable in most pediatric patients with CML. Given the differences from adult disease, these patients should probably be studied and reported separately.

CHRONIC LYMPHOCYTIC LEUKAEMIA

Trials on CLL (or Waldenstrom's macroglobulinaemia, a closely related disease), should be restricted to progressive cases and stratified according to prognosic factors. It is acknowledged that many patients with typical CLL, that is monoclonal B lymphocytosis in blood and bone marrow, have a very long lasting or stable disease. Chemotherapy in such cases does not seem to have any advantage and might produce avoidable side-effects. Moreover, a controlled trial in non- or slowly progressive disease is unrealistic, since the median survival for such cases is approximately 10 years.

Initially, required parameters are the number of lymph node areas involved, size of the largest lymph node in each area, size of splenomegaly and hepatomegaly when present, white blood cell count, and haemoglobin, reticulocyte and platelet counts. Bone marrow smears for cellularity and the percentage of lymphocytes must be checked by referees, but lymph node biopsy is not necessary. A preliminary period of about 3 months without treatment is recommended, in order to assess the natural course of the disease.

Other data can be of prognostic importance: immunoglobulin assay by electrophoresis or radial immunodiffusion method and Coombs' test. Lymphangiography and abdominal CT scan are useless in these cases.

Patients should be stratified according to clinical staging; the one most commonly employed is that described by Rai *et al.* (1975), but CLL with isolated spleen involvement should be separated (Binet, Leporrier, Dighiero, Chavron, D'Athis, Vangier, Merle, Beral, Natali, Raphael, Nizet, and Follezou 1977). The treatment protocol must be precisely defined, particularly in case of long term treatment, since there is a high risk of heterogeneity.

Response to treatment is monitored by monthly blood counts. WBC count normalization can be observed within 1 month, but clinical response is delayed and frequently only partial with persistent blood and bone marrow lymphocytosis. Complete remission is infrequent and must be documented by bone marrow study in patients with complete clinical and blood response. Bone marrow failure, manifested by anaemia and thrombocytopenia, when occuring secondarily, must be attributed to (if possible) the disease or the treatment. Therapeutic trials are difficult to conduct and analyse in advanced stages due to pancytopenia and the advanced age of most patients, thus limiting the use of cytotoxic drugs.

The low proportion of complete responses (Phillips, Kempin, Passe, Miké, and Clarkson 1977) and the usually very slow disease-progression rate make it difficult to evaluate the disease-free interval. Consequently, the most meaningful study parameter is survival of homogenous groups of patients, with long term follow-up, with few patients being lost to follow-up and causes of death recorded, related or not to disease and treatment. Unfortunately few reported studies meet these conditions, and bias in the numerator and denominator is frequent.

MULTIPLE MYELOMA

The conditions for a valid trial in multiple myeloma (MM) are very similar to those in CLL. Age, performance status, and clinical staging according to Durie and Salmon (1975) are the most important initial parameters. The immunological type of the M component, the level of urinary light chains, and assay for normal serum immunoglobulins (usually decreased) are also of importance. Moreover, the immunological type is necessary for the clinical staging. Stage 1 should be clearly differentiated from the benign monoclonal gammopathy by the usual criteria (Kyle 1978), and by the natural course of the disease observed for at least 3 months.

Complete response is unusual: a persistent small spike on electrophoresis and osteolytic skeletal lesions are usually observed in most responders. Partial responders should be characterized according to the level of serum M component as this is the main criterion for response or progression, except in cases developing renal failure. The biological response is generally preceeded by pain relief and accompanied by improvement of performance status and a rise in haemoglobin. Disappearance of osteolytic lesions is very slow and frequently absent, even in responding patients; consequently, the size of these lesions on X-ray should not be considered as a criterion of response. However, these lesions should be monitored carefully. Frank progression of some of these lesions should be considered as progression of the disease, even in patients with decreased or stable M component; such discordant progression in fact rarely occurs, and the M component is still the major criterion for evolution and definition of the disease-free interval. The best criterion seems to be the duration from the nadir of the gamma M component, to its overt progression, that is an increase by 50 per cent. Pain, performance status, and survival are also major criteria of response to treatment.

The treatment protocol must be described very precisely, as well as dose modifications according to the blood count. The degree of response should be correlated with daily and total doses per cycle and per unit of time, since, in advanced stages, intensive chemotherapy is usually more efficient but also more difficult to manage in light of the usual accompanying cytopenia.

MALIGNANT LYMPHOMAS

Theoretically the same rules which have been devised for reporting results in solid tumours apply to malignant lymphomas. However, some specific criteria have been added and must be kept in mind.

Clinical staging is determined according to the Ann Arbor staging system (Carbone and Kaplan 1971) after careful clinical examination, chest X-ray and tomography, and iliac and lumbar lymphangiography. Criteria for stage B, which include fever (more than 38°C, more than 7 days), sweats (abundant and nocturnal), and weight loss in the 6 months preceding admission, have been clearly described. Generalized pruritus and asthenia should also be recorded.

Echograms and CT scans are now widely used in many centres. The CT scan provides important information on coeliac and mesenteric areas. Mesenteric areas are frequently involved in non-Hodgkin's lymphoma, for which CT scan is frequently more useful than lymphangiography. However CT scan cannot replace lymphangiography in Hodgkin's Disease to investigate nodal structural abnormalities.

Conclusive clinical staging is sometimes the result of personal experience when faced with ambiguities: small perceptible lymph nodes in superficial areas other than the one certainly involved may or not be lymphomatous, chest X-ray can be difficult to judge when there are no anterior X-rays, and up to 20 per cent of the lymphangiographies are borderline and subject to debate. One can try to get help from adenograms of the superficial lymph nodes and from a CT scan of the internal areas.

The search for visceral involvement is frequently restricted to bone marrow biopsy. Liver biopsy, percutaneous or via laparoscopy, is sometimes recommended, mainly in non-Hogdkin's lymphoma and if the bone marrow biopsy is negative. Results of the bone marrow biopsy depend on the size of the sample. It has been shown that medullary and other visceral involvement are more frequent in stage B Hodgkin's Disease and in follicular types of non-Hodgkin's lymphoma.

Laparotomy with splenectomy results in a more precise pathological staging. It has been widely used in Hodgkin's Disease during the last decade (Kadin, Glattein, and Dorfman 1971). However, as a part of the treatment strategy, laparotomy does not appear to be useful any longer when extended field radiotherapy, with systematic infra-diaphragmatic irradiation and/or aggressive chemotherapy is used. In non-Hodgkin's lymphoma, staging laparotomy has been mainly used in the clinical stages I and II for the search of occult abdominal disease. This can be replaced by CT scan, and liver biopsy, percutaneous or via laparoscopy. One should be careful when analysing reported results, and avoid comparing trials in which patients were stratified according to pathological staging after laparotomy with patients classified by clinical staging. Special investigations should be described precisely, especially if they interfere with the therapeutic protocol.

Histological typing is also a major task in these trials. There is a general agreement for classification in Hodgkin's Disease (Lukes, Cramer and Hall 1966). However, discrepancies are often observed between pathologists, and slides should be reviewed by a referee pathology panel, with this review made prior to the randomization whenever the histological type influences the therapeutic modalities.

Histological typing of non-Hodgkin's lymphoma has been subject to heated debate between several classification systems in recent years, for example between Kiel's classification (Lennert, Mohri, Stein, and Kaiserling 1975) and the classical histological typing according to Rappaport (1966). More recently a 'working formulation' has been proposed which combines various subtypes into three different grades of malignancy (The Non-Hodgkin's Lymphoma Pathologic Classification Project 1982). These authors suggested using both one of the known classifications along with their working formula for all patients.

Criteria for evaluation of response to treatment of malignant lymphomas are close to the ones proposed by the WHO for solid tumours. Complete remission is defined as disappearance of all disease-related symptoms, and of all measurable disease, along with normalization of chest X-ray and lymphangiogram. Partial remission is a decrease of at least 50 per cent in the product of the two largest perpendicular diameters in *all* measurable lesions. 'No change' is defined when a patient does not qualify for remission or progression. Progression is defined when there is involvement of new sites, *or* recurrence in originally involved sites, *or* increase by at least 25 per cent in the original tumour masses. Early deaths, occurring before the appropriate time of remission status evaluation, should be reported and classified whether due to malignant disease, toxicity, or other causes. Toxicities must be recorded according to the WHO recommendations.

A complete remission is observed in most patients treated for Hodgkin's Disease. The rapidity of response and number of cycles necessary to achieve a complete response are probably of prognostic significance and should be reported.

Total doses of drugs used for polychemotherapy, as compared with the scheduled doses, should be clearly described, and correlated with the response. The major criterion in trials for Hodgkin's Disease is the disease-free interval, but survival duration should also be recorded. Since on relapse many patients will respond to further therapy and such responses may be prolonged, it is important to report the completeness of second and third responses to therapy. Patients who do not experience a complete remission after treatment for relapsed disease will not be cured and, though they may continue to survive, should be clearly distinguished from patients who re-enter documented complete remission. Recurrences should be confirmed by adenogram or biopsy. Long term toxicity, and the occurrence of subsequent malignancies should be carefully reported (Arsenau, Canellos, Johnson, and DeVita 1977).

Response in slowly progressive non-Hodgkin's lymphoma (nodular or diffuse well differentiated) is frequently slow, and the complete response rate is higher after prolonged treatment (Portlock *et al.* 1976); thus data should be presented, indicating the actual percentage of complete remission according to duration of treatment. Survival is long and thus many trials lack maturation of data. Trials in lymphoblastic or immunoblastic lymphomas are easier to evaluate: the response is rapid and complete response can be differentiated from partial response or failure. Duration of disease-free interval is a readily available and useful endpoint since relapses, when observed, occur early, and have rapidly developing resistance to therapy.

CONCLUSION

Recommendations have been developed recently which aim at a standardiz-ation in reporting results of cancer treatment (Miller, Hoogstraten, Staquet, and Winkler 1981). These proposed methods and rules apply chiefly to solid tumours. Haematological malignancies raise some specific problems: leuka-emia and multiple myeloma could be considered as non-measurable but evaluable tumours. However blood cell counts along with clinical symptoms and bone marrow studies in leukaemia allow a clinical staging and a precise evaluation of the course of the disease and response to treatment.

Pathological bone marrow involvement makes a clear evaluation of haematological toxicity difficult in many circumstances. Finally, it is hoped that specific recommendations for reporting treatment results of haematological tumours can be made, based on criteria already widely accepted and used.

REFERENCES

Arsenau, J. C., Canellos, G. P., Johnson, R., and DeVita, V. T. Jr. (1977). Risk of new cancer in patients with Hodgkin's Disease. *Cancer* **40**, 1912–16.

Bennett, J. M., Catovsky, D., Daniel, M. T., Flandrin, G., Galton, D. A. G., Gralnick, H. R., and Sultan, C. (1976). Proposals for the classification of the Acute Leukemias. French–American–British (FAB) Co-operative Group. *Br. J. Haemat.* **33**, 451 – 8.

Binet, J. L., Leporrier, M., Dighiero, G. (1977). A clinical system for chronic lymphocytic leukemia. *Cancer* **40**, 855–964.

Brennan, D. C., and Lewis, J. P. (1980). Remission induction regimens in acute non-lymphocytic leukemia. *W. J. Med.* **133**, 279–88.

Carbone, P. P., and Kaplan, H. S. (1971). Report of the committee on Hodgkin's disease staging classification. *Cancer Res.* **31**, 1860–1.

Choi, S. I., and Simone, J. V. (1976). Acute nonlymphocytic leukemia in 171 children. *Med. Ped. Oncol.* **2**, 119–46.

Ciampi, A., and Till, J. E. (1980) Null results in clinical trials: the need for a decision theory approach. *Br. J. Cancer* **41**, 618–29.

DeVita, V. T., Jr., Serpick, A. A., and Carbone, P. P. (1970). Combination chemotherapy in the treatment of advanced Hodgkin's disease. *Ann. intern. Med.* **73**, 881–95.

Durie, B. G. M., and Salmon, S. E. (1975). A clinical staging system for multiple myeloma. Correlation of measured myeloma cell mass with presenting clinical features. Response to treatment and survival. *Cancer* **36**, 842–54.

Durie, B. G. M., Salmon, S. E., and Moon, T. E. (1980). Pretreatment tumor mass, cell kenetics, and prognosis in multiple meyloma. *Blood* **55**, 364–72.

Frei III, E., and Canellos, G. P. (1980). Dose: a critical factor in cancer chemotherapy. *Am. J. Med.* **69**, 585–94.

Gale, R. P., and Cline, M. J. (1977). High remission—induction rate in acute myeloid leukaemia. *Lancet* **i**, 497–9.

Gehan, E. A., Smith, T. L., and Freireich, E. J. (1976). Prognostic factors in acute leukemia. *Sem. Oncol.* **3**, 271–82, 1976.

George, S. L. (1978). Design and evaluation of leukaemia trials. *Clinics in Haemat.* **7**, 227–43.

Gessner, T., Robert, J., Bolanowska, W., Hoerni, B., Durand, M., Preisler, H., and Rustum, J. (1981). Effects of prior therapy on plasma levels of adriamycin during subsequent therapy. *J. Med.* **12**, 183–93.

Golomb, H. M., Vardiman, J. W., Rowley, J. D., Testa, J. R., and Mintz, U. (1978). Correlation of clinical findings with quinacrine-banded chromosomes in 90 adults with acute non-lymphocytic leukemia. *New Engl. J. Med.* **299**, 613–19.

Hook, E. (1977). Exclusion of chromosomal mosaicism: tables of 90 per cent 95 per cent and 99 per cent confidence limits and comments on use. *Am. J. Genet.* **29**, 94–7.

Hyman, M. P., and Reiquam, C. W. (1975). Monitoring the course of chronic granulocytic leukemia with vitamin B12 binding proteins. *Am. J. clin. Path.* **63**, 796–803.

Janossy, G., Bollum, F. J., Bradstock, K. F., McMichael, Rapson, and Greaves. (1979). Terminal transferase—positive human bone marrow cells exhibit the antigenic phenotype of common acute lymphoblastic leukemia. *J. Immun.* **123**, 1525–9.

Kadin, M. E., Glatstein, E., and Dorfman, R. F. (1971). Clinico-pathological studies of 117 untreated patients subjected to laparotomy for the staging of Hodgkin's disease. *Cancer* **27**, 1277–94.

Keating, M. J., Smith, T. L., Gehan, E. A., McRedie, K. B., Bodey, G. P., Spitzer, G., Hersh, E., Gutterman, J., and Freireich, E. J. (1980). Factors related to length of complete remission in adult acute leukemia. *Cancer* **45**, 2017–29.

Kyle, R. A. (1978). Monoclonal gammopathy of undetermined significance: natural history in 241 cases. *Am. J. Med.* **64**, 814–26.

Land, V. J., Sutow, W. W., and Dument, P. G. (1976). Remission induction with L-asparaginase, vincristine, and prednisone in children with acute nonlymphoblastic Leukemia. *Med. Ped. Oncol.* **2**, 191–8.

Lennert, K., Mohri, N., Stein, H., and Kaiserling, E. (1975). The histopathology of malignant lymphoma. *Br. J. Cancer* (Suppl. II) **31**, 1–28.

Lukes, R. J., Cramer, L. F., and Hall, T. C. (1966). Report of the nomenclature committee on Hodgkin's disease. *Cancer Res.* **26**, 1311.

Marinello, J. J., Morita, M., and Sandberg, A. A. (1981). 'Masked' Philadelphia chromosome (Ph^1) due to an unusual translocation. *Cancer Genet. Cytogenet.* **3**, 227–32.

Marks, S. M., Baltimore, D., and McCaffrey, R. (1978). Terminal transferase as a predictor of initial responsiveness to vincristine and prednisone in blastic chronic myelogenous leukemia. *New. Eng. J. Med.* **298**, 812–14.

Miller, A. B., Hoogstraten, B., Staquet, M., and Winkler, A. (1981). Reporting results of cancer treatment. *Cancer* **47**, 207–14.

Non Hodgkin's Lymphoma Pathologic Classification Project (1982). National Cancer Institute sponsored study of classification of non Hodgkin's lymphomas. Summary and description of a working formulation for clinical usage. *Cancer* **49**, 2112–35.

Ohnuma, T., Rosner, F., Levy, R. N., Cuttner, J., Moon, J. H., Silver, R. T., Blom, J., Falkson, G., Burningham, R., Glidewell, O., and Holland, J. F. (1971). Treatment of adult leukemia with L-asparaginase. *Cancer Chemother. Rep.* **55**, 269–75.

Peto, R., Pike, M. C., Armitage, P., Breslow, N. E., Cox, D. R., Howard, S. V., Mantel, N., McPherson, K., Peto, J., and Smith, P. G. (1977). Design and analysis of randomized clinical trials requiring prolonged observation of each patient. II. analysis and examples. *Br. J. Cancer* **35**, 1–39.

Phillips, E. A., Kempin, S., Passe, S., Miké, V. and Clarkson, B., (1977). Prognostic factors in chronic lymphocytic leukemia and their implication for therapy. *Clinics in Haemat.* **6**, 203–22.

Portlock, C. S., Rosenberg, S. A., Glatstein, E. (1976). Treatment of advanced non-Hodgkin's lymphomas with favorable histologies: preliminary results of a prospective trial. *Blood* **47**, 747–56.

Preisler, H. D. (1978). Failure of remission induction in acute myelocytic leukemia. *Med. Ped. Oncol.* **4**, 275–6.

Preisler, H. D., and Lyman, G. H. (1977). Acute myelogenous leukemia subsequent to therapy for a different neoplasm: clinical features and response to therapy. *Am. J. Hemat.* **3**, 209–18.

Preisler, H. D., Reese, P. A., Marinello, M. J., and Pothier, L. (1983). Adverse effects of aneuploidy on the outcome of remission induction therapy for acute non lymphocytic leukemia: analysis of types of treatment failure. *Br. J. Haemat.* **53**, 459–66.

Priestman, T. J., and Baum, M. (1976). Evaluation of quality of life in patients receiving treatment for advanced breast cancer. *Lancet* **i**, 899–901.

Rai, K. R., Sawitsky, A., Cronkite, E. P., Chanana, A. D., Levy, R. N., and Pasternack, B. S. (1975). Clinical staging of chronic lymphocytic leukemia. *Blood* **46**, 219–34.

Rappaport, H. (1966). Tumors of the haematopoietic system. In *Atlas of tumour pathology*, section 3, Fasc. 8. Armed Forces Institute of Pathology, Washington.

Rowley, J. D. (1981). Do all leukemic cells have an abnormal karyotype? *New. Eng. J. Med.* **305**, 164–6.

Sakurai, M., Hayata, I., and Sandberg, A. A. (1976). Prognostic value of chromosomal findings in Ph[1] positive chronic myelocytic leukemia. *Cancer Res.* **36**, 313–18.

Sallan, S. E., Ritz, J., Pesando, J., Gelber, R., O'Brien, C., Hitchcocks, S., Coval, F., and Schlossman, S. F. (1980). Cell surface antigens: prognostic implications in childhood acute lymphoblastic leukemia. *Blood* **55**, 395–402.

Salmon, S. E., and Durie, B. G. M. (1975). Cellular kinetics in multiple myeloma. *Archs. Intern. Med.* **135**, 131–8.

Sokal, J. E. (1980). Significance of Ph[1] negative marrow cells in Ph[1] positive chronic granulocytic leukemia. *Blood* **56**, 1972–6.

Stryckmans, P., Debusscher, L., Ronge-Collard, E., Socquet, M., and Zittoun, R. (1980). The labelling index of marrow myeloblasts: predictive test of relapse of acute non-lymphoblastic leukemia. *Leuk. Res.* **4**, 79–87.

Sweet, D. L. and Golomb, H. M. (1980). The treatment of histiocytic lymphoma. *Sem. Oncol.* **7**, 302–9.

Tura, S., Baccarani, M., Corbelli, G., and the Italian Cooperative Study Group on Chronic Myeloid Leukemia. (1981). Staging of chronic myeloid leukemia. *Br. J. Haemat.* **47**, 105–21.

Vincent, P., Sutherland, R., Bradley, M., Lind, D., and Gunz, F. W. (1977). Marrow culture studies in adult acute leukemia at presentation and during remission. *Blood* **49**, 903–12.

WHO (1979). *WHO handbook for reporting results of cancer treatment*, WHO offset publication no. 48. WHO, Geneva.

Wiernik, P. H., and Serpick, A. A. (1970). Factors affecting remission and survival in adult acute nonlymphocytic leukemia. *Medicine* **49**, 505–13.

Zittoun, R., Cadiou, M., and Smadja, R. (1969). Evolution et signification pronostique des caractères cytochimiques des leucémies aigues. *Path. Biol.* **17**, 623–8.

11 Reporting treatment toxicities

Daniel L. Kisner

INTRODUCTION

The clinical evaluation of any anti-neoplastic therapy is a long complex process that begins with its initial testing in humans and continues until its acceptance or rejection as a standard therapy in a given setting of a disease. Even when a treatment becomes routinely used, it is usually continually tested in studies comparing it with newly developed treatment programmes. The key to the evaluation of any new treatment is the concept of therapeutic index, or the comparison of the benefits that the patient realizes from a given therapy with the cost of that therapy to the patient in the form of treatment-related toxicity. While therapeutic index is admittedly a concept requiring judgement decisions on the part of investigators and the scientific community, there are some basic considerations worth discussing briefly. While no clinician relishes using a therapy with a high probability of serious or potentially lethal toxicity, this therapy may, none the less, be a rational course if it provides some significant possibility of cure for a group of patients who have an otherwise uniformly fatal outcome. In general, one is willing to accept a relatively lower therapeutic index for treatment in patients with advanced malignancy who have a significant chance of meaningful palliation or prolongation of survival from that therapy. Such a therapy, however, would be considered inappropriate for use in the surgical adjuvant setting in a patient population with a high probability of surgical cure. Thus the usefulness of any treatment in a given disease depends not only on the activity of the treatment in that disease and the toxicities incurred, but also on the stage and prognosis of the specific patient population in question. If one is to make rational decisions about the value of a given therapy from the report of a clinical trial, the report must carefully detail the nature and severity of all toxicities incurred by the patients as well as discuss the patient characteristics, the precise details of the therapy, and the therapeutic responses.

An example of the need for detailed analysis of toxicity data and the clear presentation of such data in the report is the Gastrointestinal Tumor Study Group trial 8274 on locally unresectable gastric carcinoma (Schein, Stablein, Bruckner, Mayer, Ramming, Bateman, and Livston 1982). In that trial, patients with locally unresectable or locally residual gastric carcinoma were randomly allocated to chemotherapy consisting of methyl-CCNU plus 5-FU versus combined modality therapy consisting of radiotherapy (split course

5000 rads to the epigastric area) with 5-FU administered on the first 3 days of each radiotherapy course, plus maintenance chemotherapy consisting of methyl-CCNU plus 5-FU. The trial was initiated in 1974 and closed in 1976 due to a statistically superior median survival for patients randomly allocated to the chemotherapy-alone treatment arm. With further follow-up, survival curves have subsequently crossed with 15 to 20 per cent of patients receiving combined modality therapy achieving long-term disease-free survival, while patients receiving chemotherapy alone have demonstrated a continued probability for relapse and death. Thus, while median survival clearly favours chemotherapy alone, there appears to be long-term benefit for patients treated with the combined modality approach. Careful analysis of these survival curves revealed that the inferior median survival for the combined treatment arm was due to a higher probability of early death within the first 12 weeks. Examination of the case records of the patients in question revealed that the radiochemotherapy treatment was associated with serious haematological and nutritional morbidity. The investigators in the study conclude that, despite a shorter median survival, combined modality treatment for locally unresectable gastric cancer should be the current treatment of choice, as closer haematological monitoring and administration of nutritional support is quite likely to reduce the rate of early deaths associated with combined radio-therapy and chemotherapy in this setting. Thus, careful observation, analysis and reporting of treatment toxicities in this trial have permitted meaningful interpretation of the overall data and the drawing of an important conclusion which might have otherwise been lost in seemingly conflicting results.

It should be clear that the collection, organization and analysis of toxicity data is an integral part of evaluating any new therapy. The purpose of this chapter is to discuss some of the clinical and statistical issues pertinent to the collection and reporting of toxicity data. This will begin with a general discussion of issues pertinent to all forms of toxicity and will be followed by comments specific to acute and chronic toxicity.

GENERAL CONSIDERATIONS

The assessment of treatment toxicities itself is one of the most challenging aspects in clinical research. In assessing toxicity we are generally concerned with the following types of information: (1) which toxicities occur and in what percentage of patients; (2) the severity of the toxicity; and (3) when the toxicity occurs in terms of its time of onset and duration relative to therapy.

The key to the identification of a toxicity in any given patient or group of patients is a set of operational definitions for the toxicity itself. One must decide in advance what measurements or observations will be made that will enable us to identify the presence or absence of a given toxicity. For example, the assessment of hepatic toxicity may involve measurements of serum bilirubin, serum transaminases, and alkaline phosphatase. Elevations of these three parameters beyond some normal limit defines hepatic toxicity. A less clear example might be pulmonary toxicity. This is commonly reported as progressive degrees of dyspnea. An alternative approach might include measurements of plasma partial pressures of oxygen or pulmonary diffusion capacity for carbon monoxide. This example raises a relatively complex question, that is to what extent can we or should we rely on subjective information in assessing and reporting treatment toxicities. While it is clear that dyspnea may occur in a large number of pulmonary lesions, it may also be absent in a setting of quite significant abnormalities on the chest roentgenogram and with substantially altered arterial blood gases. The most objective methods of demonstrated organ dysfunction may involve invasive procedures, patient inconvenience, and additional expense. As such, they may be medically or economically inappropriate. However, within the limits of good judgement on these issues, the most objective parameters possible should be used. In any case, it is critical that the specific parameters that will be used to define a given toxicity be clearly outlined in a treatment protocol at the beginning of the trial including details of the planned observation intervals (Staquet, Sylvester, and Jasmin 1980).

Another important issue pertinent to the recognition of treatment toxicities is the problem of distinguishing toxic effects from medical complications of the cancer itself. How does one distinguish the anorexia, weight loss, and malabsorption associated with adenocarcinoma of the pancreas from the similar problems a patient might encounter undergoing combined modality therapy including irradiation of the epigastric region (Schein *et al.* 1982)? The answer in this case is not a simple one and probably relates to the progressiveness and/or reversibility of the problem. While there are many similar examples which could be discussed, it should be clear that resolution of such issues depends heavily upon the judgment of the clinicians involved as well as the investigators performing the analysis of toxicity data. No simple solutions to this problem exist, and none will be offered here.

Perhaps more difficult to estimate is the potential 'placebo effect' on toxicity in the setting of anti-neoplastic therapy. To be sure 'toxicities' ranging from emesis to alopecia to second malignancy have been seen in the 'placebo' treatment group in randomized trials (Fisher, Carbone, Economou, Frelick, Glass, Lerner, Redmond, Zelen, Band, Katrych, Wolmark, and Fisher 1975). The extent to which these are truly disease related is unclear. The increased public awareness of the toxicities of anti-neoplastic therapy may be actually producing an anticipatory conditioned response in some patients much akin to that seen in the chemotherapy patient who vomits on entering the clinic before receiving his/her treatment. Thus the 'placebo' component to treatment toxicities is an unknown but probably not an insignificant contributor.

Assessment of the severity of a given toxicity may seem a relatively simple issue but depends in some part upon how that toxicity will be represented in the scientific report of the clinical trial. In most instances, toxicity data in reports of clinical trials refer to cumulative data on the worst level of any given toxicity for each patient. For example, leukopenia is frequently reported in terms of median white blood cell (WBC) count nadirs with ranges. Herson (1980) points out that the WBC 'nadir' for any given patient will tend to be lower the more frequently the WBC count is measured during the period after the administration of therapy. For example, if the true nadir for the WBC count occurs on day 10 with a given chemotherapy agent, the reported 'nadir' for a patient will be lower if the WBC count is measured on days 5, 10, 15, and 20 than if it is measured on days 7, 14, and 21. Thus, in general terms if a toxicity is to be reported in terms of its worst severity manifested, increasing the frequency of observations will tend to assure detection and subsequent reporting of worse degrees of toxicity. In any case, this potential effect of the frequency of observations on the severity of toxicity observed makes it imperative that the intervals for measuring the parameters which will identify and grade toxicities be clearly defined in the treatment protocol and adhered to.

Another problem pertinent to the assessment of the severity of toxicity relates to the overall duration of therapy. If one assumes that a patient has an unspecified risk of manifesting a toxicity with a given dose of a given therapy then it is possible that a patient's overall probability of demonstrating that toxicity during his or her course may depend upon the total number of doses given, even if one excludes the possibility of cumulative toxic effect. In designing clinical trials, it should be kept in mind that comparisons of toxicity between two therapies may be affected if the protocol calls for unequal durations of therapy or total number of doses.

The time of onset and the duration of a toxicity are also critical to the assessment of its importance. As treatment programmes have become more complicated by the combining of two or more modalities, linking a toxicity to a given specific therapy requires precision regarding the time at which the toxic effect begins. In phase I chemotherapy trials, for example, time to onset of leukopenia, time to nadir, and time to recovery are important parameters that will play a role in the development of optimum scheduling for the agent and how it is to be used in combination chemotherapy or combined modality treatment programmes. As Vietti (1980) has pointed out, there are some instances in which the duration of a given toxicity may be of equal or greater importance than the absolute magnitude of that toxicity. A WBC nadir of less than 500 cells per microlitre may be of no clinical importance if its duration is less than 1 week, but may produce profound infectious complications should the duration be significantly longer. This may represent a potential weakness in toxicity grading systems that have the magnitude of toxicity as their principal end-points. It should also be clear that the issue of the frequency of observation outlined above regarding nadirs applies equally to the precision of determining day of onset and recovery for a therapy. The higher the frequency of observations, the more precisely those dates will be determined. If observations are made at 7-day intervals, the toxicity seen at day 14 and found to have resolved on day 28 may have a true duration of from 8 to 20 days. With this frequency of observation, the accurate determination of duration for relatively short-lived toxicities is impossible. Thus in the development of a treatment protocol, there must be thoughtful planning of the observation intervals taking into consideration the precision required.

THE ANALYSIS OF DRUG TOXICITY DATA

Simply reporting the severity and duration of toxicities observed in a clinical trial should be considered inadequate use of potentially valuable data. As outlined above, toxicity data play an important role in assessing the therapeutic index for a treatment and frequently teach us valuable lessons about the biology of the disease treated. In a thoughtful discussion of these issues, Herson (1980) has pointed out that in analysing toxicity data one should be seeking to learn whether the induction of toxic effects was required to produce a favourable anti-neoplastic response, and whether the combining of two or more treatments may tend to enhance or reduce toxicity (for example radiation plus chemotherapy in the GITSG locally unresectable gastric carcinoma trial; Schein *et al.* 1982, cited above). The first question is a matter of some considerable debate and concern not only to investigators but to the lay public. Since the question of the need of toxicity in cancer treatment is really at the core of the issue of therapeutic index, it seems an appropriate part of the analysis of any clinical trial. The second question is also of considerable interest in light of the progressive trend towards combination chemotherapy and combined modality treatments. Therapies with differing mechanisms of action may well have toxicities that are not synergistic or even additive, and as such may demonstrate a substantially improved therapeutic index when given in combination. This question is also, therefore, a critical part of data analysis for trials with combined therapies.

A special part of the analysis of toxicity data requires sequential examination of observations made in each patient to determine whether a toxicity recurs with repetitive dosing and whether or not it is cumulative in nature. The conclusion of cumulative toxicity requires the demonstration of progressive worsening of toxicity with repeated dosing. It should be apparent that patients receiving dose escalations in a trial are appropriately excluded from this type of analysis.

Two additional general points should be made regarding the appropriate analysis of toxicity data. One must be continually aware of factors that introduce bias in such analyses. One example of such a factor briefly discussed above is the increased risk of a patient manifesting a toxicity with repeated dosing or longer durations of therapy. This factor might become important, for example, in comparing the toxicities of two chemotherapy regimens compared in a randomized phase III trial. Should one regimen produce a significantly higher response rate than the other, it is highly likely that the median number of courses of therapy will be greater for the more active regimen, giving patients in that regimen a higher probability of experiencing toxic effects. If not properly analysed, the toxicity reporting of such a study might inappropriately emphasize the toxic effects of the more therapeutically active regimen. Comparisons of toxicities for the two regimens should involve comparisons of patient groups with equal numbers of doses or courses of treatment.

A second potential for bias in data analysis in general refers to the question of which patients are to be included in the analysis. It should be kept in mind that a patient may be fully evaluable for toxicity analysis while being inevaluable for response or even survival analysis. In general, any patient receiving therapy should be included in a toxicity analysis. The obvious problem with that approach is the question of what to do about patients lost to follow-up after initial treatment but before any post-treatment observations for toxicity assessment. This is a difficult problem since a patient may remove himself from treatment and follow-up because of the toxicities from the first course of therapy that he found to be unacceptable. Apparent changes in toxicity data over time may be due to the difference in the number of patients included from course to course. It should be clear that unaggressive pursuit of such patients may introduce a bias in the analysis of toxicity data. It is true that even with aggressive follow-up some patients are truly lost (for purposes of collecting toxicity information). The number of patients that fall in this category should be clearly delineated and discussed when reporting toxicity results. Certainly a drug that produces a very high rate of 'lost to follow-up' after the first dose should be regarded with suspicion in terms of its toxicity.

A similar point should be made regarding the issue of dosage modifications necessitated by toxicities. If a treatment can be administered in adequate antineoplastic doses to only a small fraction of patients because of concomitant toxicity, its therapeutic index is poor. Dose reductions or postponements may reduce the severity of reported toxicities, but may well render the therapy ineffective. Patients in whom toxicity-related dose modifications have been made should be analysed separately regarding therapeutic response. Likewise the toxicity of a treatment regimen must be analysed in such a way as to relate toxic effects with dose and interval of treatment.

An additional issue in examining toxicity data is the determination of what types of patients experience a given toxicity. Put another way, the risk factors for development of specific toxicities should be identified. In large randomized trials with a heterogeneous patient population, this may be a complex process requiring considerable statistical capabilities. Linear logistic regression may be used for example to determine which patient factors are related to the appearance of a given toxicity (Kisner and Sylvester 1980). None the less, it is critical to the selection of patients for subsequent treatment with the therapy in question and to therapeutic efforts aimed at preventing or ameliorating the toxicity in future studies.

Lastly, it should be pointed out that comparisons of toxicities between two therapies must be carried out between patient populations which are similar with regards to known prognostic factors for response and survival for the disease in question. In large randomized trials, this may be accomplished prospectively by stratifying the randomization in order to balance the distribution of the major known prognostic factors between treatment groups. This process is key to the analysis of toxicity data if prognostic factors for the development of specific toxicities are to be discovered.

Having concluded a brief review of the general issues involved in assessment and analysis of treatment toxicity, the issues specifically pertinent to acute and chronic toxicities will now be discussed.

ACUTE TREATMENT TOXICITIES

Since the majority of toxic manifestations caused by anti-neoplastic therapies are acute or subacute in nature, there tends to be a large volume of data collected at multiple time points. For data management purposes, the co-operative groups have found it convenient to create scalar grading systems allowing investigators to simply indicate a grade [0 to 4] for a given toxicity on the forms submitted to the central data centre (Vietti 1980). Standardizing such a scale of grading system within a co-operative group permits simple comparison of toxicities between treatment programmes and facilitates computerized storage and analysis of toxicity data. Additionally, the use of a standardized grading system for toxicity facilitates treatment modifications within a therapeutic trial (WHO 1979). In a discussion of the grading system in use in the clinical co-operative groups in the United States, Vietti (1980) compared the specifics of systems from three co-operative groups. While the three systems were similar in content and design, there were variations in the definitions of grades for several important toxicities. Thus in examining reports of different co-operative groups, one is unable to assume equivalent toxicity when both groups report grade 2 azotemia for example. This is a serious limitation in the current use of toxicity grading systems. It would seem that if grading systems were worth using, they should be worth standardizing between clinical groups in an attempt to make data generated by those groups comparable. With that goal partially in mind, the World Health Organization convened two meetings in 1978 and 1979 in an attempt to standardize the reporting of cancer treatment results in general. A significant part of that effort was directed at standardizing toxicity reporting. Representatives from 13 eastern and western nations participated in this effort. The recommended grading system for acute and subacute toxicities resulting from those two meetings is displayed in Table 11.1.

In reviewing the WHO criteria, there are two points worth making. Firstly,

Table 11.1. *Recommendations for grading of acute and subacute toxic effects*

	Grade 0	Grade 1	Grade 2	Grade 3	Grade 4
Haematological (adults)					
Haemoglobin	≥ 11.0 g/100 ml	9.5–10.9 g/100 ml	8.0–9.4 g/100 ml	6.5–7.9 g/100 ml	<6.5 g/100 ml
	≥ 110 g/l	95–109 g/l	80–94 g/l	65–79 g/l	<65 g/l
	≥ 6.8 mmol/l	5.6–6.7 mmol/l	4.95–5.8 mmol/l	4.0–4.9 mmol/l	<4.0 mmol/l
Leucocytes (1000/mm³)	≥ 4.0	3.0–3.9	2.0–2.9	1.0–1.9	<1.0
Granulocytes (1000/mm³)	≥ 2.0	1.5–1.9	1.0–1.4	0.5–0.9	<0.5
Platelets (1000/mm³)	≥ 100	75–99	50–74	25–49	<25
Haemorrhage	None	Petechiae	Mild blood loss	Gross blood loss	Debilitating blood loss
Gastrointestinal					
Bilirubin	$\leq 1.25 \times N^*$	1.26–$2.5 \times N^*$	2.6–$5 \times N^*$	5.1–$10 \times N^*$	$>10 \times N^*$
Transaminases (SGOT/SGPT)	$\leq 1.25 \times N^*$	1.26–$2.5 \times N^*$	2.6–$5 \times N^*$	5.1–$10 \times N^*$	$>10 \times N^*$
Alkaline phosphatase	$\leq 1.25 \times N^*$	1.26–$2.5 \times N^*$	2.6–$5 \times N^*$	5.1–$10 \times N^*$	$>10 \times N^*$
Oral	No change	Soreness/erythema	Erythema, ulcers; can eat solids	Ulcers; requires liquid diet only	Alimentation not possible
Nausea/vomiting	None	Nausea	Transient vomiting	Vomiting requiring therapy	Intractable vomiting
Diarrhoea	None	Transient <2 days	Tolerable, but >2 days	Intolerable, requiring therapy	Haemorrhagic dehydration
Renal					
Blood urea nitrogen or blood urea creatinine	$\leq 1.25 \times N^*$	1.26–$2.5 \times N^*$	2.6–$5 \times N^*$	5–$10 \times N^*$	$>10 \times N^*$
Proteinuria	No change	1+ <0.3% <3 g/l	2–3+ 0.3–1.0 g% 3–10 g/l	4+ >1.0 g% >10 g/l	Nephrotic syndrome
Haematuria	No change	Microscopic	Gross	Gross + clots	Obstructive uropapthy
Pulmonary	No change	Mild symptoms	Exertional dyspnea	Dyspnea at rest	Complete bed rest required
Fever with drug	None	Fever <38°C	Fever 38°–40°C	Fever >40°C	Fever with hypotension

Table 11.1. *(continued)*

	Grade 0	Grade 1	Grade 2	Grade 3	Grade 4
Allergic	No change	Oedema	Bronchospasm; no parenteral therapy needed	Bronchospasm; parenteral therapy required	Anaphylaxis
Cutaneous	No change	Erythema	Dry desquamation, vesiculation, pruritis	Moist desquamation, ulceration	Exfoliative dermatitis; necrosis requiring surgical intervention
Hair	No change	Minimal hair loss	Moderate, patchy alopecia	Complete alopecia but reversible	Non-reversible alopecia
Infection (specify site)	None	Minor infection	Moderate infection	Major infection	Major infection with hypotension
Cardiac					
Rhythm	No change	Sinus tachycardia, >110 at rest	Unifocal PVC, atrial arrhythmia	Multifocal PVC	Ventricular tachycardia
Function	No change	Asymptomatic, but abnormal cardiac sign	Transient symptomatic dysfunction; no therapy required	Symptomatic dysfunction responsive to therapy	Symptomatic dysfunction non-responsive to therapy
Pericarditis	No change	Asymptomatic effusion	Symptomatic; no tap required	Tamponade; tap required	Tamponade; surgery required
Neurotoxicity					
State of consciousness	Alert	Transient lethargy	Somnolence <50% of waking hours	Somnolence >50% of waking hours	Coma
Peripheral	None	Paresthesias and/or decreased tendon reflexes	Severe paresthesias and/or mild weakness	Intolerable paresthesias and/or marked motor loss	Paralysis
Constipation**	None	Mild	Moderate	Abdominal distention	Distension and vomiting
Pain‡	None	Mild	Moderate	Severe	Intractable

*N, upper limit of normal value of population under study.   **This does not include constipation resultant from narcotics.
‡Only treatment-related pain is considered, *not* disease-related pain. Use of narcotics may be helpful in grading pain depending on the patient's tolerance level

the recommendations reject the notion of attaching vague terms of clinical significance to specific toxicity grades (for example mild, moderate, severe, life-threatening). Instead there has been an attempt to objectify wherever possible the definitions of a given grade in order to reduce reporting error and bias (WHO 1979). A second observation is that for the parameters bilirubin, transaminases, alkaline phosphatases, blood urea nitrogen, and serum creatinine the various grades are defined in terms of multiples of the normal value. This is important because the laboratory techniques for measuring these parameters may vary as to the normal values and the units in which they are reported from institution to institution and from country to country. For these reasons, grading systems that rely on absolute values of these parameters for defining their grades are doomed to limited use.

Despite the value of a standardized scale system for reporting treatment toxicities, one must be mindful of the limitations of such a system. The system addresses only severity of toxicity. It does not answer questions regarding time of onset, duration, or recovery from toxic effects. Considerably more detail may be necessary in organizing toxicity data for publication. As an example, one can consider the situation of phase II chemotherapy trials. The format in Table 11.2 for haematological toxicity partially illustrates the appropriate level of detail necessary.

Additionally, it may be appropriate to display median nadirs for each course given at full doses to demonstrate any cumulative toxicity. If appropriate, toxicity data should also be compared for responding and non-responding patients in order to assess the therapeutic index. Similarly, toxicity

Table 11.2. *Phase II toxicity reporting: haematology sample data—drug X (100 patients)*

	Leucocytes (1000/mm³)		Granulocytes (1000/mm³)		Platelets (1000/mm³)	
Median pretreatment level (range)	4.8	(3.7–5.2)	2.1	(1.8–2.6)	159	(127–264)
WHO grade	0		0		0	
Median nadir (range)	2.4	(0.9–4.1)	1.2	(0.3–2.1)	96	(27–240)
WHO grade	2		2		1	
Median day onset (range)	8	(8–15)	8	(8–15)	15	(8–22)
Median day nadir (range)	15	(15–22)	15	(15–22)	22	(15–28)
Median day recovery (range)	22	(15–28)	22	(15–28)	28	(15–28)
Number of patients without toxicity (grade 0)	20	(20%)	15	(15%)	35	(35%)
Number of patients with grade 4 toxicity (%)	10	(10%)	12	(12%)	5	(5%)
Number of patients (%) hospitalized with: (1) Fever			5	(5%)		
(2) Hemorrhage			2	(2%)		
Number of patients (%) requiring dose modifications: 31 (31%)						

data may be displayed comparing two or more patient groups (that is normal versus abnormal renal or hepatic function, age groups, etc.).

This example is in no way complete, but it should demonstrate the limitations of scalar grading systems while putting them into perspectives as a valuable component in toxicity reporting.

While one can examine the WHO grading criteria and most certainly find individual definitions with which there is disagreement, it should be pointed out that with few exceptions this system is not substantially different from other systems currently in use. For the reasons outlined above and for the sake of improved comparability between clinical trials, the WHO system should be uniformly adopted. The clinical trials performed under the aegis of the European Organization for Research on Treatment of Cancer (EORTC) have already been converted successfully to the use of this grading system, and I hope that with time the system will receive greater acceptance.

CHRONIC AND LATE TOXICITIES

A detailed discussion of the nature and etiology of chronic or late toxicities is beyond the purpose of this chapter. It should be pointed out that late effects and chronic toxicities are not suitably approached using grading systems such as the ones that have been developed for acute and subacute toxicities.

These chronic and late toxic effects have become an increasing problem as treatment modalities in advanced disease have resulted in improved long-term survival. Identification and accurate estimation of the relative risk of late effects are becoming progressively more critical as we enter an era of increasing use of surgical adjuvant anti-neoplastic therapy in patients with a likelihood of surgical cure. Patients that are cured surgically are also exposed to other anti-neoplastic therapies such as chemotherapy and radiotherapy and the development of late effects in this patient population is of considerable concern. For these reasons observation of long-term survivors in advanced disease studies and the patients remaining free of disease on adjuvant therapy trials must be aggressively performed at regular intervals for the detection of late toxic effects.

There are at this time no standardized formats or systems for reporting chronic or late toxicities. The WHO (1979) has recommended that the following seven items be included in any report of such toxicities: (1) organ site or system affected; (2) timing in relation to presumed causative therapy; (3) nature of toxicity or disability (this includes second malignancies); (4) magnitude of symptoms; (5) impact on ambulatory performance status; (6) therapy required; and (7) response to therapy.

While these criteria are in no way precise, they do encompass the principal information necessary to the evaluation of such toxicities. As anti-neoplastic therapy becomes more efficacious and larger numbers of patients are placed on surgical adjuvant chemotherapy trials, late toxicities may become a more important part of the reporting of treatment results. In that event, it is likely that more standardized formats for reporting such toxicities will be developed in the future.

SUMMARY AND CONCLUSIONS

An attempt has been made to discuss the principal issues pertinent to the assessment of toxicity, analysis of toxicity data, and the reporting of that data for clinical trials. No attempt has been made to exhaustively discuss biological aspects of toxicity or specific statistical methods used in analysis. Emphasis has been placed upon concepts that should be considered by the clinician as he/she designs a clinical experiment and writes the treatment protocol. It cannot be stated too strongly that the written protocol should be the bible of the clinical researcher. Observations not required in the protocol are most often never made. Once the clinical trial is finished, it is frequently too late to go back and retrieve information that should have been specified in the protocol. Even a well-designed clinical experiment is unlikely to succeed if it is poorly described in the written protocol.

Even though the discussion of the analysis of toxicity data was general in nature, it should be viewed with the idea firmly in mind that the accurate determination of the toxicity of a treatment is as important in determining the therapeutic index for a treatment as is the anti-tumour activity. A highly active therapy may produce inferior survival results because of excessive toxicity. In such cases, adequate characterization of the risk factors for toxicity, the nature of the toxicity and its onset and duration frequently provide clues to more appropriate treatment schedules for the therapy or interventions designed to prevent the toxicity.

A plea has been made for standardization of toxicity grading systems for acute and subacute toxicities with the specific proposal being the recently published World Health Organization criteria. The system is proposed with the caveat that all such grading systems are limited in their value because they address solely the severity of toxic effects and not their duration. Despite this, these systems have been found to be valuable and arguments in opposition to using a standardized approach are relatively shallow.

The collection and reporting of data on chronic or late toxic effects represents a significant challenge to research clinicians and statisticians alike. This issue is assuming greater importance as more patients who are clinically disease-free after surgical therapy are being placed on adjuvant treatment. In these patients perhaps more than any other group, we should be mindful of our obligations and responsibilities as physicians to weigh carefully the risks and potential benefits of any treatment.

REFERENCES

Fisher, B., Carbone, P., Economou, S. G., Frelick, R., Glass, A., Lerner, H., Redmond, C., Zelen, M., Band, P., Katrych, D. L., Wolmark, N., and Fisher, E. R. (and other cooperating investigators) (1975). 1-Phenylalanine mustard (L-PAM) in the management of primary breast cancer. A report of early findings. *N. Engl. J. Med.* **292**, 117–22.

Herson, J. (1980). Evaluation of toxicity: statistical considerations. *Cancer Treat. Rep.* **64**, 463–8.

Kisner, D. L. and Sylvester, R. J. (1980). Guidelines for reporting cancer clinical trials. In *Bases Scientifiques et Reglementaires de L'Evaluation des Medicaments*, pp. 477–87. INSERM, Paris.

Schein, P. S., Stablein, D. M., Bruckner, H. N., Mayer, R., Ramming, K., Bateman, J., and Livstone, E. (1982). A comparison of combination chemotherapy and combined modality therapy for locally advanced gastric carcinoma. *Cancer* **49**, 1771–7.

Staquet, M., Sylvester, R., and Jasmin, C. (1980). Guidelines for the preparation of EORTC cancer clinical trials protocols. *Eur. J. Cancer* **16**, 871–5.

Vietti, T. J. (1980). Evaluation of toxicity: clinical issues. *Cancer Treat. Rep.* **64**, 457–61.

WHO (1979). *WHO Handbook for Reporting Results of Cancer Treatment.* WHO Offset Publication no. 48. WHO, Geneva.

Part IV
Drug and dose selection

12 Experimental bases for drug selection

Federico Spreafico, Mark B. Edelstein, and Peter Lelieveld

INTRODUCTION

The last decade has witnessed significant progress in the success rate of clinical anti-cancer therapy as best exemplified by the fact that a proportion, albeit small, of human neoplasms can now confidently be considered as curable, in the sense that the patient's life expectancy approaches that of normal individuals. Although advances in each of the three classical approaches to cancer treatment, that is surgery, radiotherapy and chemotherapy, together with improvements in related areas (for example diagnosis, supportive care) have all been instrumental in this progress, it can reasonably be stated that chemotherapy has played the dominant role. It is abundantly clear however that the progress achieved in cancer chemotherapy is still very far from being satisfactory, both qualitatively and quantitatively. In fact, the categories of responsive neoplasms do not include a large number of the most frequent clinical malignancies. In addition, the toxicity (immediate, delayed, long-term) of presently available anti-cancer agents, which are not completely specific for transformed cells, imposes a stiff price to the patient and sets relatively rigid limits for the clinician. The large number of 'precurable'[12.1] and 'subcurable'[12.2] clinical neoplasms and the limitations of presently employed drugs render obvious, therefore, that the search for both more effective strategies in the use of available cancer chemotherapeutic compounds and for better and novel agents, should continue. A retrospective analysis of the development of cancer chemotherapy shows that both these philosophies have been important for the progress obtained in this field. However, the lesson of history makes it clear also that the true corner-stone of advancement in this, as in many other areas of therapeutics, has been represented by the discovery of novel and better drugs.

Excluding from this discussion secondary-type anti-cancer agents, such as biological response modifiers, radiosensitizers or protectors, which would require a largely *ad hoc* analysis, the general philosophies and open problems of the search and selection of novel cytotoxic cancer chemotherapeutics will form the major issues to be dealt with in this chapter.

[12.1] Not presently curable.
[12.2] Presently poorly curable.

It is evident that the choice of a compound for initial phase I and II clinical testing is the last step in a complex, multi-phase process whose major stages are, very schematically, the following: acquisition, identification of activity, production and formulation, pharmacotoxicology, and clinical testing. As with any other type of therapeutic agent, the main elements which determine the selection of an anti-tumoral are: (i) the characteristics of its activity compared with existing compounds, taking into consideration both quantitative (for example level of potency, width of spectrum) as well as qualitative (for example mode of action) aspects; and (ii) its pharmacotoxicological properties. Because of its crucial importance to selection, it is therefore appropriate to first review and discuss the current procedures for the preclinical identification of anti-neoplastic activity, that is the process commonly referred to as screening.

SCREENING: IDEALS AND REALITIES

Because of its widespread use in the development of drugs and other industrial materials, this term is frequently given somewhat different meanings. With regard to anti-tumorals, the ideal screen is that which selects only those products which will be effective in one or more clinical neoplasms, while eliminating the clinically inactive materials. In other words, the ideal screen should possess both 100 per cent predictive capacity for both true positives (that is clinically active) and true negatives, and 100 per cent discriminative capacity between true and false positives or negatives. False positives are those compounds which are active in pre-clinical conditions but not in man. In addition to general predictiveness for animal–man extrapolation, the screen should ideally allow the recognition of active anti-tumorals whatever their mode of action while being entirely specific, in the sense that the effect observed should reflect exclusively an anti-neoplastic activity. Ideally, the screening should also possess specific predictiveness thus allowing the recognition of effectiveness for one or more of the over 100 types of human neoplastic diseases. In theory, specificity should also apply to other properties of the drug which can be major determinants of its clinical activity, for instance revealing those toxic characteristics of the agent which will be important or limiting in the clinic. In addition to a screen's specificity, predictiveness, the quantitative nature of the results obtained and their reproducibility, another essential requirement for an ideal screening is that all such objectives should be attainable within the frame of a reasonable time–cost effectiveness.

Given these requirements and considering that pre-clinical systems are just models of clinical conditions, with all the implicit limitations of the term 'model', it will not be surprising that actual screens are far from the ideal since only some of the above-listed objectives can be reached with confidence. In practice, screening systems not only select false positives but can also be expected to miss a number of clinically active but experimentally inactive agents (false negatives). Although in principle of great concern, the validity of a screen in discriminating true and false negatives is difficult to evaluate since compounds inactive in pre-clinical testing are seldom, if ever, clinically investigated. It is evident that the risk of false negatives is inversely related to the number and quality of models employed with regard to their capacity to reveal the value of the different philosophies aimed at cancer therapy. The problem is thus ultimately dependent on the level of fundamental knowledge of the intimate nature of the transformed state, the type of possible anti-tumorals being sought (that is anti-proliferative agents versus compounds with other modes of action such as differentiation promoters), and the practical feasibility, also in terms of costs and time requirements, of the large-scale use of such multi-model screens. It should be noted however that no existing programme of anti-tumour drug development is so rigid as to exclude from clinical testing compounds showing activity in other relevant models or conditions. Thus so far the validity of a particular screening programme is evaluated essentially in terms of its capacity to identify positives and their activity in subsequent clinical testing, thus permitting a retrospective analysis of the discriminative power between true and false positives of the procedures employed.

False-positive compounds should receive special attention in the evaluation of screening effectiveness. Various reasons can account for an experimentally active compound not being useful in the clinic: (1) following adequate testing in several neoplastic conditions, no significant clinical effectiveness may be observed (the true false positives, *sensu strictu*); (2) pharmacological differences between the screening model(s) and man, whether dependent on the host and/or the tumour, may prevent obtaining, in the latter, sufficiently high or prolonged active drug levels to exert effectiveness; (3) a drug may be active in a human tumour but its toxicity may be higher than for agents already in use with no increase in response rate; (4) even if human activity is observed, the type of toxicity seen may prevent its clinical exploitation; (5) it may prove impossible to produce a clinically-usable formulation of the compound; (6) for whatever reason, a drug may never be adequately tested in the clinic. In examining the reasons for the exclusion from further clinical use of several agents selected in experimental animals, the occurrence of severe, unpredictable, or irreversible toxicity was found to be the rationale in the majority of cases (Johnson and Goldin 1975). However, it is also relevant to note that, at least for the past, a relatively high proportion (exceeding 40 per cent) of compounds considered worthy of testing in a clinical trial were not adequately investigated in man, frequently for unclear reasons (Von Hoff, Rozencweig, and Muggia 1979).

In practice, screening has lately been subdivided in stages, with a primary screening step representing the very first test of a material for activity, or lack thereof, and a secondary screening stage comprising tests aimed at obtaining the elements necessary for deciding whether the product warrants further investigation, with the ultimate objective of obtaining indications on its clinical potential. Primary screening assays can be *in vivo*, comprising either animal tumours (generally long-transplanted rodent neoplasms) or human tumours xenografted in experimental animals, or *in vitro*. The latter approach has relied upon the use not only of human or animal cells derived from fresh explants or maintained as long-term cultures, but also of prokariotic cells as well as of biochemical assays aimed at measuring the effect on selected subcellular functions such as the activity of certain enzyme systems (Weisenthal 1981). Since the objectives of primary and secondary screening are different (identification of activity versus obtaining an extended rationale for clinical potential), at least in part the requirements for assays in the two stages can be considered different. It is in fact at the second stage that the type of compound under investigation can be of greater importance and may require a more flexible study approach. It is evident that the requirements for deciding on the clinical potential of an entirely new structure can be different in part from those of an analogue of an already known substance, as discussed at greater length below. In connection with such aspects, and having stated that actual-life screening is far from the ideal, a brief description of the historical development of screening procedures is necessary for analysing the current state of the art.

SCREENING: PAST AND PRESENT

Since the initial demonstrations in the 1940s that the use of chemicals (that is nitrogen mustard and subsequently aminopterin) could influence beneficially the course of some human neoplasms, a progressively increasing effort aimed at searching for other active anti-tumorals was launched in various countries, especially in the USA where this programme was developed with greater intensity and organization (see Johnson and Goldin 1975). At first, reflecting the individualistic nature of the effort, many experimental systems were developed including *in vivo* tumour systems and *in vitro* assays with mammalian cell lines, fungi, bacteria, and subcellular systems. Results from an early comparative analysis (Gellhorn and Hirschberg 1955) of the data obtained in as many as 74 diverse pre-clinical assays for drugs of known clinical effectiveness, established essentially that an *in vivo* tumour system could not be replaced by a non-tumour system, and that no single *in vivo* tumour model could select all useful drugs known at the time, and therefore a spectrum of tumours should have been employed for screening. Accordingly, a panel of three murine tumours (L1210 leukaemia, sarcoma 180, and adenocarcinoma 755) was employed systematically for a decade together with an incidental parallel testing in a much larger spectrum of animal tumours.

Goldin, Serpick, and Mantel (1966), in a retrospective analysis of the predictiveness of over 100 tumour models, concluded that all but one of the clinically active drugs known at that date (Mithramycin) would have been selected by the use of the mouse L1210 system and the rat Walker 256 carcinoma. The latter system (more sensitive than L1210) was then replaced by another murine tumour, the P388 leukaemia, cheaper than the rat model, and more sensitive than L1210 leukaemia to various DNA binders, antibiotics, and plant products (Venditti 1975). Through such an approach approximately 30 000 to 40 000 compounds were screened annually in various American, European, and Japanese centres under the aegis of the NCI sponsored screening programme.

The principal factors in model selection are represented by the emergence of biological principles of treatment from fundamental investigation, clinical feedback, and feasibility of large-scale exploitation. Accordingly, because one possible limit of the previously described approach could have been a preferential selection of compounds active on rapidly growing rather than on the slower, solid neoplasms, a new procedure was adopted in 1975 by the NCI (Venditti, Goldin, Miller, and Rozencweig 1978). This newer version includes a first 'pre-screen' step and a second phase relying on a panel of transplantable tumours representing the major histological types of cancer in the western world. The panel thus consists of mouse colon, breast and lung tumours, human tumours of the same types xenografted in athymic nude mice, and two mouse tumours (L1210 and B16 melanoma) which have been found of demonstrable value in the past. If justified by prior information, other *ad hoc* systems are obviously employed (for example a tumour of a given organ in the case of a compound having shown selective toxicity for that organ).

A scheme of the flow of substances as was policy in 1981 is presented in Fig. 12.1. As depicted this scheme also comprises the *in vitro* human tumour stem-cell clonogenic assay as described by Hamburger, Salmon, Von Hoff, and

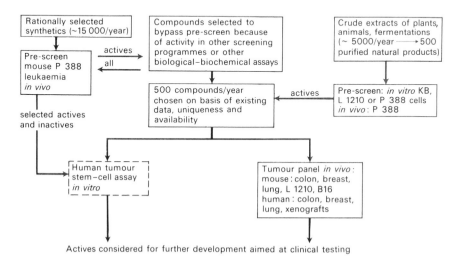

Fig. 12.1. Current flow of drugs in the NCI screening programme.

their associates (Salmon and Von Hoff 1981). This technique is, however, still in an experimental phase, as discussed below. The costs of using a tumour panel had as a consequence a decrease in the total number of substances which could be screened and a selection of compounds was thus necessary. Hence the pre-screen step was devised for compounds with no prior biological, biochemical, or pharmacotoxicological data relevant to anti-neoplastic activity, the P388 leukaemia being the best available compromise between sensitivity to known anti-tumorals and sufficient restrictiveness to avoid overloading of the panel.

SCREENING: LESSONS LEARNT

As mentioned, the screening procedures described have been the most extensively adopted internationally; it is, therefore, appropriate to examine the main lessons which have emerged from this endeavour. Firstly, the system has a degree of validity as revealed by the fact that since the programme's inception the number of clinically active drugs identified through the screen has steadily increased. Of the approximately 36 anti-tumorals currently available commercially, two-thirds were developed in the frame of this programme. However, the question of its relative validity in respect to other systems cannot be answered since no other screening philosophy has been tested on a large enough basis to permit comparisons.

A second lesson learnt is that, as it might easily have been expected, no single model would have selected all currently known drugs possessing established clinical effectiveness. For instance, l-Asparaginase was introduced in the clinic because of its activity in animal systems other than those included in the screen at that time, and o, p-DDD was tested against adrenocortical carcinoma on the basis of its selective toxicity for this organ in normal animals. More recently, 2-Deoxycoformycin was selected on the basis of its activity in biochemical assays while being inactive in the screening panel. Whether the newer screening approach relying on a greater number of model systems is more effective than previous methodologies adopting a smaller number of assays also cannot be formally established since the clinical testing of a sufficient number of compounds selected through the new procedure has not yet been completed. The relative effectiveness in terms of the true:false positive ratio cannot thus be assessed.

Thirdly, high and especially broad spectrum activity in experimental tumours is associated with a greater chance that the compound will show at least minimal clinical activity in one or more human neoplasms. This point has been confirmed in recent retrospective comparative analyses (Goldin and Venditti 1980; Goldin, Venditti, Macdonald, Muggia, Henney, and DeVita 1981) of the activity in the current NCI screening panel of approximately 30 drugs having recognized clinical effectiveness. Considering in fact the entire screening panel in its animal and human xenografts models, all known clinically established drugs, except l-Asparaginase, are active in at least half of the systems, with values ranging from 46 per cent for drugs such as Doxorubicin, methotrexate, bleomycin, and 6-Mercaptopurine, to over 80 per cent for cyclophosphamide, cis-platinum, melphalan, and CCNU. Related to this point, an additional lesson learnt from the collective screening experience is that pre-clinical predictiveness in terms of activity for specific tumour types in humans is only modest.

Although the experience is still limited in terms of both the number of agents evaluated and the tumours tested, and thus cautions against possibly premature general conclusions, the xenograft models employed so far in the NCI panel have shown also only partial correspondence between pre-clinical sensitivity and known clinical activity for a number of well-established compounds (Goldin *et al.* 1981). For instance, the MX-1 breast xenograft model failed to identify Doxorubicin as active in contrast to the known activity of this compound in human mammary cancer. The same reviews also indicated that whereas products active on human xenografts are, in general, also active in one or more murine models, the converse is not necessarily true, as there exists a larger percentage of compounds active in the mouse than in the 'human' systems employed. Just as solid tumours can select compounds which would not have been selected in the L1210 model, human tumour xenografts appear to be capable of selecting a few compounds otherwise not selected by the murine models. Furthermore, human xenografts and murine tumours of the same organ and general histological type can select different types of compounds (see Skipper 1981). The problem of whether 'xenograft positives' are more active in the clinic than 'mouse positives' cannot be solved without further information on the clinical efficacy of the newer compounds. If confirmed on a larger scale, the reduced sensitivity of the xenografts may be important in the selection of clinical candidate substances since it would be expected to result in a decrease in the proportion of false positives. The fact, however, that a long transplanted fragment derived from a single human tumour has been at the basis of the xenograft models employed, coupled with the well-known heterogeneity in responsiveness which exists within neoplasms of similar histology in animal tumours in animals, human tumours in humans or cultures of tumour cells, must be taken into account when the poor predictiveness for specific tumour types is considered. As recently discussed by Venditti (1981), marked variations in responsiveness exist not only among subclones of human tumour xenografts but also for at least some long-transplanted murine tumours. The fact that heterogeneity in cellular composition appears to be a fundamental property of neoplasms and that metastases may vary among themselves as well as differ *vis-à-vis* the primary tumour (Spreafico, Mantovani, Giavazzi, Conti, and Anaclerio 1982), clearly indicates that the pre-clinical use of just one animal tumour and one human tumour of each major histological type will have a poor chance of specific predictiveness and that new approaches are needed. Thus, a multi-step screening system appears to be the most productive methodology. Such an approach should comprise a first level with systems aimed at identifying activity, coupled with a second stage relying on a series of less responsive animal and/or human models mimicking the low responsiveness of many clinical neoplasms. A third phase, consisting of a relatively large number of individual tumours of each histological type to establish priorities for phase II trials, emerges as the objective for the future.

Because of its relevance to what is discussed above (that is the panel of five to six tumours currently employed being the conceptual equivalent of testing a new drug in only five to six patients, each with a different type of cancer), the potential of the human tumour stem-cell assay in drug selection should be considered. An in-depth analysis of the advantages and limits of such an approach is beyond the scope of this chapter. Essentially, this procedure involves the culturing of freshly explanted human tumours in soft agar and determining the inhibition of colony growth after exposure *in vitro* to a range of drug concentrations. The reader is referred to a number of recent reviews of this specific methodology as well as of other *in vitro* assays for drug screening (Salmon and Von Hoff 1981; Venditti 1981; Weisenthal 1981) for more detailed discussions.

Basically, two general questions have been asked of the human tumour stem-cell assay. Namely, whether this approach can predict the response of an individual patient's tumour to a given drug, and whether a series of human tumours of a particular type can be used to predict efficacy, or lack thereof, of a compound in subsequent phase II trials. Although experience is still relatively limited and requires validation on a much larger scale, available results suggest that at least in certain laboratories and for a number of tumour types, an interesting degree of correlation exists between results in the clinic and in the assay (Salmon and Von Hoff 1981). A positive predictive ability in the 60 per cent range and a negative predictive capacity (that is accuracy in predicting ineffective drugs in a given individual) of approximately 90 per cent has been reported. It is important to note, however, that these interesting results have been obtained in retrospective studies, whereas the true value of the clonogenic assay in terms of guiding the choice of drugs will have to be established in prospective randomized trials that may be difficult to conduct. In fact the objective therapeutic results, in terms of response rate, duration of response, and survival and/or toxicity obtained through the use of treatments chosen according to the assay, will have to be compared in equivalent populations of patients with those seen with the use of traditional therapy for that given disease (Carter 1981).

With regard to the usefulness of the tumour stem-cell assay in screening, the question cannot yet be answered since a number of conceptual and feasibility problems are still open and prevent the advancement of even tentative judgments on the value of this approach for the screening of totally unknown substances. For instance, drug concentrations and exposure times of the unknown compound to be screened must be chosen arbitrarily. The relative selectivity of the compound for neoplastic and normal cells is obviously difficult to assess with confidence in *in vitro* systems. The need for freshly explanted cells will create practical difficulties in terms of reproducibility of the test. Although as discussed by Venditti (1981), theoretically valid solutions can be envisaged for at least some of these problems (for example the use of the P388 model to pre-screen for specificity and as a guide for the choice of drug concentrations), the human tumour stem-cell assay is still too much at an experimental stage to allow conclusions on its comparative practicality and merit in screening. A NCI-supported project aimed at the evaluation of this approach, together with a host of studies currently underway in many centres, should provide in the not too-distant future answers to at least a number of the open questions concerning this interesting methodology.

SELECTION CRITERIA AND THE PROBLEM OF ANALOGUES

As briefly examined in the preceeding section, more than two decades of experience with screening, while re-emphasizing the imperfect nature of the process (ultimately the consequence that a scaled-down pre-clinical counter-part of the cancer patient does not exist), have provided a short series of general points of help in guiding the selection of potentially clinically active compounds. Before a further discussion of some selection criteria for clinical candidate products, two interrelated general aspects should be considered in view of their direct relevance to this process. The first aspect is concerned with the type of drugs which appear to be the most desirable in order to increase the present effectiveness of cancer chemotherapy. The second point is related to the already stated fact that screening can be expected to deal with different broad categories of substances. Very schematically, one may subdivide the input to the screening into: (a) products for which no prior basis for expecting activity exists; (b) compounds synthesized *ad hoc* on the basis of hypotheses, or suggestive evidence, on basic mechanisms of cancer cell function, transformation or neoplastic progression; (c) products entering the screening because of enlightened observations in other biological conditions; and (d) analogues or derivatives of molecules known for their activity in human and/or animal cancer. As will be examined below, somewhat different selection criteria can apply to these various categories.

With regard to the first point, though the limits of any such categorization are obvious, the most desirable new cancer chemotherapeutics in the 1980s can be listed in the following classes: (1) substances having novel mechanisms of cytointerfering action; (2) compounds effective on presently non-responsive or minimally responsive human cancers; (3) agents with better therapeutic indices than existing ones; and (4) agents with non-cross-resistance *vis-à-vis* currently available drugs. In other words, the aims are thus to identify agents permitting the transfer of precurable neoplasms into the subcurable category and of the latter type of cancers into the curable class, as well as to increase the effectiveness of current therapy both by extending current possibilities of combination chemotherapy and by reducing the limits imposed by available drugs (Skipper 1981).

These objectives have consequences on the selection criteria for clinical candidate products. For instance, compounds possessing a novel chemical structure (that is not previously explored with regard to anti-neoplastic activity), even if not exhibiting very high activity in a spectrum of pre-clinical assays, may nevertheless be considered more favourably for clinical testing than other molecules (for example congeners of known actives) on the presumption of an at least partially different mode of cytotoxic action and/or resistance mechanisms. In both animal and human neoplasms, combinations of non-cross-resistant drugs have in general been found to be more effective than single-drug treatments. Moreover, the presence of multi-drug-resistant cells is by many regarded as a critical limitation to a better effectiveness of current therapy. Accordingly, the resistance mechanisms and cross-resistant characteristics of a novel agent could be advocated as one of the priority criteria for drug selection. It is fair to say that current screening procedures have so far given low or no emphasis to this aspect whereas it can be reasonably argued that it should receive more attention. Also poorly considered thus far in drug selection is the potential of the novel agent to interact favourably with other known actives and to be integrated into combined modality treatment approaches. Since adjuvant chemotherapy has proven superior in a variety of advanced animal neoplasms and evidence exists for its greater effectiveness in at least some human tumours, an enlargement of the model conditions used in secondary screening to assess for this potential could thus be advocated.

Remembering one of the most important lessons learnt from over 20 years of screening, a further critical selection criterion consists in the width and level of activity in a spectrum of pre-clinical tumour assays. Because of the generalization that broad spectrum activity, even if restricted to murine tumours, appears to be associated with a greater chance for clinical activity, the EORTC strategy in secondary screening has been somewhat different from that of the NCI over the past few years. Briefly, compounds found active in the primary screen and considered worthy of interest, because of their chemical structure or origin, level of activity, and/or initial pharmacological data, are tested in a larger panel (up to over 20 systems) of secondary assays encompassing murine tumours, human tumour xenografts and, more recently, of human tumour cells in culture. Approximately 3000 substances are collected annually, also with NCI support, by the EORTC Screening and Pharmacology Group (SPG), from pharmaceutical and chemical industries, or academic research centres. These compounds are subjected to primary screening (essentially, but not exclusively, in the P388 system) in various SPG-member institutions (in Belgium, France, England, Hungary, Italy, Germany, Ireland, Yugoslavia, and Holland) yielding about 100 compounds with confirmed minimal activity. In general, the minimal level of activity in primary screening considered of interest for further testing is set at higher level than in the standard NCI primary screen. Approximately 20 substances are judged worthy of more in-depth evaluation and are tested for broad spectrum activity (with emphasis for the animal systems on solid, slow growing, metastasizing, poorly-responsive tumours), proliferation and schedule-dependency, cross-resistance, synergism with clinically established active compounds, etc. Annually, the SPG offers two to three agents for clinical testing to the EORTC groups involved in phase I and II trials and in pharmacokinetics-clinical pharmacology, these groups being thus involved in the selection process at an early stage. Although only a partial predictive correspondence for specific tumour types exists between animal and human cancers, the use of a large tumour panel increases the possibility of establishing the specific predictivity of the various systems. High activity of a new compound in pre-clinical models of neoplasms, for which no significantly effective treatment exists in the clinic, can thus be an additional reason for selection.

The selection of analogues or congeners of known active compounds, and especially of drugs with established effectiveness in humans and for which a large clinical experience has been gathered, poses somewhat different problems from those encountered in the selection of a 'new' compound. Schematically, selection in this case involves five general aspects. The first consists in the fact that the analogue must possess a significantly superior activity with respect to the parent compound. Indeed, with certain classes of chemicals, for instance the nitrosoureas, for which many very active analogues have recently been synthesized, the superiority should be very marked and in general observable in a number of pre-clinical assays. A second self-explanatory criterion is the demonstration by the new analogue of a different spectrum of activity in the pre-clinical tests from that of the parent compound of the same chemical class or with regard to other agents having the same mechanism of action. The third aspect is represented by the existence in the new compound of significantly more favourable pharmacological properties, such as oral absorption, different persistance in the organism or tissue distribution (for example penetration into the CNS), or different metabolic pathways (for example lack of requirement for bioactivation). The cost effectiveness of the novel analogue in terms of potential human use can also represent a basis for selection.

One further very important criterion is obviously the demonstration by the analogue of quantitatively and/or qualitatively different toxicological characteristics. For instance, a novel platinum derivative showing significantly lower nephrotoxicity or an anthracycline analogue with reduced cardiotoxicity, even if possessing quantitatively similar activity to the parent drug, could be considered as priority agents for clinical testing. In view of the fact that a high proportion of false positives have been so categorized because of their unacceptable toxicity in man and that for various classes of anti-tumorals relatively large numbers of analogues have been produced, the toxicological aspect of screening has received progressively more emphasis in the last years at least in certain screening programmes. This has been true for the EORTC screening, in which toxicity evaluation has become an integral part of the secondary screening, particularly for analogues and congeners of drugs having acute or subacute toxicity to one particular organ which is clinically limiting. This implies that, for instance, for a new platinum derivative or bleomycin analogue, assessment of animal renal and lung toxicity, respectively, can represent one of the very first testing steps in secondary screening. It is obvious in fact that comparative results obtained *vis-à-vis* the 'parent' drug may heavily influence the decision on whether or not to further investigate such products. Since the toxicity of oncostatic agents is unfortunately of multiple origin and, accordingly, complete testing is long, difficult, and expensive, targeted toxicity assessment is obviously more difficult for novel molecules for which no previous experience exists for helping in the selection of 'specific' testing. For such type of compounds (and obviously also for analogues chosen as clinical candidates) more standard acute and subacute animal testing is thus carried out, results being obviously important for ultimate drug selection in addition to being requested by regulatory agencies prior to human testing.

ANIMAL TOXICOLOGY IN RELATION TO PHASE I TESTING

In addition to being instrumental in the selection of clinical candidate drugs, pre-clinical toxicity studies serve two other general functions. Namely it provides an indication of the toxicity that a new substance may be expected to have in humans also in terms of investigating whether drug-induced toxicity is reversible, cumulative, delayed, manageable, and/or predictable. Secondly, it serves to provide a reasonable starting dose for phase I clinical trials. Exploration of efficacy of anti-cancer drugs usually takes place at a dose approaching the maximum tolerated dose (MTD), that is the dose which is associated with tolerable and reversible side-effects when administered with a given treatment schedule in a given patient population. Although anti-cancer drugs are allowed 'more' toxicity than the average newly introduced compound, the corollary of this statement is that more attention should, in principle, be given to the definition of toxicity for anti-cancer agents than for new drugs in general. However, the current lack of entirely reliable pre-clinical models of human cancer in terms of chemotherapeutic responsiveness, implying that a drug's potential can be assessed with certainty only after testing in humans, is a strong argument for adopting a minimum of animal toxicology consistent with safety so that rapid progression to the clinic of promising candidates occurs. Since the animal toxicity data forms the basis for the choice of the phase I starting dose, the question of the quantitative predictiveness of animal toxicity for humans should be addressed firstly. Since this topic has been recently discussed in detail (Goldin, Rozencweig, Guarino, and Schein 1980; Rozencweig, Von Hoff, Staquet, Schein, Penta, Goldin, Muggia, Freireich, and DeVita 1981), it will be examined here only briefly.

Historically, the first model for the study of the pre-clinical toxicology of anti-tumorals has been a detailed protocol developed at NCI (Prieur, Young, Davis, Cooney, Homan, Dixon, and Guarino 1973). This protocol involved the use of dogs and monkeys which were given either single or repeated doses in a number of schedules, and (since 1974) single-dose toxicity in mice to determine LD_{10}, LD_{50}, and LD_{90} and the slope of the dose–response curve. In addition, to seek information on the major organ toxicities in both species, their predictability, and the reversibility of acute or delayed toxic side-effects, a major aim of the studies in dogs and monkeys has been to determine the toxic dose low (TDL) for single and repeated treatments, since 1/3 TDL[12.3] in the most sensitive of the two species has been a widely employed starting dose for phase I trials. This choice was based, on one hand, on the consideration that too low an initial dose leads to a time-consuming clinical trial and a delay in actual human testing of the drug's effectiveness, and, on the other hand, on a series of findings obtained analysing retrospectively animal–human quantitative correlations in terms of toxicity. The initial results were produced by Freireich, Gehan, Rall, Schmidt, and Skipper (1966) who, by evaluating 18 agents, determined that on a mg/m² basis, the MTD was on the average, that is for groups of drugs, similar in man and in each of the five animal species considered. Similar results have been obtained in later analyses using additional drugs (Goldsmith, Slavik, and Carter 1975; Schein 1977; Penta, Rozencweig, Guarino, and Muggia 1979). On the basis of the MTD for 37 agents, Homan (1972) estimated that the probability of exceeding the human MTD using 1/3 MTD in dogs or monkeys carried a similar risk of 10 per cent and the use of the MTD in the more sensitive between the two species decreases this risk only minimally, to 6 per cent. Using 1/10 MTD, the risk was 1 per cent with either species and 0.5 per cent employing the data of the most sensitive species. In subsequent studies (Goldsmith *et al.* 1975; Penta *et al.* 1979; Goldin *et al.* 1980) it was demonstrated that the mouse could be as good or better a predictor for quantitative toxicity as larger animals. Moreover, the mouse permits the establishment in both normal and tumour-bearing hosts of more accurate dose–response curves with respect to routes and schedules of administration, and other parameters of potential clinical interest, at a lower

---

[12.3] TDL is defined relative to the highest non-toxic dose (HNTD; the highest dose at which no haematological, chemical, clinical, or morphological drug-induced alteration occurs, TDL corresponding to twice HNTD); toxic dose high (TDH = 2 × TDL) is a dose that produces any such changes but, at variance with TDL, doubling this dose produces death, thus TDH × 2 = LD (lethal dose).

cost, and in shorter time periods than is possible in other species. In view, also, of the overpredictiveness of the monkey with regard to a number of qualitative toxicities, there appears, thus, to be no advantage offered by the monkey in pre-clinical studies over the combination of mouse and dog, a conclusion recently accepted also by the US Food and Drug Administration (FDA).

In a more recent study conducted on 21 agents for which the data permitted a well-founded comparative analysis, it has been found (Rozencweig *et al.* 1981) that both the $1/6$ LD_{10} in the mouse and $1/3$ TDL in dogs gave tolerated starting doses in man. It was also determined that, on average, there was no significant difference in terms of the number of dose-escalating steps to reach MTD in man (it is usually considered that phase I trials optimally should not require more than six to seven escalation steps) when selecting the lowest between $1/6$ LD_{10} in the mouse and $1/3$ TDL in dogs, or selecting $1/10$ LD_{10} in the mouse, provided this dose is tolerated in dogs. The second alternative is obviously faster since it does not require determining specific toxicity levels in the dog. Although it is evident that if the most sensitive species determines the human starting dose, the greater the number of species, the greater the probability of choosing a starting dose below the human MTD. These findings suggest that using a sufficiently low fraction of a specific toxic-dose level in a single animal species (that is $1/10$ LD_{10} in the mouse) is a satisfactory approach to determine the initial dose for clinical testing, especially when its safety is assessed in another species such as the dog. Thus, such an approach has recently been adopted in the USA where under the revised, FDA-approved protocol, phase I trials can begin upon completion of a minimum 28-day observation period in the mouse at two dose schedules and a 60-day observation in dogs at $1/10$ LD_{10} dose in the mouse.

The question of quantitative toxicity extrapolation is intimately connected with that of the predictability of qualitative toxicity of anti-cancer drugs. This is an area in which an active debate is currently open, not only as to what type of tests in which animal species should be performed to obtain information which may assist the clinician in the conduct of human testing, but also whether relatively in-depth efforts in this direction should be undertaken at all. The matter is more complicated than for interspecies quantitative extrapolation, taking into account that the types of toxicities which may be induced by anti-tumorals are numerous, some of them posing relatively arduous problems for their routine detection (for example cardio- or pulmonary toxicity). In addition, marked interspecies variations exist in the sensitivity for certain side-effects. While testing in animals for a reasonably large number of qualitative toxicities, encompassing not only the most common ones (for example a haematotoxicity) but also relatively rare ones, would be difficult to perform and would impose a high financial and time burden, it has to be considered also that for at least certain human toxicities a number of curative measures exist. Consequently, a number of iatrogenic toxicities do not in practice constitute an overriding problem for experienced investigators.

As mentioned above, at variance with previous practices exploiting dogs and monkeys, the most recent pre-clinical toxicology NCI protocol relies only on mice and dogs and does not require that histopathology be performed prior to phase I but only prior to phase II. This change was spurred by studies (Goldin *et al.* 1980) which showed that (in the conditions exploited in the older protocols) the monkey provided no advantage over the dog, that both species had failed to predict for certain important toxicities (for example cardiotoxicity for anthracyclines) while overpredicting for others (for example liver and kidney damage), thus giving a relatively high proportion of both false positive and negative results. It would appear that large animals (whether dogs alone or in combination with monkeys) can be useful predictors for toxicities which are commonly encountered with cytotoxic drugs and to which clinicians are, therefore, already alerted. At variance, the predictiveness of these species for rare toxicities is low, at least when standard protocols are adopted.

Considering that a series of important side-effects have not emerged from past studies in dogs so that qualitative toxicity data are of only relative use to experienced clinical investigators who anticipate the worse, the question is still open as to the value of using two species (that is dog and mouse), or only the mouse, as currently under discussion in some countries (for example England). In this regard it should be noted that the comparative predictive value of rodents, with respect to other species for qualitative toxicity, is still formally undetermined, and there is no a priori rationale for expecting that murine data would be more relevant intrinsically to man than those of other species. However, the fact that a large number of quantitative results in conditions more relevant to the clinic (for example tumour-bearing hosts) can be obtained in rodents in a relatively short time, thus also allowing flexibility, selectivity, and cost effectiveness in the possible use of other species, is an aspect which cannot be overlooked.

Since, in spite of its limitations, toxicity assessment in animals can nevertheless be of use, it is evident that an active research effort is needed to devise faster and more relevant toxicology procedures in small animals. Possibly, emphasis should be placed on the detection of the rarer and the less-treatable side-effects, and to obtain information which can be of assistance to the physician on whether the iatrogenic toxicity is cumulative, reversible, delayed, predictable, and/or manageable (Rall 1973). However, it can also be argued (Rozencweig *et al.* 1981) that safety in phase I trials may be more dependent on the attention given to monitoring toxicity during the trial and the availability of adequate treatment facilities, than on the procedure of dose escalation and the pre-clinical data. Just as at the current 'state of the art' animals can provide only indications of anti-tumour activity and of specific tissue response in man, pre-clinical toxicology studies similarly give only indications of maximal drug doses with which to commence human testing. Considering both past experience in such clinical testing and the increasing refinement in clinical methodology, there seems to be a reasonable case against the use of long, so-called exhaustive, standard pre-clinical toxicology studies, especially in large animals. More flexible approaches using rodents appear to be more productive.

CONCLUDING REMARKS

From what has been discussed above the conclusion emerges that the search for and evaluation of novel anti-tumorals is not simple and still far from having reached most of the ideal objectives considered in the Introduction. In spite of the many inadequacies and limitations of the current strategy and approaches, which render the whole screening process as one by definition requiring constant improvement and rethinking in response to advancements in fundamental knowledge, it cannot be denied that the effort has been productive. Although only human testing can provide the true answer with such compounds, as is true for other therapeutic agents, a number of novel approaches towards testing have appeared in recent years and justify a degree of optimism in the expectation of more effective identification of anti-cancer drugs.

REFERENCES

Carter, S. K. (1981). Predictors of response and their clinical evaluation. *Cancer Chemother. Pharmac.* **7**, 1–4.

Freireich, E. J., Gehan, E. A., Rall, D. P., Schmidt, L. H., and Skipper, M. E. (1966). Quantitative comparison of toxicity of anticancer agents in mouse, rat, hamster, dog, monkey and man. *Cancer Chemother. Rep.* **50**, 219–44.

Gellhorn, A., and Hirschberg, E. (1955). Diverse systems for cancer chemotherapy screening, I. Summary of results and general correlations. *Cancer Res.* (Suppl. 3), 1–13.

Goldin, A., Rozencweig, M., Guarino, A. M., and Schein, P. S. (1980). Quantitative and qualitative prediction of toxicity from animals to humans. In *Controversies in cancer treatment* (eds. H. J. Tagnon and M. J. Staquet) pp. 83–104. Masson, Paris.

—— Serpick, A. A., and Mantel, N. (1966). A commentary. Experimental screening procedures and clinical predictability value. *Cancer Chemother. Rep.* **50**, 173–218.

—— and Venditti, J. M. (1980). Progress report on the screening program at the Division of Cancer Treatment, National Cancer Institute. *Cancer Treat. Rev.* **7**, 167–76.

—— Venditti, J. M., Macdonald, J. S., Muggia, F. M., Henney, J. E. and DeVita, V. T. (1981). Current results of the screening program of the division of cancer treatment. National Cancer Institute. *Eur. J. Cancer* **17**, 129–42.

Goldsmith, M. A., Slavik, M., and Carter, S. K. (1975). Quantitative prediction of drug toxity in humans from toxicology in small and large animals. *Cancer Res.* **35**, 1354–64.

Homan, E. R. (1972). Quantitative relationships between toxic doses of antitumor chemotherapeutic agents in animals and man. *Cancer Chemother. Rep.* **3**, (pt 3, no. 3), 13–19.

Johnson, R. K. and Goldin, A. (1975). The clinical impact of screening and other experimental tumor studies. *Cancer Treat. Rev.* **2**, 1–31.

Penta, J. S., Rozencweig, M., Guarino, A. M., and Muggia, F. M. (1979). Mouse and large animal toxicology studies of twelve antitumor agents: relevance to starting dose for phase I clinical trials. *Cancer Chemother. Pharmac.* **3**, 97–101.

Prieur, D. J., Young, D. M., Davis, R. D., Cooney, D. A., Homan, E. R., Dixon, R. L., and Guarino, A. M. (1973). Procedures for preclinical toxicologic evaluation of cancer chemotherapeutic agents: protocols of the laboratory of toxicology. *Cancer Chemother. Rep.* **4**, (pt 3), 1–30.

Rall, D. P. (1973). General principles of the toxicologic investigation of anticancer drugs. In *Cancer medicine* (eds. J. F. Holland and E. Frei III) pp. 675–81. Lea and Febiger, Philadelphia.

Rozencweig, M., Von Hoff, D. D., Staquet, M. J., Schein, P. S., Penta, J. S., Goldin, A., Muggia, F. M., Freireich, E. J., and DeVita, V. T. (1981). Animal toxicology for early clinical trials with anticancer agents. *Cancer clin. Trials* **4**, 21–8.

Salmon, S. E. and Von Hoff, D. D. (1981). *In vitro* evaluation of anticancer drugs with the human tumor stem cell assay. *Sem. Oncol.* **8**, 377–85.

Schein, P. S. (1977). Preclinical toxicology of anticancer agents. *Cancer Res.* **37**, 1934–7.

Skipper, H. S. (1981). *Some thoughts on screening for new anticancer drugs. Past, present and future.* Southern Research Institute, Birmingham, Alabama.

Spreafico, F., Mantovani, A., Giavazzi, R., Conti, G., and Anaclerio, A. (1982). Metastatic potential of metastases, tumor cell heterogeneity and therapeutic implications. *Recent Res. cancer Res.* **80**, 1–8.

Venditti, J. M. (1975). Drug evaluation branch program. Report to screening contractors.*Cancer Chemother. Rep.* **5** (pt 2), 1–4.

—— (1981). Preclinical drug development: rationale and methods. *Sem. Oncol.* **8**, 349–61.

—— Goldin, A., Miller, I., and Rozencweig, M. (1978). Experimental models for antitumor testing in current use by the National Cancer Institute USA. Statistical analysis and methods for selecting agents for clinical trials. In *Advances in cancer chemotherapy* (eds. S. K. Carter, A. Goldin, K. Kuretan, G. Mathé, Y. Sakurai, S. Tsukagoshi, and H. Umezawa) pp. 201–19. University Park Press, Baltimore.

Von Hoff, D. D., Rozencweig, M., and Muggia, F. M. (1979). The evaluation of cytotoxic drugs. *Cancer Treat. Rev.* Suppl. **6** 1–8.

Weisenthal, L. M. (1981). *In vitro* assays in preclinical antineoplastic drug screening. *Sem. Oncol.* **8**, 362–76.

13 Design and conduct of phase I trials

Daniel D. Von Hoff, John Kuhn, and Gary M. Clark

INTRODUCTION

There is no doubt that the first administration of a new anti-cancer agent to the man (the phase I trial) represents one of the most important steps in the development of that new agent. The purpose of the phase I trial is to determine a safe dose for further studies for therapeutic activity and to define the qualitative organ system toxicity associated with the compound. This initial phase I experience with the agent largely determines the interest in the agent. Excessive toxicity and even lack of activity are frequently grounds for discontinuation of development of the agent (Von Hoff, Rozencweig, Soper, Helman, Penta, Davis, and Muggia 1977b). Therefore, a careful thoughtful approach to the design and execution of the phase I trial is essential.

As we explore the various aspects of the phase I clinical trial of a new anti-cancer agent it will become clear that the methods for performing phase I trials are based both on hard scientific facts as well as on clinical experience. It will also become clear that there is room for innovative approaches to the goals of the phase I trial.

GOALS OF THE PHASE I TRIAL

Most authors and investigators have agreed that there are basically three goals in the phase I trial (Carter 1977; Gottlieb 1974; Schein 1977; Carter, Selawry, and Slavik 1977; Williams and Carter 1978; Karon, Sieger, Leimbrock, Finkelstein, Nesbit, and Swaney 1973).

(a) To establish a maximum tolerated dose (safe dose) for a new drug on a given schedule via a given route of administration.

(b) To determine the qualitative (which organ system involved) toxicity as well as the quantitative (predictability, extent, duration and reversibility) toxicity of the drug.

(c) To look for evidence of anti-tumor activity of the new drug.

A possible additional goal of the phase I trial might be to investigate some of the basic clinical pharmacology of the drug. This basic clinical pharmacology could include uptake, metabolism, excretion, and organ distribution of the new drug. Each one of the major goals will be discussed in some detail below.

MAJOR ISSUES IN DESIGN AND CONDUCT

While the goals and concepts of a phase I trial appear simple there are, in reality, several major issues in the design and conduct of these trials. These issues fall into four major categories: (a) patient selection factors; (b) drug starting dose, escalation, and schedules; (c) patient requirements; and (d) determination of maximal tolerated dose.

Patient selection factors

Certainly the type of patient entered in a phase I study is of prime importance since a phase I trial is a human toxicology study. The selection of patients for the phase I trial includes many important factors (Carter 1977; Gottlieb 1974; Woolley and Schein 1979; Carter *et al.* 1977; Williams and Carter 1978; Karon *et al.* 1973). These include the following factors:

1. All patients must have microscopically confirmed diagnosis of disseminated cancer which is no longer amenable to treatment with more established forms of treatment. The investigator must be certain that patients have no other more effective treatment alternatives than what could be provided by a phase I agent. The precise definition of when a patient's tumour is no longer amenable to established forms of treatment may be very clear in some instances. For example, a patient with breast cancer who has failed surgery, chemotherapy with cyclophosphamide, methotrexate, 5-fluorouracil, Prednisone, tamoxifen, Adriamycin, mitomycin C, vinblastine, and radiotherapy could be a candidate for a phase I trial. However, a patient with disseminated colorectal carcinoma who has not received any chemotherapy might be considered a good candidate for a phase I trial by one investigator while another investigator might feel the patient should be given 5-fluorouracil first and offered a phase I agent only if the patient fails to respond to 5-fluorouracil. At present, Dr Paul Woolley has put it best when he said: 'Care must be taken that patients do not relinquish their rights to established effective therapy, while insuring that the terminally ill are not subjected the needless toxicity' (Woolley and Schein 1979).

2. Distinctions should be made between solid tumour and acute leukaemia patients. The major problem here is that patients with acute leukaemia have a defective organ system which is the subject of toxicological evaluation of the drug (the haemopoietic system). In addition, acute leukaemia patients usually tolerate as much or higher doses of drugs than patients with solid tumours (Karon *et al.* 1973). The quickest solution to this problem is to perform phase I trials in two separate groups of patients—patients with solid tumours and patients with acute leukaemias. The patient entered in a phase I trial need not have measurable disease. Measurable disease is definitely required in a phase II efficacy trial with a new agent.

3. Patient age is a consideration for patient selection. Retrospective analyses

have shown that pediatric patients (< 18 years of age) may tolerate higher doses of a drug than patients ≥ 18 years of age (Von Hoff, Rozencweig, and Muggia 1977a). In addition, there are some data which indicate that younger patients' tumours (patients < 50 years) may be more sensitive to chemotherapy than older patients' tumours (≥ 50 years) (Rosenblum, Gerosa, Dougherty, Reese, Barger, Davis, Levin, Strike, and Wilson 1982; Von Hoff, Osborne, Neuenfeldt, and Clark 1982). Phase I designs should, therefore, call for separate phase I trials in children and adults. However, safety and dose escalation data from one group may be used as the basis for the starting dose for the other group.

Pregnant patients are generally excluded from phase I studies because of potential teratogenic risks.

4. Life expectancy of the patient is also a consideration. Performance status of the patient can be an indicator of that life expectancy. It is routine to indicate that a patient's life expectancy should be at least 12 weeks (as judged by the investigator) before the patient can be eligible for the phase I trial. This time period would assure a minimum period of observation after drug administration to allow for observation of drug-related effects. It should, however, be remembered that physicians frequently overestimate survival (Woolley *et al.* 1979; Parker 1972).

5. Intervals between prior treatment and institution of the phase I drug should be enough to ensure that the toxic effects of previous therapy have passed. This interval is usually 1 month but at least 6 weeks should be allowed for patients who have just received prior nitrosoureas or mitomycin C (Wasserman, Slavik, and Carter 1974; Moertel, Reitemeier, and Hahn 1969).

6. Patients must have normal organ function including normal bone marrow, hepatic, renal, and cardiac function. Metabolic parameters such as glucose, electrolytes, calcium, and phosphorus should also be within normal limits. Specific explorations of drug doses in patients with compromised major organ function should be relegated to later stages of the phase I trial with careful pharmacokinetic studies in those patients.

7. Patients considered for phase I trials should ideally be on no concomitant drugs (pain medications, etc.). Such a patient is difficult to find but concomitant medication should always be considered.

8. Obtaining the informed consent of the patient is of utmost importance. This is an area that has recently created some controversy. If a strict definition of the phase I trial being a toxicology trial is followed, then patients must understand they are volunteering for the sake of other cancer patients who may benefit from the results of the study. They must understand that they may develop serious toxicity or even death without a definite prospect for personal benefit (Woolley *et al.* 1979). In addition, most patients have had and failed prior surgery, radiotherapy, and chemotherapy. Therefore, the chances of any therapy benefiting the patient are small. However, the phase I clinical trial is not only a toxicology trial. It is a trial with a therapeutic intent. The drug was

selected because of some expectation of anti-tumour activity in man. Therefore, it is always possible a patient might benefit by having a remission in a phase I trial with a new agent. Responses have indeed been noted in a number of phase I trials (Von Hoff, Houser, Gormley, Bender, Glaubiger, and Young 1978; Von Hoff, Pollard, Kuhn, Murray, and Coltman 1980; Von Hoff, Myers, Kuhn, Sandbach, Pocelinko, Clark, and Coltman 1981c). The choice for the patient is often no further therapeutic intervention versus a phase I agent. In summary, before a patient enters a phase I trial he needs to have a detailed understanding of the therapeutic options. He should be fully informed that the prospects of therapeutic benefit from the phase I drug are very small (but not non-existent). He should be aware also that he may withdraw from the phase I trial at any time and that withdrawal will in no way prejudice his future care.

Starting dose, schedule, escalation

Selection of starting dose

Most phase I trials in the past have utilized a starting dose selected by taking one-third of the toxic dose low (TDL) in the most sensitive large animal species (in mg/m^2) (Carter 1977; Carter *et al.* 1977; Prieur, Young, Davis, Cooney, Homan, Dixon, and Guarino 1973; Schein 1977; Homan 1972; Goldsmith Slavik, and Carter 1975). A number of studies have shown that a better correlation exists between toxic doses among various animal species and man when the dose is expressed per body surface area units (mg/m^2) rather than by body weight units (mg/kg) (Homan 1972; Freireich, Gehan, Rall, Schmidt, and Skipper 1966; Penta, Rozencweig, Guarino, and Muggia 1979).

The toxic dose low is defined as the lowest dose which produces alteration in the animal including haematologic, chemical, clinical, or morphological drug-induced alteration, and doubling the TDL does not produce lethality. A great deal of experience has proven both the safety and usefulness of this method of selecting the starting dose for man (Carter 1977; Carter *et al.* 1977; Prieur *et al.* 1973; Schein 1977; Homan 1972; Goldsmith *et al.* 1975).

More recently there has been a major re-evaluation of the method for selecting a starting dose in man. The first relevant detailed study was conducted by Freireich and colleagues in 1966 (Freireich *et al.* 1966). They compared the qualitative toxicity of 18 anti-cancer agents in the mouse, rat, hamster, dog, monkey, and man. All animal species in that analysis proved to be equally relevant for predicting the maximally tolerated dose in humans. These initial observations were confirmed in subsequent retrospective analyses using additional anti-cancer agents by Goldsmith *et al.* (1975), Homan (1972), and Penta *et al.* (1979).

Some authors, including Penta *et al.* (1979), have reviewed the early work of Freireich *et al.* (1966), as well as performed other retrospective studies and determined that an equally safe methodology for determining the starting dose for a new drug in man would be to take one-third of the LD_{10} in mice (the dose that is lethal for 10 per cent of mice receiving that dose), expressed in mg/m^2, as a starting dose for phase I trials in man. Proponents of this approach point to the finding that this method might require a lesser number of dose escalations to reach the human maximally tolerated dose (Penta *et al.* 1979). A more recent analysis by Rozencweig, Von Hoff, Staquet, Schein, Penta, Goldin, Muggia, Freireich, and DeVita (1981) suggests a similar number of dose escalation steps would have been required in phase I clinical trials if the starting dose had been based on one-tenth the LD_{10} in the mouse and one-third the TDL in the dog. Other authors caution that occasionally LD_{50} and LD_{10} determinations in mice may vary by as much as 100 per cent (Guarino, Rozencweig, Kline, Penta, Venditti, Lloyd, Dolzworth, and Muggia 1979). Therefore, recognition of factors responsible for differences of toxic dose levels in mice would enhance the proper utilization of that approach.

The use of one-tenth the LD_{10} in mice as a starting dose for phase I trials in man is just beginning in prospective phase I trials sponsored by the National Cancer Institute. Results of those trials should help to determine whether that method has any advantage over the traditional one-third of the TDL starting dose.

Schedule

The choice of schedule for a phase I study has been guided by a variety of pieces of information and factors including schedule dependence in animal tumours, proposed mechanisms of anti-tumour action, patient convenience, desire to perform clinical pharmacology studies, pre-clinical animal pharmacokinetic information, and other properties of the drug (such as solubility). The usual approach is to perform phase I trials on a variety of schedules which at least include a daily and an intermittent every 3 to 4 week schedule.

At the present time there is some doubt as to what impact the schedule has on the ultimate anti-tumour activity of a drug. In leukaemia, cytosine arabinoside has had more activity as a continuous infusion or with doses given at close intervals (Frei, Bickers, and Hewlett 1969). However, it has yet to be proven that different schedules of administrations of any drug gives an advantage in terms of anti-tumour effect for patients with solid tumours. The toxicities of anti-cancer agents can, however, definitely be modified by adjusting the schedule (for example mucositis as a dose-limiting toxicity for 5-fluorouracil given as a continuous infusion as opposed to leukopenia as a dose-limiting toxicity for an intermittent schedule of administration).

Dose escalation

The escalation methodology for phase I trials has been developed empirically. The most accepted methodology utilizes a dose escalation scheme designated the modified Fibonacci search scheme (Carter *et al.* 1977; Hansen 1970) whereby dose escalations are initially rapid, with smaller increments the closer one approaches the toxic range (see Table 13.1). Utilizing this scheme, the maximally tolerated dose of a new agent has usually been reached in from 2 to 12 (median = 6) dose escalations (Carter *et al.* 1977; Penta *et al.* 1979). Thus, this method has been safe and effective. Critics of this methodology point to the possibility that patients are wasted in unnecessarily slow escalation patterns. An alternative method of escalation proposes standard increments of 50 per cent of the original dose with decreases to 25 per cent increments when toxicity is reached (Gottlieb 1974). However, this practice has not been as widely tested prospectively as the modified Fibonacci scheme. Overall, the modified Fibonacci search scheme approach remains the standard method for escalation in phase I clinical trials.

Table 13.1. *Idealized modified Fibonacci search scheme approach to dose escalation in a phase I study*

Drug dose	Percentage increase above preceding dose level
n^*	—
2.0 n	100
3.3 n	67
5.0 n	50
7.0 n	40
9.0 n	33
12.0 n	33
16.0 n	33

* Starting dose $= n(mg/m^2)$

Patient requirements

The usual practice is to enter three patients with solid tumours not previously treated with the study drug at each non-toxic dose level. The first patient should be entered at each level and observed for at least 4 weeks. If no toxicity is noted the other two patients may be entered at that dose level 1 week apart. All patients are observed for 3 to 4 weeks before proceeding to the next dose escalation. When any toxicity is reached, six patients are entered at that dose level and at subsequent dose levels showing any toxicity up to and including the maximally tolerated dose level (Carter 1977; Gottlieb 1974; Woolley and Schein; Carter *et al.* 1977; Williams and Carter 1978). In addition, it is desirable that when the maximally tolerated dose level is reached that at least three more patients are entered at that level and kept on therapy (tumour response permitting) to determine chronic or cumulative toxicity.

It should be a general policy not to re-enter a patient at a higher dose escalation level. This philosophy is based on the feeling that any observed toxicological effects of the drug should reflect the effects of a single dose or a defined number of repeated doses at a specific dose level. Escalation within the same patient may mask the presence of cumulative toxicity.

Determination of a maximal tolerated dose (MTD) in man

The definition of a MTD may be different among clinical investigators. Some investigators describe it as 'maximum deliverable dose which is not associated with lethality while for others it represents the *first* evidence of treatment-limiting toxicity' (Woolley and Schein).

Reasonable definitions of toxic levels in man have been set down by Carter *et al.* (1977) and are shown in Table 13.2.

Table 13.2. *Definitions of toxic levels in man*

Term	Definitions
Subtoxic dose	A dose that causes *consistent* changes of haematologic or biochemical parameters and might thus herald toxicity at the next higher dose level or with prolonged administration
Minimal toxic dose	The smallest dose at which one or more of three patients show consistent, readily reversible drug toxicity
Recommended dose for therapeutic (phase II trial)	The dose that causes moderate, reversible toxicity in most patients
Maximum tolerated dose	The highest safely tolerable dose

In actual practice, the MTD recorded is often a function of the degree of prior therapy to which patients on the study have been exposed. 'When analyzing the results of a phase I study it is imperative to be cognizant of this patient selection factor before deciding the dose for further clinical investigation' (Carter *et al.* 1977).

PRACTICAL EXAMPLE OF A PHASE I TRIAL

There are a large number of phase I trials which have been reported in the literature. As an example on how a phase I trial is performed we have chosen the recently reported phase I trial of dihydroxyanthracenedione (Mitoxantrone, NSC 301739) in patients with solid tumours (Von Hoff *et al.* 1980).

Mitoxantrone was selected for clinical trial because of excellent anti-tumour activity in a variety of animal tumour systems including the L1210 mouse leukaemia and B16 mouse melanoma. The drug also exhibited anti-tumour activity in the human tumour cloning system (Von Hoff, Coltman, and Forseth 1981*a*).

The toxic dose low for Mitoxantrone in the most sensitive animal species (the beagle dog) was 3.6 mg/m^2 on a single dose schedule. Therefore the starting dose in man was one-third of the 3.6 mg/m^2 or 1.2 mg/m^2. A single dose every 4 weeks schedule was chosen for study because there was no evidence of schedule dependency for the drug in any pre-clinical tumour system.

The clinical trial was begun at 1.2 mg/m^2 given every 4 weeks. The patient characteristics are noted in Table 13.3. Note that all patients had received prior chemotherapy and all had solid tumours.

Table 13.3. *Phase I Mitoxantrone study: patient characteristics*

Characteristics	
Total no. of patients	25
Men/women	24/1
Age (years)	
Median	57
Range	30–68
No. of patients with prior treatment	25
Chemotherapy	25
Radiotherapy and chemotherapy	14
Tumour type	
Lung	
Squamous	6
Adeno	7
Small cell	1
Melanoma	3
Pancreas	2
Bladder	1
Prostate	1
Hepatoma	1
Colon	1
Esophagus	1
Head and neck	1

Three patients were entered at each dose level. Doses were escalated according to the modified Fibonacci search scheme detailed in Table 13.1 above. As noted in Table 13.4 the blood counts (and other toxicities) were recorded at each dose level. As detailed in Table 13.4, leukopenia was clearly the dose limiting acute toxicity. Thrombocytopenia was uncommon. The maximal tolerated dose in this trial was 14 mg/m^2 while the dose recommended for therapeutic phase II trials was 12 mg/m^2. No other major non-

Table 13.4. *Myelosuppression by Mitoxantrone at each dose level*

Dose (mg/m^2)	No. of patients/ no. of courses	Median (cells × 10^3/μl) WBC	Platelets
1.2	4/4	9.0 (7.2–12.8)*	165 (130–323)
2.4	3/5	9.4 (7.0–12.9)	143 (27–331)
4.0	3/5	16.4 (13.6–19.4)	204 (193–235)
6.0	3/6	7.1 (6.0–15.2)	374 (322–445)
8.0	3/7	3.1 (2.9– 3.3)	274 (236–335)
10.0	3/4	2.4 (2.2– 2.4)	110 (96–116)
12.0	5/9	2.1 (1.3– 3.8)	124 (46–331)
14.0	1/1	0.2	6

* Numbers in parentheses, range.

haematological toxicity (nausea and vomiting, alopecia, cardiotoxicity, or phlebitis) was noted in that study.

Overall, the phase I clinical trial with Mitoxantrone was straightforward and was accomplished in a reasonable time period (6 months) with the minimum number of patients needed to arrive at the maximal tolerated dose.

PHASE I TRIALS DIRECTED BY *IN VITRO* AND *IN VIVO* SYSTEMS

It has been the goal of a number of investigators to design some *in vitro* or *in vivo* system which might predict for response of an individual patient's tumour to a particular chemotherapeutic agent. Such a system would be a specific help for phase I clinical trials. Not only could the patient be pre-selected for a maximal chance for a response but the level of drug which needed to be achieved in a particular patient might be extrapolated from *in vitro* results.

At present there are two systems which look promising for predicting the response of a patient's tumour to a particular drug. Both these systems look promising also for use as a screen for detecting new anti-neoplastics.

The first system is an *in vitro* mouse system called the subrenal capsule assay. This assay was developed by Bogden, Cabl, and Le Page (1981). The second system was developed by Hamburger and Salmon and is called the human tumour cloning system (Hamburger and Salmon 1977). If the initial *in vitro in vivo* correlations found for these systems are verified they could restrict phase I trials only to patients who had a reasonable chance for responding (Salmon, Hamburger, Soehnlen, Durie, Alberts, and Moon 1978; Von Hoff, Casper, Bradley, Jones, and Makuch 1981b). This would indeed be a boon to patients and clinical investigators. Prospective trials integrating these assay systems with phase I trials are now being undertaken in a number of institutions.

SUMMARY

The phase I clinical trial has evolved over the years to a fairly standard procedure based on clinical experience with a number of methodologies. It is clear that new approaches to the performance of the phase I trial are required in the future. These approaches should maximize the chances for a rapid, safe determination of toxicities as well as maximize the chances of a therapeutic effect for the patient.

ACKNOWLEDGEMENT

This work was supported by grant 2–R10 CA 22433–05 of the Southwest Oncology Group and contract NCI-CM-27509-19.

REFERENCES

Bogden, A. E., Cabl, W. R., and LePage, D. J. (1981). Chemotherapy responsiveness of human tumors as first transplant generation xenografts in the normal mouse. *Cancer* **48**, 10–20.

Carter, S. K. (1977). Clinical trials in cancer chemotherapy. *Cancer* **40**, 544–57.

—— Selawry, O., and Slavik, M. (1977). *Methods of development of new anticancer drugs.* US Department of Health, Education, and Welfare, Bethesda.

Frei, E., III, Bickers, J. N., and Hewlett, J. S. (1969). Dose schedule and antitumor studies of arabinosyl cytosine (NSC–63878). *Cancer Res.* **29**, 1325–30.

Freireich, E. J., Gehan, E. A., Rall, D. P., Schmidt, L. H., and Skipper, H. E. (1966). Quantitative comparison of toxicity of anticancer agents in mouse, rat, hamster, dog, monkey and man. *Cancer chemother. Res.* **50**, 219–44.

Goldsmith, M. A., Slavik, M., and Carter, S. K. (1975). Quantitative prediction of drug toxicity in humans from toxicology in small and large animals. *Cancer Res.* **35**, 1354–64.

Gottlieb, J. A. (1974). Phase I and phase II clinical trials: a critical reappraisal. In *The pharmacologic basis of cancer chemotherapy. Williams and Wilkens, Baltimore.*

Guarino, A. M., Rozencweig, M., Kline, I., Penta, J. S., Venditti, J. M., Lloyd, H. H., Dolzworth, D. A., and Muggia, F. M. (1979). Adequacies and inadequacies in assessing mouse toxicity data with antineoplastic agents. *Cancer Res.* **37**, 2204–10

Hamburger, A. W. and Salmon, S. E. (1977). Primary bioassay of human tumor stem cells. *Science* **197**, 461–3.

Hansen, H. H. (1970). Clinical experience with 1-(2-chloroethyl)3-cyclohexyl-1-nitrosourea (CCNU, NSC 79037). *Proc. Am. Ass. cancer Res.* **11**, 43.

Homan, E. R. (1972). Quantitative relationships between toxic doses of antitumor chemotherapeutic agents in animals and man. *Cancer chemother. Rep.* **3**, 13–19.

Karon, M., Sieger, L., Leimbrock, S., Finkelstein, J., Nesbit, M. F., and Swaney, J. J. (1973). Azacytidine: a new active agent for the treatment of acute leukemia. *Blood* **42**, 359–65.

Moertel, C. G., Reitemeier, R. J., and Hahn, R. G. (1969). Mitomycin-C therapy in advanced gastrointestinal cancer. *J. Am. med. Ass.* 204, 1045–7.

Muggia, F. M. (1970). Phase I study of 4'–diethyl–epipodophyllotoxin–β–Dithenylidene glycoside (PTG, NSC 122819). *Proc. Am. Ass. cancer Res.* **11**, 58.

Parker, C. M. (1972). Accuracy of predictions of survival in later stages of cancer. *Br. med. J.* **2**, 29–31.

Penta, J. S., Rozencweig, M., Guarino, A. M., and Muggia, F. M. (1979). Mouse and large animal toxicology studies of twelve antitumor agents: relevance to starting dose for phase I clinical trials. *Cancer Chemother. Pharmac.* **3**, 97–101.

Prieur, D. J., Young, D. M., Davis, R. D., Cooney, D. A., Homan, E. R., Dixon, R. L., and Guarino, A. M. (1973). Procedures for preclinical toxicologic evaluation of cancer chemotherapeutic agents: protocols of the laboratory of toxicology. *Cancer chemother. Rep.* **4**, 1–30.

Rosenblum, M. L., Gerosa, M. A., Dougherty, D. V., Reese, C., Barger, G., Davis, R., Levin, V. A., Strike, T., and Wilson, C. B. (1982). Stem cell sensitivity is the reason for younger patients with malignant gliomas surviving longer than older patients. *Third Human Tumor Cloning Conference Number 11.* Tucson, Arizona.

Rozencweig, M., Von Hoff, D. D., Staquet, M. J., Schein, P. S., Penta, J. S., Goldin, A., Muggia, F. M., Freireich, E. J., and DeVita, V. T., Jr. (1981). Animal toxicology for early clinical trials with anticancer agents. *Cancer clin. Trials* **4**, 21–8.

Salmon, S. E., Hamburger, A. W., Soehnlen, B., Durie, B. G., Alberts, D. J., and Moon, T. E. (1978). Quantitation of differential sensitivity of human tumor stem cells to anticancer drugs. *N. Engl. J. Med.* **298**, 1321–7.

Schein, P. S. (1977). Preclinical toxicology of anticancer agents. *Cancer Res.* **37**, 1934–7.

Von Hoff, D. D., Coltman, Jr, C. A., and Forseth, B. (1981a). Activity of Mitoxantrone in a human tumor cloning system. *Cancer Res.* **41**, 1853–5.

—— Rozencweig, M., and Muggia, F. M. (1977a). Variation in toxicities of anticancer drugs in children and adults. *Clin. Pharmac. Ther.* **21**, 121.

—— Osborne, C. K., Neuenfeldt, B., and Clark, G. M. (1982). Effect of patient age on sensitivity of human breast cancer in the human tumor cloning system. *Third Human Tumor Cloning Conference number 12.* Tucson, Arizona.

—— Casper, J., Bradley, E., Jones, D., and Makuch, R. (1981b). Association between human tumor colony forming assay results and response of an individual patient's tumor to chemotherapy. *Am. J. Med.* **70**, 1027–32.

—— Pollard, E., Kuhn, J., Murray, E., and Coltman, Jr, C. A. (1980). Phase I clinical trial of dihydroxyanthracenedione (NSC 301739). *Cancer Res.* **40**, 1516–18.

—— Houser, D., Gormley, P., Bender, R., Glaubiger, D., and Young, R. C. (1978). Phase I study of methanesulfonamide, N-4-(9acridinyl-amino)-3-methoxy penyl-(m-AMSA) using a single dose schedule. *Cancer treat. Rep.* **62**, 1421–6.

—— Myers, J. W., Kuhn, J., Sandbach, J. E., Pocelinko, R., Clark, G., and Coltman, Jr, C. A. (1981). Phase I clinical trial of 9–10 anthracenedicarboxaldehyde bis ((4,5-dihydro-1*H*-imidazol-2yl)hydrazone) dihydrochloride (CL216,942). *Cancer Res.* **41**, 3118–21.

—— Rozencweig, M., Soper, W. T., Helman, L. J., Penta, J. S., Davis, H. L., and Muggia, F. M. (1977b). Whatever happened to NSC ——? An analysis of discontinued anticancer agents. *Cancer treat. Rep.* **61**, 759–68.

Wasserman, T. N., Slavik, M., and Carter, S. K. (1974) Methyl-CCNU in clinical cancer therapy. *Cancer treat. Res.* **1**, 251–69.

Williams, D. J. and Carter, S. K. (1978). Management of trials in the development of cancer chemotherapy. *Br. J. Cancer* **37**, 434–47.

Woolley, P. V. and Schein, P. J. (1979). *Methods in cancer research.* Academic Press, New York.

Part V
Phase II trials

14 Clinical aspects in the design and conduct of phase II trials

Stephen K. Carter

INTRODUCTION

It takes years of work and a great deal of expense to develop a drug for clinical study. The decision about whether a new drug has enough efficacy to warrant large-scale studies is made based on the phase II study results. Phase II is in essence an efficacy screen. Cancer is not one, but a multiplicity of diseases, each with its own potential responsiveness to a new anti-cancer drug. New drugs are placed into the clinic based, for the most part, on anti-tumour activity observed in transplantable murine tumour systems. These tumour systems are at best predictive for some level of human anti-cancer activity. They do not have the ability to be disease specific in their prediction. In addition, responsiveness or lack thereof, in one human tumour type in no way enables the clinical investigator to predict whether a drug will or will not be found active in another tumour type. Therefore, a new anti-cancer drug must have phase II studies in individual diseases with a specific decision about further trials made on a disease-oriented basis.

When a new drug enters phase I trial the clinical research strategy is completely modality oriented. A variety of advanced diseases are used and the type is not of critical importance. In phase II studies the disease-oriented strategy becomes of equal importance to the modality-oriented strategy (Fig. 14.1). The protocol will be labelled a phase II study of the given drug in lung cancer, breast cancer or colon cancer, etc. The disease-oriented strategy determines several critical factors in the trial design including: (1) where in the treatment course of the disease it is appropriate to do a phase II study of a new agent; and (2) what end result, in terms of efficacy, will be deemed as positive in relation to what the general drug responsiveness of the tumour is and has been.

The phase II study concept, and the appropriate design and strategy considerations, has various applications within clinical oncology. The classic phase II approach involves the evaluation of new anti-cancer drugs. There is in addition the unique aspect of the phase II study as it relates to the following: (1) analogues of known active agents; (2) combination chemotherapy regimens; (3) biological response modifying agents; (4) radiation sensitizing and protector drugs; and (5) predictors of drug response.

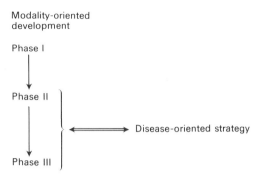

Fig. 14.1. Interaction of modality-oriented development and disease-oriented strategy.

PHASE II OF A NEW DRUG

The phase II evaluation of a new anti-cancer drug is a screen to determine whether the compound has anti-tumour activity worthy of further clinical evaluation (Carter 1977). The crucial decision at the end of the phase II study is whether more widespread (phase III) trials with the drug are indicated or not. The phase II evaluation must be a disease-oriented one in which the decision concerning phase III study is made individually for each tumour type evaluated. The reason why the phase II evaluation is described as a screen is because it is rarely possible to perform a phase II study in every tumour type for which a new drug might be hoped to be active. Therefore, it is usual to select a representative sample of tumour types for phase II study. Within the drug development programme of the Division of Cancer Treatment there has evolved the concept of signal tumours. The concept of signal tumours is that a new drug, as a minimum, will be tested in each of the signal tumours. If the drug is negative it can be reasonably assumed that most likely the drug would not be meaningfully active in other tumour types. The signal tumours include breast cancer, colo-rectal cancer, lung cancer, melanoma, acute leukaemia, and lymphoma.

At the start of phase II study the drug is used at the recommended dose level which has evolved from the phase I study. In most cases this is a close approximation to the maximum tolerated dose (MTD) with modifications appropriate to the extent of prior therapy as learnt from the phase I experience. It is common to choose a single schedule, although occasionally multiple schedules will be used when interest in the drug is extensive. At the current time intermittent schedules are dominant in cancer chemotherapy and the two most common schedules used for new drugs are either five times daily or a single dose every 3 to 4 weeks, depending upon the recovery time from myelosuppression. It is highly unlikely that these intermittent schedules are optimal for every drug, but it has not yet been possible to rationally design an optimal schedule for a new drug from the pharmacokinetic data which may be obtained in phase I study.

The end-points of a phase II study are response rate and toxicity data. Efficacy is determined by a denominator made up of the number of patients treated and/or evaluable and a numerator, which is the number of responding patients utilizing the criteria of the study (Hayward *et al.* 1979). The decision to be reached is whether the agent could be effective in x per cent of patients or more, or is unlikely to be effective in x per cent of patients or more (Gehan and Schneiderman, 1973). Since the number of patients in a phase II study is relatively small and the prognostic heterogeneity within tumours great there is a probable error factor in phase II decision-making which has only been partially elucidated. A positive phase II study will obtain confirmation, or the lack thereof, in subsequent trials. A negative phase II study is repeated rarely, however. Therefore, we have some sense of the false-positive rate in phase II studies but little, if any, about the false-negative rate. This is unfortunate, since a false-negative phase II study is a much more damaging error in drug development and clinical oncology than is a false-positive evaluation.

There are two predominant designs for phase II studies. The first is a drug-oriented approach in which a large number of patients with a variety of diseases are treated with a particular drug. This has been the classical phase II investigation through which the active drugs such as 5-fluorouracil, cyclophosphamide, methotrexate, and, more recently, Adriamycin (O'Bryan, Luce, Talley, Gottlieb, Baker, and Bonadonna 1973) have been detected. Although the total patient numbers are sometimes quite large, there are often relatively few patients in each disease category. In addition, little information is obtained concerning the disease and patient characteristics that affect response.

Actually, there are many parameters of disease and patient population that influence the ability of a drug to induce objective response or to favourably alter survival. For example, the performance status of the patient has a marked effect on survival in lung cancer (Zelen 1974), and on response rate in colon cancer (Moertel, Schutt, Hahn and Reitemeier 1974). Prior chemotherapy affects the objective response rate in solid tumours (Mathe 1973) as well as in the haematological malignancies (Frei, Luce, and Gamble 1973). Various metastatic sites respond differently within the same disease category, such as soft tissue versus visceral disease in breast cancer (Broder and Tormey 1974) and malignant melanoma (Carter and Freidman 1976). The list of significant variables is often unique for each major disease. It is not surprising, therefore, that patient selection factors could significantly alter the results of a small uncontrolled drug-oriented trial.

These considerations have led to the second major type of phase II trial, the disease-oriented study. The critical factor in this approach is that the prognostic variables which may affect response are accounted for in the study design. Currently, these studies are being performed in either a controlled randomized fashion or a non-randomized sequential manner. The principle purpose of randomization is to eliminate conscious or unconscious bias on the part of the investigator in assigning treatments.

In the non-randomized phase II study consecutively entered patients are given a single treatment. The trial is directed to a specific disease category or subcategory, that is pancreatic cancer versus all gastrointestinal cancer, or squamous cell carcinoma of the lung as opposed to all lung cancer. Restrictions on patient entry may be imposed to limit the study to groups with specific prognostic variables or, in large studies, specific prognostic groups may be analysed separately after completion of the study. If possible, most studies should include patients with defined host and disease parameters that may make them likely to respond to a reasonably active agent. The study design, priorities for drug testing, and the type of patients to be treated depend upon the therapy currently available for a given disease.

There are certain malignancies against which most of the standard and investigation agents have been evaluated and for which specific drugs have some effectiveness, albeit limited. Examples of such situations include the use of cyclophosphamide in lung cancer, 5-fluorouracil in colon cancer, and dacarbazine in malignant melanoma. Although none of these agents offer significant benefit for most patients, a small but significant number of objective responses occur. Since a new agent would probably not receive adequate evaluation if all patients had far advanced and refractory disease, a randomized study using the standard agent as a control might be an appropriate means of detecting agents of equal or greater effectiveness.

Two phase II study designs that employ a standard treatment control are illustrated in Fig. 14.2 (designs A and B). Stratification of patients is performed in both studies and randomization to standard therapy accomplishes two purposes. Firstly, it allows testing of the new regimen in previously untreated and relatively good risk patients. Secondly, at least half of the patients will be given what is considered standard treatment. In fact, on design A the cross-over design ensures that most of the patients will receive the standard treatment at some point in their therapy.

The cross-over phase of the design may occur at a fixed time or when disease progression occurs. When the latter point is used, effectiveness of the agents as secondary therapy can be evaluated, possibly some information on the cross-resistance of the two compounds may be obtained, and time to progressive disease can be used as an additional parameter of treatment evaluation. Also, specification of secondary therapy in the overall study design standardizes subsequent treatment and facilitates evaluation of overall survival.

There are some situations in which a standard agent control would be inappropriate. These obviously include diseases where chemotherapy is of no known benefit or so few agents have been tested that no 'standard' treatment can be recommended. At the opposite end of the spectrum are diseases against which initial chemotherapy is so effective that use of an untested agent as primary treatment would be unethical.

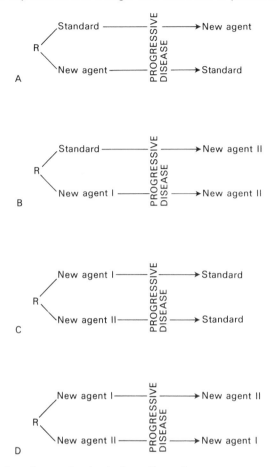

Fig. 14.2. Designs for randomized phase II studies.

The disease-oriented decision, about whether phase III studies with a new drug are indicated, depends upon the efficacy observed in phase II against the background of what chemotherapy can accomplish in the particular tumour in question. In unresponsive tumours such as large bowel cancer, non-oat-cell lung cancer, malignant melanoma and pancreatic cancer, almost any level of activity can be considered as a positive phase II study. In responsive tumours in contrast this is not the case. Not only must the response rate be in general higher, but toxicological considerations are of greater importance. In responsive tumours combination chemotherapy will be the general rule and a new drug should have toxicological characteristics which would not preclude easy combination with other active drugs. An outline of my own personal criteria which would warrant phase III studies with a new structure are given in Table 14.1.

Table 14.1. *Phase II studies in adult tumours: criteria which would warrant phase III studies with a new structure*

Tumour	Can phase II be performed in previously untreated patients	Objective response rate which would warrant further study (%)	Comment
Colo-rectal	Yes	20–30	Drugs of equal activity to 5-FU have not given successful combinations
Breast	No	30–40	A response rate of 20–30% would be acceptable if toxicity spectrum was positive for combination, for example lack of myelosuppression
Pancreas	Yes	20–30	Same as for colon
Gastric	Yes	20–30	Greater potential for combination regimens
Non-small-cell lung	Yes	20–30	Should be more active than current agents since combinations of current 'active' agents have not been successful in impacting upon survival
Small cell lung	No	30–40	Same as for breast
Ovary	No	30–40	Same as for breast
Cervix	Yes	20–30	
Bladder	Yes	20–30	
Prostate	Yes	20–30	
Testis	No	30–50	
Malignant melanoma	Yes	20–30	Drugs as active as DTIC and nitrosoureas have not been successful building blocks for combinations
Squamous cell carcinoma head and neck	Yes	30–40	

Table 14.1. *Phase II studies in adult*

Tumour	Can phase II be performed in previously untreated patients	Objective response rate which would warrant further study (%)	Comment
Hodgkin's Disease	No	30–50	Toxicological characteristics which favour ease of combination would push criteria toward lower response rate
Non-Hodgkin's lymphoma	No	30–50	Same as above
Acute myelocytic leukaemia	No	20–30	Same as above
Multiple myeloma	No	30–40	Same as above

PHASE II TESTING OF ANALOGUES

Analogues pose specific problems in phase II study because their evaluation must be made in comparison with what can be accomplished with the parent structure and in relation with what the rationale was in choosing the analogues for test (Carter 1978). An analogue can be superior to its parent structure in five different ways; (1) it can have a superior efficacy in responsive tumours; (2) it can have efficacy in unresponsive tumours (broader spectrum); (3) it can have efficacy in tumours resistant to the parent drug, this resistance manifested by failure after treatment with the parent structure; (4) it can have diminished acute toxicity; or (5) it can have diminished chronic toxicity. The end-point for a positive phase II with an analogue depends upon which of the five potential ways the analogue's superiority is hoped for.

If the oncological strategy hopes for superior efficacy in a responsive tumour to the parent compound, then the phase II trial must show enough evidence of that possibility to make phase III trials indicated. This approach can be complicated if the parent structure is part of a highly active primary combination. An example would be the evaluation of a vincristine analogue in Hodgkin's Disease. There are two approaches to solving the problem. One solution is to test the analogue after failure on a non-vincristine containing combination, such as MVPP (nitrogen mustard, vinblastine, procarbazine, and prednisone) and ABVD (Adriamycin, bleomycin, vinblastine, and dacarbazine). The second approach is to substitute the analogue for vincristine in the MOPP combination (mechlorethamine, oncovin, pro-carbazine, and prednisone). The major difficulty with this second approach is it takes a phase III study to achieve the answer and in essence assumes a positive phase II.

The evaluation of an analogue in an intrinsically unresponsive tumour to the parent structure is a great deal easier. In this situation the evaluation becomes almost identical to that of a new structure, since any level of meaningful activity is indicative of the need for phase III study.

The strategy for a lack of cross-resistance to the parent structure is also relatively simple. A positive phase II only requires any level of significant activity in patients who have developed progressive disease while under treatment with the parent structure. This type of phase II evaluation by definition must occur as at least second line drug treatment. This must be kept in mind in the analysis of a negative study. A negative study may be due to far advanced disease beyond the hope of any response rather than true resistance. This problem can be handled by close attention to the performance status and other important response variables in the analysis.

Analogues developed in the hope of diminished toxicity have increased in importance in recent years. This has been true particularly with the analogues of: (1) Adriamycin (cardiac toxicity); (2) bleomycin (pulmonary toxicity); (3) cis-platinum (renal toxicity); and (4) nitrosoureas (marrow toxicity). If the desired end-point for an analogue is diminished toxicity then the phase II study evaluation has two components: (a) in terms of efficacy there should be presumptive evidence of at least comparable activity with the parent structure; and (b) in terms of toxicity there should be presumptive evidence of diminished toxicity in the critical parameter. The toxicity end-point in phase II is difficult if chronic toxicity is the hope. An example would be in the case of an anthracycline analogue of Adriamycin designed with the hope of diminished cardiac toxicity. The lack of cardiac toxicity in a phase II study can be attributed to the fact that chronic dosing has not occurred. Evidence of cardiac toxicity in phase II however would be highly damaging to the potential for phase III study.

PHASE II TRIALS OF COMBINATION CHEMOTHERAPY

Combinations of drugs are used in order to maximize cell kill and to overcome resistance. Successful combinations involve using drugs active when used alone against the tumour in question. A combination chemotherapy regimen also has a phase I and II concept, but it is usually telescoped into a combined study which is often labelled as a pilot study. The phase I aspect of the pilot study involves establishing the dose levels of the various drugs in the combination. The phase II component involves an evaluation of the efficacy in the tumour type being studied. In most cases combination chemotherapy regimens are disease-oriented and are made up of drugs active against the disease in question when used alone. Because of this, activity at some level is almost always observed and the phase II evaluation is a comparative one as it is in single agent phase II studies. The evaluative comparison that is made with a combination varies depending upon the effectiveness of chemotherapy in general against the specific tumour. For example, a combination against colorectal cancer should show enough activity in a pilot (phase II) study to indicate that it may be superior to 5-fluorouracil used alone, which gives an objective response rate of about 20 per cent. In advanced breast cancer the phase II evaluation would involve potential superiority to an overall response rate of 50 to 70 per cent and a complete response rate of 10 to 20 per cent as primary chemotherapy treatment. If the combination regimen is being tested as second line chemotherapy, then a potential response rate in excess of 20 to 30 per cent would be the end-point. In responsive tumours, therefore, the phase II evaluation comparison is complex depending on where, in the course of advanced disease, it is being tested and where it is hoped that it will be ultimately used.

Toxicological considerations will also be an important part of the phase II evaluation of a new combination. The toxicity will be looked at from two potential viewpoints. One will be the viewpoint of toxicity when used in a palliative mode for advanced disease. The second viewpoint will be the toxicity when used in a curative mode as part of adjuvant or combined modality therapy.

PHASE II TRIALS WITH BIOLOGICAL RESPONSE MODIFYING AGENTS

Biological response modifying (BRM) agents are materials designed to affect host response to tumours in a way which will result in a positive therapeutic benefit. Examples currently under clinical study include interferon and thymosin.

With a BRM agent it may well be true the MTD may not be the optimal dose for achieving the hoped for therapeutic gain. Despite this, it would appear to be prudent to establish the MTD in phase I study so as to ultimately relate the maximally effective dose to the dose–response effect for toxicity. It must be assumed that there will be a dose level which will achieve optimal modification of host biological response to the tumour. This could be called the maximum effective dose (MED). Depending upon the toxicity potential of the BRM agent and its mechanism of action it may be that the MED and MTD will be identical as it is for most chemotherapeutic agents. This might not occur for one of two basic reasons. The first would be if the toxicity occurs at relatively low dose levels before the absolute MED can be reached. The second reason, which is related, would be if there is a very wide dose–response effect which extends up to very high doses. It is hard to imagine that any biologically active material would not cause effects on normal cells at some dose level.

As indicated earlier, the phase II study for a chemotherapeutic agent is an efficacy screen to determine whether there is enough evidence of anti-tumour effect to warrant large-scale phase III studies. It is known that the activity, or lack thereof, in one tumour type with cytotoxic drugs will not predict for another type. Therefore a series of disease specific phase II studies are undertaken.

With a BRM it must be assumed, until proven otherwise, that effectiveness will differ in different tumour types. This may be caused by any one of the following facts: (1) different tumours may elicit different host response; (2) different tumours may be more or less amenable to therapeutic benefit from a BRM effect; (3) differential tumour cell burdens may respond differently to BRM effects; (4) pharmacological sanctuaries or privileged sites may exist for BRM effect. Because of this it would be prudent to design a series of disease-oriented phase II studies for BRM agents.

With cytotoxic drugs the therapeutic end-point for phase II study is objective regression of tumour. What is not known is whether this will be feasible for BRM agents. It was not deemed appropriate for immune modulating agents such as BCG, *C. parvum*, levamisole, etc. It is being used for current trials of human leucocyte interferon. It may therefore differ with different BRM agents. If objective regression is obtainable with a BRM, then the phase II strategy is simple; but if it is not, it will be more complicated.

If objective response cannot be used as an end-point for phase II study, there are two broad possibilities for phase II design. One approach would be to add the BRM to standard therapy and use as the judgement parameter a prolongation of response duration or survival. This has the disadvantage of requiring a control group for comparison. With immunomodulating agents many groups attempted to use historical controls without a great deal of success. It is difficult to control for all important prognostic variables and there are potential differences in diagnostic work-up and care delivery which are very difficult to control for.

In addition early actuarial estimation may give one an early false positive, since there is a longer follow-up time for the historical control. If a prospective randomized control is used, then the problem becomes the use of a phase III methodology to give a phase II answer. In such a phase II study a statistically significant difference in survival may not be needed but just enough comparability or a suggestion of superiority to warrant a phase III study. Obviously if such a study design is used, the rubric of phase II–III study might be the most applicable.

Another approach would be to look for only a consistent modulation of host response, which would be assumed to be intrinsically valuable. Armed with this consistency of implied biological response impact, appropriate phase III studies could then be considered justifiable. This approach has the attraction of clinical decision-making based on presumed mechanisms of action, but has the drawback of not attempting to demonstrate evidence of true biological impact prior to commitment of large-scale clinical trial resources.

If a BRM agent's effect can only be measured by a positive influence on survival this strategy may be the only one it is feasible to contemplate.

If the phase II concept for a BRM is indirect measurement of host response through some laboratory or clinical examination, then a controlled design seems to be essential. What has been shown with measurement of immune reactivity, such as skin tests, lymphocyte blastogenesis assays, etc., is a high degree of intrinsic biological variability. A double-blind study at the Mayo Clinic of two dose levels of methanol extraction residue of BCG (MER) with placebo revealed comparable enhanced immunological reactivity with both drug and placebo (O'Connell, Moertel, Ritts, Frytak, and Reitemeir 1979). Such could be the case with a BRM.

A phase II design could involve a double-blind evaluation of the BRM and a placebo with the end-point being impact on a group of clinical and laboratory assays presumed to be indications of modulated host biological response to the tumour. If a difference that favoured the BRM was observed large-scale adjuvant or phase III trials would be justified. This would involve a phase II study that was both more complex in design and more expensive than a classic phase II study with a cytotoxic compound. This would be worthwhile, however, if it could effectively screen for the potential value of a long-term and highly expensive adjuvant trial. In addition, the phase II concept should be flexible enough to encompass a wide range of biological materials.

PHASE II TRIALS WITH RADIATION SENSITIZERS

A new emphasis in clinical oncology has been the development of drugs designed with the purpose of sensitizing cells to kill with radiation therapy. Currently under test are a series of electron affinic drugs which experimentally can enhance the radiation sensitivity of hypoxic tumour cells to make them act as if they were oxic in relation to X-ray effect. The first of these to have been tested clinically was metronidazole. Currently misonidazole and desmethyl-misonidazole, which are second and third generation analogues, are in the clinic with newer analogues soon to follow.

The phase II evaluation of these drugs must be performed in combination with the delivery of radiation therapy. The efficacy end-point must be evidence of enough activity with the drug + X-ray to indicate a reasonable possibility that a controlled study against X-ray alone would be positive. At the same time the toxicity of the drug + X-ray must be compared with historical background of X-ray alone in order to develop a preliminary therapeutic index.

The phase II studies with misonidazole were designed to be cancer site and stage specific (Wasserman, Stetz, and Philips 1981). They were estimated to require between 30 and 40 patients per study using a fixed dose schedule of radiation and misonidazole. These studies were designed to be preparatory for phase III studies and there were five defined goals: (1) to establish the tolerance of any modifications in the dose schedule of radiation that were necessary in order to use misonidazole; (2) to establish the tolerance of misonidazole in a large number of patients with a given cancer site and stage; (3) to increase the clinical familiarity of multiple investigators with misonidazole; (4) to establish the reproducibility of the ultraviolet pharmacological assay; and (5) to look for information on the frequency of tumour clearance compared with the historical clinical experience of radiation alone in the specific sites and stages under test. The schedules of radiation and misonidazole in these studies differed in three ways study by study: (1) conventional fractionation of radiation therapy with two fractions in 18 hours, with misonidazole being given once or twice per week; (2) intermittent fractionation of radiation therapy and intermittent misonidazole with the sensitizer being given prior to every fraction of radiation; and (3) a large weekly dose of radiation plus misonidazole and conventional fractionation without the sensitizer for the rest of the week.

PREDICTORS OF RESPONSE

The clinical evaluation of predictors of response will require a specific strategy which is only now in evolution (Carter 1981). The experience that has been gained with the estrogen receptor (ER) assay and the stem cell assay will, hopefully, lay the groundwork for a more expeditious and efficient clinical evaluation of future potential predictors.

The evaluation of a predictive assay goes through two broad stages of study. The first stage involves retrospective correlation and the second involves prospective correlation. The initial clinical study of a potential predictive assay takes place within a single institution where patients are treated empirically and their response, or lack thereof, is correlated with the prediction made by the assay in question. In a small number of patients, the true-positive and true-negative rates are calculated to see whether larger-scale studies are indicated. This initial study could be described as the phase I evaluation. In this study, a preliminary estimate of cost effectiveness is made and an initial determination of a cut-off point for positivity can be made.

If this initial study is encouraging, then a larger scale retrospective evaluation (phase II) is the next step. This may involve data from many institutions or just wider scale investigation within a smaller number. The design of the study is still to treat patients empirically, independently of the assay, and afterwards correlate the effect with the assay results. The end-point is still a calculation of the sensitivity and specificity, as demonstrated by the true- and false-positive and true- and false-negative rates. The economics and the reproducibility of the assay on a large scale, particularly in different institutions, becomes an important part of the evaluation. Another critically important aspect of this study is a final determination of what the cut-off point will be for positivity in the large scale prospective studies to come.

The phase III aspect of the evaluation becomes a prospective study of the value of the assay. In this kind of study, the assay is performed first and therapy is determined by the result. The clinical results of treating by the assay must be shown to be superior to the results of treating *a comparable group of patients* independently of the assays. This comparison will involve the standard efficacy end-points (response, duration of response, and survival) in relationship to the toxicity of therapy. If superiority is found, then the cost of the assay must be factored into the analysis to determine whether the increase in the therapeutic index, demonstrated in a selected clinical research population, will be cost effective in large-scale general patient use.

The Phase IV evaluation of the predictive assay will be a study of the assay in a large-scale population to see whether the results obtained in the clinical research setting can be translated into a cost effective manner to the general population.

The prospective stage of the clinical evaluation has been the most neglected in terms of clinical trial methodology development. For example, a truly prospective evaluation of the ER assay has still to be performed, and only now are investigators beginning to think about how to evaluate prospectively the stem cell assay.

SOME GENERAL CONSIDERATIONS

The proper selection of patients for phase II studies is a critically important aspect of the proper design and execution of these trials. The patients chosen should be those that have a reasonable potential of responding to an active compound. The prognostic variable, which cuts across all disease lines and is one of the most potent in any phase II trial, is the performance status. Whether the scale used is the Karnofsky (KPS) (Karnofsky and Burchenall 1949), or the Zubrod modification (also called the ECOG performance scale) (Zubrod *et al.* 1960), patients with poor performance status have a lower response score to most therapies than do those with a high score. Ideally, patients for phase II trials should be chosen with a reasonable performance status, such as $KPS \geq 60$. In the interpretation of phase II trials careful attention should be paid to the performance status of the patients along with other important prognostic variables. Among these other variables, extent of disease and prior therapy are both ones that usually cut across disease lines.

Another important aspect of selecting patients for phase II trials is the choice of patients with measurable disease. Objective regression is far from a perfect measuring tool for drug effect, but it is the best available to us at this time. In the past, many attempts have been made to utilize criteria other than objective regression in measuring effect. The most intelligent and complex approach was the criteria developed by the late David Karnofsky. These criteria attempted to objectify the subjective along with measuring the shrinkage of measurable lesions. This approach has lost favour since it has become recognized that investigator bias can play too strong a role with these criteria and that there is a lack of comparability from investigator to investigator.

There exist some tumour situations in which fully measurable lesions are not commonly found. The prime examples are lung cancer and prostate cancer, but the problem exists in bladder cancer, cervix cancer, and head and neck as well. In lung cancer many patients present with masses arising out of the mediastinum and which, therefore, are not fully measurable in a bidimensional way. These lesions tend to be called 'evaluable' as apart from measurable. These patients are often included in phase II trials with the demand being made that these 'evaluable' lesions must shrink by more than 75 per cent to qualify as a response. Eagan, Fleming, and Schoonover (1979), at the Mayo Clinic, have developed response criteria for these evaluable masses and have shown, at least in their hands, that the response rates and survival are comparable in patients with measurable and evaluable lesions.

Prostate cancer is a particular challenge for phase II study because the majority of patients present solely with bone lesions which are impossible to clearly measure. This has led to various response criteria, which allow for stability of disease, pain relief, and the diminishing of elevated acid phosphatase in determining a response. Unfortunately, different groups use different mixes of criteria, which makes the prostate chemotherapy literature a minefield of difficult to interpret data.

A possibility for phase II study that has been entertained only occasionally is to use survival as the end-point. Survival has the advantage of being a clean end-point and reflecting the impact of therapy on all patients. Survival has many difficulties however. One of these is the heterogeneity of starting points which can be chosen. The starting point of initiation of chemotherapy can be an extremely heterogeneous one in diseases such as breast cancer, where many therapies are administered in a range of sequences. Other problems include the fact that survival can be influenced by therapy after relapse on the phase II treatment and the difficulty of developing a criteria for 'activity'. Determining that the survival of a cohort of patients treated with a phase II agent indicates activity, assumes the ability to relate that survival to a reliable historical control for a comparable cohort either on no therapy or on a standard therapy. This historical control does not exist at this time, and so only a prospective concomitant control is usable. This requires a phase III methodology to answer a phase II question.

An important consideration in phase II studies is who should undertake them. Given the investigative nature of the phase II study and the critical importance of optimal delivery of the therapy in question, they should only be performed by oncological teams experienced in clinical research. Some phase II studies are performed by single institutions, others by multi-centre co-operative groups. Ideally a single institution study is preferable because of the tighter quality control and the relative consistency of overall therapeutic approach. Multi-centre trials are needed when single institution resources will not suffice in a reasonable time frame. Large-scale co-operative phase II studies are worrisome for the following reasons: (1) there is a tendency for some institutions to place only a small number of cases on the study, leading to concerns about effectiveness of therapy delivery and case selection bias; and (2) there is a tendency for an excessive number of patients to be placed on the study, which raises ethical concerns, if the study turns out to be negative.

CONCLUSION

The phase II study is one of the most important junctions in the clinical development of any new therapy. For a new drug it is the critical decision point as to whether widespread studies are indicated or the compound should be dropped from further consideration. The phase II concept exists for all new therapies, be they combination chemotherapy regimens, new radiation oncology approaches, new surgical approaches, new biological response modification approaches or combined modality thrusts. The common denominator for all is that after a relatively small number of patients have been treated, a decision must be made as to whether more study is indicated. The relatively small number of patients in a phase II study raises the spector of a high false-positive and false-negative rate. A false negative is the most undesirable of all end-points, since a negative study is repeated rarely and, therefore, in such a study a good therapy is lost. A positive study will be repeated and so a false positive will ultimately be discovered with only a loss of time and resources as the price to pay.

The phase II strategy and methodology, and an end-point cut-off for positivity, should be well worked out prior to placing a new drug into the clinic or launching trials with a new therapy. Too often in oncology, new drugs and new therapies are placed into the clinic with the hope of achieving a magic bullet type of breakthrough. This finding of a 'penicillin for cancer' will be easy to evaluate since the historical data base will easily suffice as a control. Most of the advances in cancer treatment have *not* come through such dramatic breakthroughs but rather have come through the establishment of building blocks of active drugs and therapeutic approaches. To uncover these building blocks requires a careful strategy and methodology of clinical work-up with the phase II aspect being pivotal. Clinical oncology is full of new drugs, particularly analogues, which exist for years in the limbo of investigative studies without a clear decision as to what their role, if any, actually is.

The essence of any good phase II study, as with any clinical trial, is quality control and comparability. Clinical oncology needs to address the issues of quality control, response criteria, and data reporting techniques with the degree of rigour and co-operation that has led over the years to the establishment of accepted systems of histological classification and staging. The oncology literature is a jungle of free enterprise approaches to clinical trial interpretation and data reporting. The reader must approach the literature with a *caveat emptor* philosophy. The literature is ever growing and unless order is brought out of the chaos we may lose good new treatments and may expose our patients to inferior treatments unnecessarily.

REFERENCES

Broder, L. and Tormey, D. (1974). Combination chemotherapy of carcinoma of the breast. *Cancer Treat. Rev.* **1**, 183–205.

Carter, S. K. (1977). Clinical trials in cancer chemotherapy. *Cancer* **40**, 544–57.

—— (1978). The clinical evaluation of analogues. I. The overall problem. *Cancer Chemother. Pharmac.* **1**, 69–72.

—— (1981). Predictors of response and their clinical evaluation. *Cancer Chemother. Pharmac.* **7**, 1–4.

—— and Freidman, M. A. (1976). 5-(3,3-dimethyl-1-triazeno)-imidazole-4-carboxamide (DTIC, DIC, NSC 45388)—a new antitumor agent with activity against malignant melanoma. *Eur. J. Cancer* **8**, 85–92.

Eagan, R. T., Fleming, T. R., and Schoonover, B. S. (1979). Evaluation of response criteria in advanced lung cancer. *Cancer* **44**, 1125–8.

Frei, E., III, Luce, J. K., and Gamble, J. F. (1973). Combination chemotherapy in advanced Hodgkin's disease: induction and maintenance of remission. *Ann. intern. Med.* **79**, 376–382.

Gehan, E. A. and Schneiderman, M. A. (1973). Experimental design of clinical trials. In: *Cancer medicine* (Eds. J. F. Holland and E. Frei, III). Lea and Ferbiger, Philadelphia.

Hayward, J. L., Carbone, P. P., Henson, J. C., Kumaoka, S., Segaloff, A., and Rubens, R. D. (1979). Assessment of response to therapy in advanced breast cancer. *Cancer* **39**, 1289–94.

Karnofsky, D. A. and Burchenall, J. H. (1949). The clinical evaluation of chemotherapeutic agents in cancer. In *Evaluation of chemotherapeutic agents* (ed. M. C. Macleod) pp. 199–205. Columbia University Press, New York.

Mathé, G. (1973). Clinical examination of drugs, a scientific and ethical challenge. *Biomedicine* **18**, 169–72.

Moertel, C. G., Schutt, A. J., Hahn, R. G., and Reitemeier, R. S. (1974). Effects of patient selection on results on phase II chemotherapy trials in gastrointestinal cancer. *Cancer Chemother. Rep.* **58**, 257–60.

O'Bryan, R. M., Luce, J. K., Talley, R. W., Gottlieb, J. A., Baker, L. H., and Bonadonna, G. (1973). Phase II evaluation of Adriamycin in human neoplasia. *Cancer* **32**, 1–8.

O'Connel, M. J., Moertel, C. J., Ritts, Jr, R. E., Frytak, S., and Reitemeir, R. J. (1979). A comparative clinical and immunological assessment of methanol extraction residue of Bacillus Calmette–Guerin *vs.* placebo in patients with advanced cancer. *Cancer Res.* **39**, 3720–4.

Wasserman, T. H., Stetz, J., and Phillips, T. L. (1981). Radiation Therapy Oncology Group clinical trials with misonidazole. *Cancer* **47**, 2382–90.

Zelen, M. (1974). Keynote address on biostatistics and data retrieval. *Cancer Chemother. Rep.* **4**(3), 31–42.

Zubrod, G. C., Scheidemann, M., Frei, E. III, Brindley, C., Gold, L. G., Schnider, B., Oviedo, R., Gorman, J., Jones, R. Jr, Johnson, U., Colsky, J., Chalmers, T., Ferguson, B., Derick, M., Holland, J., Selawry, O., Regelson, W., Lasagna, C., and Owens, A. H. Jr (1960). Appraisal of methods for the study of chemotherapy of cancer in man: comparative therapeutic trial of nitrogen mustard and triethylene thio phosphoramide. *J. chron. Dis.* **11**, 7–33.

15 Statistical aspects in the design and analysis of phase II clinical trials

Jay Herson

INTRODUCTION

Research with a new chemotherapeutic agent generally progresses through several levels as described by Williams and Carter (1978). Firstly, pre-clinical or animal studies are performed to establish the agent's mode of action and evidence of acute toxicity. The first-level clinical trial is the phase I study. Here, consecutive patients are treated with the new agent and 'non-toxic' dosage schedules determined. The recommended dose is then used in the phase II or efficacy study. The purpose of the phase II trial is to determine if the new agent is of sufficient effectiveness to be worthy of further study. Once it is determined that a minimum level of effectiveness has been attained, randomized phase III comparative trials involving the new agent, usually in combination with other agents, are conducted.

Phase II trials are carried out in either a single institution or in a multi-institutional setting. In most settings, patients whose disease is first diagnosed as a particular malignancy are treated on the current phase III trial for that malignancy. Patients who relapse on a phase III trial are then offered treatment on a phase II trial. When several phase II, phase I, or pilot trials are being conducted for a given tumour type concurrently, an agreed upon priority list determines the order of trials on which patients are entered. Unless otherwise specified, it will be assumed in what follows that all patients on a phase II trial have the same tumour type.

GENERAL SPECIFICATIONS

Measure of effectiveness

To evaluate a new treatment, a measure of effectiveness must be selected. A common measure is the response proportion (represented by θ)—the proportion of all patients on the phase II trial judged to have responded to treatment with the new agent. The principal investigator classifies each patient as a responder or non-responder to therapy using previously agreed upon objective criteria at some fixed time after the start of therapy. Appropriate clinical measures of response have been discussed by Muggia, Rozencweig, Staquet, and McGuire (1980) and reported by the WHO (1979).

Response proportion threshold (θ_0)

To answer the fundamental question asked in a phase II trial, 'Does the new agent have sufficient efficacy to be worthy of further study?' investigators must specify a threshold value of the response proportion (represented by θ_0) as well as a decision-making strategy.

The threshold is the cut-off point between values of θ that indicate efficacy and those that indicate inactivity. It is selected by investigators at the commencement of the trial and varies according to the type of malignancy and type of chemotherapeutic agent under investigation. Values of θ_0 between 0.20 and 0.30 are common. θ_0 is set at this fairly low level because in this era of combination chemotherapy, a single agent is not expected to have high efficacy when used alone. Moreover, phase II patients have relapsed at least once and thus have fairly advanced disease. Their malignant cells may be resistant to 'state of the art' agents.

The position of the new agent in the priority list and the nature of the preceding treatments certainly affects the magnitude of θ_0. Suppose a phase II trial of anguidine for remission induction in acute lymphocytic leukaemia in children was conducted with the priority list shown in Table 15.1 in effect. In

Table 15.1. *Hypothetical priority list for clinical trials for remission induction in childhood acute leukaemia*

Patient status	Remission induction treatment
Newly diagnosed	Vincristine + prednisone
First relapse	Vincristine + prednisone + L-asparaginase
Second relapse	Rubidazone
Third relapse	Anguidine

this setting, by the time patients are entered on the anguidine trial, not only are they in their third relapse but their disease is resistant to conventional therapy (vincristine + prednisone or vincristine + prednisone + L-asparaginase) and to a fairly successful new agent (rubidazone). One would expect θ_0 to be chosen lower for anguidine in this case than if anguidine were used for first-relapse patients right after they had received vincristine + prednisone.

For convenience, two additional values of the response proportion will be defined; θ_1, the largest value of θ for which the treatment will be considered highly ineffective, and θ_2, the smallest value of θ for which the treatment will be considered highly effective $(\theta_1 < \theta_0 < \theta_2)$.

Types of error

In deciding on the disposition of a new agent, two types of error can be made: false positives (recommending an ineffective agent for further study) and false negatives (declaring an effective agent ineffective). The use of statistical strategies that control these two types of error is of paramount importance and will be discussed later. Investigators must decide which type of error is more important to minimize. Many believe the false negative is the more serious error (Williams and Carter 1978) because, when committed, it may discourage further use of an effective agent. Although the importance of a false-positive error is also conceded, it is believed that in this case the ineffectiveness of the agent will be discovered in further study.

It is difficult to generalize on the consequences of false-positive and false-negative errors on future patients. Much depends on the precise nature of the future use of the new agent. If, after passing the phase II level, the new agent is to be used in combination with other drugs of known effectiveness, the risk of a false-positive conclusion might be less than if the new agent were to be used in single-agent therapy. However, if the particular combination in which the new agent was incorporated offered considerable toxicity to the patient, then the false-positive consequences might exceed the false-negative consequences. Similarly, if future use of the new agent is as a single agent, there might be fewer consequences of a false positive if the new agent is to be used in an adjuvant trial in which patients are essentially tumour-free at the time chemotherapy is initiated than if the new drug is to be used in a trial for patients with metastatic disease.

The magnitude of the false-positive error must be taken into account. If $\theta_0 = 0.30$ and a false-positive error is made when the true underlying response rate (θ') equals 0.27, the consequences of further testing are not as great as when the error is made when $\theta' = 0.10$. The decision-making error issues can be at least partially resolved by conducting phase II trials that seek to eliminate the clearly ineffective drugs (for example a response proportion of $\theta' \leq 0.15$ when $\theta_0 = 0.30$).

In interpreting the consequences of decision errors in phase II trials, it must be understood that a new agent neither automatically appears in a future phase III trial nor is automatically eliminated from further research solely on the basis of the outcome of a phase II trial. Future research is dependent on the availability of alternative new agents that show promise, concurrent research by other institutions, the necessity for new agents in phase III research, clinical judgement, and of course, funding.

Hypothesis testing

The false-positive and false-negative errors may be related to type I and type II errors in statistical hypothesis testing (Colton 1974). Let

$$H_0: \theta < \theta_0 \text{ (null hypothesis)}$$
$$H_1: \theta \geq \theta_0 \text{ (alternate hypothesis)}.$$

Here, a type I error, rejecting the null hypothesis when true, is equivalent to a false-positive error, and a type II error, accepting the null hypothesis when false, is equivalent to a false-negative error. The power of the hypothesis test is the probability that the null hypothesis is rejected for a given value of θ under the alternative hypothesis. The power may be computed for any value of θ under the alternative hypothesis. Thus, the significance level of a hypothesis test is equivalent to the probability of a false-positive error and the complement of the power of the test is equivalent to the probability of a false-negative error.

Sample size determination and expected trial duration

The greater the sample size, the greater the precision in estimation of θ and the greater the power of the hypothesis test (the smaller the false-negative-error probability) against a given alternative. Biostatisticians can compute the minimum sample-size requirement on the basis of investigator specifications for precision and false-positive and false-negative-error probabilities.

The expected duration of the trial is estimated on the basis of required sample size and an estimate of annual patient accrual. The patient pool for a phase II trial consists of patients who relapse on a phase III trial or phase II trial of higher priority. Thus, accrual estimates can be obtained from the relapse experience on these 'feeder' trials.

A phase II trial should generally be completed within 2 years. Longer trials are usually accompanied by dwindling interest on the part of investigators. A decision on maximum tolerable duration is normally made on the basis of funding, how many other groups are doing research with this new agent, and the rapidity with which new agents are needed for incorporation into phase III clinical trial protocols.

When estimated 2-year patient accrual falls short of required sample sizes for control of false-positive and false-negative errors, frequently investigators either compromise their specifications of maximum allowable errors or commence the trial under the false security that ultimate patient accrual will be much greater than was estimated at the outset of the trial. When unacceptable accrual is expected, investigators would be better advised to negotiate a joint venture with another institution in order to take advantage of the larger combined accrual rate.

DESIGNS

A design is a plan of action for carrying out the trial and for deciding whether a treatment is likely to be active or inactive.

Single-stage design

In a single-stage design, the new agent is classified as either effective or ineffective on the basis of a fixed sample size (N) which is reached regardless of whether the early trial results exhibit evidence of effectiveness or ineffectiveness. If $\leq C$ (critical value) responders are observed in N patients, the treatment is classified as ineffective, whereas $>C$ responders results in a conclusion of treatment activity. The parameters N and C constitute the single-stage design specification.

To determine the minimum required sample size and C, investigators must specify: (1) θ_0; (2) the required precision in $\hat{\theta}$ (usually in terms of maximally tolerated coefficient of variation); (3) the maximally tolerated significance level; (4) an alternative, θ_2, for which rejection of H_0 is desired; and (5) minimally tolerated power against $\theta = \theta_2$.

In general, sample sizes of 20 to 30 usually suffice for $0.20 \leq \theta_0 \leq 0.30$, coefficient of variation ≤ 30 per cent, $0.30 \leq \theta_2 \leq 0.50$, significance level of 0.05, and power 0.80.

Sequential and multi-stage designs

Motivation

In recent years, investigators have become aware of the need for early termination of phase II trials for ethical reasons when early data tend to support the hypothesis of treatment ineffectiveness, and for early reporting of results when the early data favour the hypothesis of treatment effectiveness. Early termination, either with or without a data-motivated statistical hypothesis test, has the effect of increasing either the false-positive or false-negative-error rate (depending on how the hypothesis is formulated) usually above tolerable limits (Armitage, McPherson, and Rowe 1969).

Strictly sequential designs

In the search for designs that permit early termination of the trial while maintaining overall control of false positive and false negative errors, a final choice might be strictly sequential designs (Wald 1947). Here, no fixed sample size is specified and investigators make a decision whether to terminate or continue accruing patients after each new patient is entered. The methods allow for control of overall false-positive and false-negative-error probabilities. Several papers have been written regarding the problems in conducting strictly sequential trials of cancer therapy (Byar, Simon,

Friedewald, Schlesselman, De Mets, Ellenberg, Gail, and Ware 1976; Pocock, 1978; George 1980). The chief drawbacks are the administrative burdens of maintaining a constant vigil over the data, and the delays between patient entry and response determination, and between response determination and the reporting of response to the trial co-ordinator.

Multi-stage designs

A compromise between the strictly sequential and the single-stage design is the multi-stage design. Although a 'full' sample of size N is declared, patients are entered in k batches of sample size $n_1, n_2, \ldots, n_k$ where $n_1 + n_2 + \ldots + n_k = N$. After each batch is accrued, a decision is made either to terminate the trial or to continue to the next stage on the basis of the number of responding patients observed up to that point. Multi-stage methods allow for control of overall false-positive and false-negative-error rates.

The major disadvantage of the multi-stage design lies in the administrative problems in monitoring the trial so as to properly order the incoming observations and to minimize non-randomness in the sequence of incoming patient data. Herson (1983) has presented procedures for dealing with these problems.

The general structure of multi-stage designs is depicted in Table 15.2. Some

Table 15.2. *General structure of the multi-stage design*

Stage	Sample size	Cumulative sample size	Cumulative critical values	Cumulative observed number of responders	Action
1	n_1	N_1	C_1, D_1	R_1	Terminate trial for ineffectiveness if $R_1 \leq C_1$. Terminate for effectiveness if $R_1 > D_1$.
2	n_2	N_2	C_2, D_2	R_2	Terminate trial for ineffectiveness if $R_2 \leq C_2$. Terminate for effectiveness if $R_2 > D_2$.
...	...	...	...	...	
...	...	...	...	...	
k	n_k	$N_k = N$	C_k, D_k $(C_k = D_k - 1)$	R_k	Trial terminates. Data support ineffectiveness if $R_k \leq C_k$ and effectiveness if $R_k > C_k$.

multi-stage designs proposed for phase II trials vary slightly from this structure, and these differences will be pointed out below. The parameters k, N_i, C_i, D_i, for $i = 1, \ldots, k$ constitute the multi-stage design specification.

Some multi-stage designs may be called early termination rules. In this type of design, N, C, and D are selected on the basis of a single-stage design and the various intermediate stages are derived from them. In the general multi-stage situation, N_i, C_i, and D_i are chosen by other considerations and N, C, and D are not necessarily related to any specific single-stage design.

Multi-stage designs may also be classified by their ultimate purpose. Hypothesis testing constitutes only one of three ways multi-stage designs may be classified by purpose. Some multi-stage designs seek only to estimate θ rather than to present a formal method for reaching a conclusion on treatment effectiveness. Finally, some designs are for risk minimization. These designs are based on decision theory. Instead of concentrating on false-positive and false-negative-error rates, decision theory methods establish formulas for computing the 'loss' inherent in correct and incorrect decisions. The loss is generally expressed as a function of θ. By assigning a probability distribution to θ, based on prior knowledge of its likely magnitude, a decision rule that minimizes the expected loss, known as the risk, can be found.

The ability to incorporate pre-trial beliefs about the magnitude of θ through a prior probability distribution is another means of classifying multi-stage designs. Investigators will probably have some idea of the likely magnitude of θ from animal studies, and previous phase I and II trials for the same tumour type with pharmacologically similar drugs and for the same drug with embryonically related tumours. When prior information is not available, investigators may specify a 'non-informative' prior distribution (Box and Tiao 1973). A popular non-informative prior is the uniform distribution in which the probability of θ falling into any interval (for example 0.20 to 0.30) is dependent only on the width of the interval. Herson (1979b) gives advice regarding the quantification of prior beliefs in phase II trials.

Review of multi-stage designs proposed for Phase II trials

Table 15.3 presents a summary of nine multi-stage phase II designs. The summary characteristics are:

(i) Purpose—estimation (E), hypothesis testing (HT), or risk minimization (RM).

(ii) Mathematical foundation—classical statistical inference (CSI), Bayesian inference (BI), or decision theory (DT).

(iii) Trial terminates—some schemes terminate patient entry when early data support either treatment ineffectiveness or effectiveness (I/E), and some terminate only on evidence of ineffectiveness (I).

(iv) Early termination rule—yes or no.

(v) Number of stages—some designs allow only two stages and some allow any number of stages (k).

(vi) Prior information—yes or no.

(vii) Source of designs—indicates how an investigator selects a design to meet his/her needs by computation using formulas, trial and error, or computer programs.

The following is a summary of the rationale and some special features of these designs.

Table 15.3. *Summary of multi-stage designs for phase II trials*

Name	Reference	Purpose	Mathematical foundation	Trial terminates for	Early termination rule	No. of stages	Prior information	Derivations of designs
(a) Gehan's rule	Gehan (1961)	E	CSI	I	Yes	2	No	Tables or computation
(b) Play the winner	Stanley (1981)	E	CSI	I	Yes	k	No	Simple computation
(c) Generalized multi-stage	Schultz et al. (1973)	HT	CSI	I/E	No	k	No	Trial and error computer program available
(d) One sample multiple testing	Fleming (1981)	HT	CSI	I/E	Yes	k	No	Computation
(e) Predictive probability	Herson (1979b)	HT	CSI/BI	I	Yes	k	Yes	Iteration computer program available
(f) Repeat significance testing	Pocock (1977)	HT	CSI	I/E	No	k	No	Computation
(g) Two-stage decision theory	Sylvester and Staquet (1977, 1980)	RM	DT	I	Yes	2	Yes	Trial and error
(h) Chemical screening	Elashoff and Beal (1976)	RM	DT	I/E	No	2	Yes	Trial and error
(i) Limited accrual	Lee et al. (1979)	Error control	CSI	I/E	No	2	No	Trial and error

Purpose: E, estimation; HT, hypothesis testing; RM, risk minimization.
Mathematical foundation: CSI, classical statistical inference; BI, Bayesian inference; DT, decision theory.
Trial terminates for: I, ineffectiveness; E, effectiveness.

(a) *Gehan's rule* (Gehan 1961) In this scheme, the trial is discontinued if no responses are observed in a preliminary sample of n_1 patients. If at least one response is observed in the preliminary sample, an additional n_2 patients are sampled. Sample size n_1 is determined by the specified significance level for the hypothesis test and n_2 represents the number of additional patients needed to estimate the response rate with required precision (in terms of standard error).

For example, if $\theta_0 = 0.20$, to maintain a false-negative rate of 0.05 the investigator selects $n_1 = 14$. To produce a 5 per cent standard error $45 \leq n_2 \leq 86$ and for a 10 per cent standard error $1 \leq n_2 \leq 11$. In each case, n_2 is determined by the number of responses in the first 14 patients. For the 10 per cent standard error design when the treatment under investigation is effective ($\theta = 0.20$), the expected sample size is 21 and the probability of not taking a second sample is 0.04. For an ineffective treatment ($\theta = 0.05$), the average sample size is 15 and the probability of taking a second sample is 0.51.

Unfortunately, Gehan's rule has been greatly misunderstood by clinicians. Most believe that the rule is a hypothesis testing procedure rather than an estimation procedure and that for $\theta_0 = 0.20$, 14 patients is sufficient for a clinical trial. Rarely is the second sample mentioned.

(b) *Play the winner* (Stanley, personal communication) The Eastern Cooperative Oncology Group has modified the 'play the winner' rule originally designed for phase III trials (Colton 1963) for use in phase II trials (Stanley, personal communication). Twenty patients are treated initially. Thereafter, five patients are added for each response in the first 20 patients treated (up to a maximum of 20 additional patients). The ultimate goal is estimation of θ with a sample size ethically commensurate with early results.

When the treatment is effective ($\theta = 0.20$), the expected sample size for this scheme is 36 and the probability of no further sampling past the initial 20 patients is 0.01. When the treatment is ineffective ($\theta = 0.05$), the expected sample size is 25 and the probability of sampling more than 20 patients is 0.64.

(c) *Generalized multi-stage design* (Schulz, Nichol, Elfring, and Weed 1973) These authors presented formulas for computing false-positive and false-negative-error probabilities and average sample sizes for an arbitrarily chosen multi-stage design.

(d) *Generalized multi-stage design with calculation of critical values* (Fleming 1982) This author extended the work of Schultz *et al.* (1973) by presenting formulas for the calculation of critical values that correspond to an investigator's selected false-positive and false-negative error rates. Fleming also restricted consideration to early termination rules.

Table 15.4 presents a two-stage plan for testing the hypothesis: $H_0: \theta \leq 0.05$ versus $H_1: \theta \geq 0.20$. With a full sample size of 25 patients, a false-positive probability of 0.03 and a false negative probability of 0.24 would be attained.

Table 15.4. *Generalized multi-stage design with calculation of critical values (H_o: $\theta \leq 0.05$ vs H_1: $\theta \geq 0.20$, $\theta_1 = 0.05$, $\theta_2 = 0.20$)*

Stage	Cumulative sample size	Cumulative critical values
1	15	0, 4
2	25	3, 4

False-negative probability (when $\theta = 0.20$) = 0.24.
False-positive probability (when $\theta = 0.05$) = 0.03.
Average sample size (when $\theta = 0.05$) = 20.3.

(e) *Predictive probability* (Herson 1979*b*)   By either the Schultz *et al.* (1973) or the Fleming (1982) approach, many designs can be specified that meet selected false-positive and false-negative-error requirements. Herson (1979*b*) proposed that investigators concentrate on that subset of admissible multi-stage designs that are not only early termination rules but also are consistent with a 'predictive probability' requirement.

Predictive probability methods use the principles of Bayesian inference (Box and Tiao 1973) to enable investigators to answer the question: 'Given that R_i responses have been observed in N_i patients, what is the probability that $\leq C(=C_k)$ responses will be observed in N patients?' This probability is called the predictive probability. A large predictive probability (for example ≥ 0.80), indicates that early termination is advisable. In such case early evidence indicates that if the trial continued to the end, rejection of the (null) hypothesis of drug activity (that is $\leq C$ responses) is likely.

Herson's hypotheses are as follows:

$$H_0: \theta \geq \theta_0$$
$$H_1: \theta < \theta_0$$

Thus, the null hypothesis (H_0) is one of activity and the alternate hypothesis (H_1) is one of inactivity. By this method the power of the test can be used to control rejection of highly ineffective treatments. Although this formulation is the opposite of most approaches, false-positive and false-negative errors are still controlled.

An interactive computer program known as KSTAGE is available to assist the user in selecting predictive probability designs (Atkinson, Brown, and Herson 1981).

Table 15.5 presents an example of a predictive probability design for testing the hypothesis H_0: $\theta \geq 0.20$ versus H_1: $\theta < 0.20$ using a uniform prior distribution for θ. A full sample size of 26 patients is used, and the false-positive and false-negative rates are 0.13 and 0.10, respectively. The table indicates that if 0 responders are observed in the first 15 patients, the predictive probability is 0.94 that ≤ 2 responders will be observed in the first 26 patients.

Table 15.5. *Predictive probability design (*H_0*:* $\theta \geq 0.20$ *vs* H_1*:* $\theta < 0.20$*)*

Stage	Uniform prior distribution Cumulative sample size	Cumulative critical values	Predictive probability
1	15	0, ∞	0.94
2	26	2, ∞	1.00

False-negative probability (when $\theta = 0.20) = 0.10$.
False-positive probability (when $\theta = 0.05) = 0.13$.
Average sample size (when $\theta = 0.05) = 20.9$.

(f) *Repeated significance testing* (Pocock 1977) Armitage, McPherson, and Rowe (1969) showed that repeated significance testing of accumulating data using standard significance tests with usual significance levels (for example 0.05) has the effect of increasing the overall significance level of the test. Armitage (1975) showed that repeat significance testing can be a useful method for analysing sequential clinical trials: a significance level is chosen for a significance test that is to be performed after each observation up to a fixed maximum sample size. The overall significance level is preserved. Pocock (1977) extended this concept to multi-stage designs. Pocock's main application was for comparative two-treatment trials, but advice is given on application to single-treatment trials.

(g) *Two-stage decision theory* (Sylvester and Staquet 1977; 1980) These authors have introduced decision theory to phase II trials. Table 15.6

Table 15.6. *Sylvester and Staquet: loss function for phase II clinical trial*

True therapeutic effectiveness	During phase II trial Treat N patients	At conclusion of phase II trial Accept drug for further study	Reject drug from further study
$\theta < \theta_0$	$k(\theta_0 - \theta)N$	$k(\theta_0 - \theta)m$	0
$\theta = \theta_0$	0	0	0
$\theta > \theta_0$	$k(\theta_0 - \theta)N$	$k(\theta_0 - \theta)t$	$k(\theta - \theta_0)t$

N, Full sample size.

θ, True response proportion.

θ_0, Lowest acceptable response proportion to justify further study.

m, The number of patients treated with the new drug in the subsequent study if the drug is found to be active in the phase II study.

t, The average number of patients who are treated with an effective new drug after completion of the phase II trial before a second new drug which is at least as good is found.

k, The difference in (ethical) cost of further treatment (with a possibly different treatment regimen) between a patient who does not respond to the new drug and a patient who does respond. Assume $k > 0$.

presents a description of the loss function along with various factors considered in establishing the loss function. The authors assume a two-point prior probability distribution for θ, that is $\theta = \theta_1$, with probability w and $\theta = \theta_2$ with probability $1 - w$ for $\theta_1 < \theta_0 < \theta_2$, $0 < w < 1$.

Sylvester and Staquet (personal communication, 1980) extended these designs to two-stage designs by adding an early termination rule. Table 15.7

Table 15.7. *Two-stage decision theory design.* [$\theta_0 = 0.20$, $\theta_1 = 0.05$, $\theta_2 = 0.25$; m (estimated number of patients exposed to new treatment on phase III trial) = 50; w (probability $(\theta = \theta_1)$) = 0.50.]

Stage	Cumulative sample size	Cumulative critical values
1	18	0, ∞
2	23	2, ∞

False-negative probability (when $\theta = 0.25$) = 0.05.
False-positive probability (when $\theta = 0.05$) = 0.10.

exhibits a decision theory design for the case where $\theta_0 = 0.20$, $\theta_1 = 0.05$, and $\theta_2 = 0.25$; prior beliefs are summarized in what might be called a two-point uniform distribution, that is θ_1 and θ_2 are equally likely ($w = 0.50$); and where 50 patients will encounter this new treatment in a phase III trial. The design shown minimizes risk and yields false-positive and false-negative probabilities of 0.10 and 0.05, respectively.

(h) *Chemical screening* (Elashoff and Beal 1976)
A decision theory application was designed for use in animal studies in screening chemicals for carcinogenicity. The structure is quite similar to that of Sylvester and Staquet, differing mainly in the loss functions used. For chemical screening, loss functions were determined solely on the basis of the number of animals killed. With some modification, these designs could be applied to phase II trials.

(i) *Limited accrual* (Lee, Staquet, Simon, Catane, and Muggia 1979)
The limited accrual design is for the situation in which investigators are unable to select sample size N because of limited accrual, the likely case in single-institution trials. It is a two-stage design, but the authors do not restrict $C_2 = D_2 - 1$ (Table 15.2). Instead $C_2 < D_2$. Thus, at the end of the trial, the drug may be declared ineffective (number of responses $\leq C_2$) or effective (number of responses $> D_2$), or the trial may be declared inconclusive (number of responses lies between C_2 and D_2). In the face of small sample sizes and in an

attempt to control false-positive and false-negative errors, the authors believed it necessary to allow for inconclusive results.

Investigators evaluate potential two-stage plans on the basis of false-positive and false-negative rates, as well as on the probability of an inconclusive result when the new agent is in fact either highly effective or highly ineffective, and on the probability of recognizing a highly effective or highly ineffective drug. A computer program prints a list of criteria for several different designs and one is chosen that meets specifications.

Table 15.8 presents an example of a limited accrual design for testing $H_0: \theta \leq 0.20$ versus $H_1: \theta > 0.20$ (that is $\theta_0 = 0.20$) with $\theta_1 = 0.10$ and $\theta_2 = 0.30$. The full sample size of 25 allows for a false-positive rate of 0.46, a false-negative rate of 0.05, and a probability of an inclusive result of 0.38. Due to the limited accrual, the authors are willing to accept relatively high probabilities of false-positive and inconclusive results in order to maintain a low false-negative probability.

Table 15.8. *Limited accrual design (*$H_0: \theta \leq 0.20$ vs $H_1: \theta > 0.20$, $\theta_1 = 0.10$, $\theta_2 = 0.30$)*

Stage	Cumulative sample size	Cumulative critical value
1	15	0, 4
2	25	1, 6

False-negative probability (when $\theta = 0.30$) = 0.05.
False-positive probability (when $\theta = 0.10$) = 0.46.
Probability of an inconclusive result = 0.38.

(j) *Discussion*

The reader will note that most of the multi-stage plans reviewed above appeared in the literature during 1977–81. It is safe to say that not enough experience exists with these plans to adequately advise investigators on their relative merits. In the examples of two-stage plans for $\theta_0 = 0.20$ presented above, the plans are remarkably similar in that the required full sample size is generally about 25 patients and that the first stage terminates because of ineffectiveness with zero responders in the first 15 to 18 patients. Thus, any of these plans would terminate for a poor early performance and the appearance of one responder would be sufficient to send the trial to the second stage. With false-negative errors considered more serious than false-positive, this generally accepted strategy makes sense.

Four of the seven hypothesis testing/decision theory designs presented are defined for $k > 2$ (as well as $k = 2$) stages. For the sake of comparison only two-stage designs were considered here. With false-positive and false-negative-error rates held constant an increase in the number of stages tends to result in a decrease in average sample size.

Early termination plans have greater practical appeal than multi-stage plans not based on this principle. By the definition of an early termination rule, investigators perform the same statistical test at the end of the trial as they would if they were following a single-stage design. Thus, early termination avoids the incongruous situation of an investigator specifying an overall significance level of 0.05, finding a p value of 0.03 when the full sample size is reached, and being told by a statistician that a statistically significant result had not occurred because a p value of 0.001 was required at the kth stage to assure an overall 0.05 significance level.

In most phase II trials in oncology, there do not appear to be good reasons to terminate a trial when early data support the hypothesis of treatment effectiveness. Investigators should accrue the full sample size in this case. The larger sample size allows for the estimation of θ with greater precision than would be possible with early termination. The larger sample size might allow also for estimation of the response proportion in logical subgroups of patients defined on the basis of site, histology, stage, number of prior relapses, etc. Moreover, the larger sample size provides for more experience with the new agent. There are many benefits to be gained from greater experience, especially knowledge of toxicity. Although Fleming's design (1982) allows for early termination for treatment effectiveness, the author concedes this point and proposes a compromise whereby this type of termination is allowed only in extreme cases (for example see Table 15.4), which occur infrequently in practice.

The introduction of decision theory and incorporation of prior information in phase II trials is exciting, but more developmental work is needed on the specification of appropriate loss functions and on quantifying prior knowledge.

One important feature of all multi-stage designs is the control of overall false-positive and false-negative-error probabilities. Although the limited accrual method of Lee *et al.* (1979) allows for the computation of false-positive and false-negative rates, the significance of these computed rates is questionable due to the relatively high percentage of trials that terminate in inconclusive results.

More work is needed on helping investigators select a specific design once they have decided which multi-stage strategy they want to use. Interactive computer programs must be developed, written in exportable code, and made available to interested users.

The 'several-disease' problem

Until now, it has been assumed that all patients in the phase II trial have the same tumour type. In practice, patients with a wide spectrum of tumour types may be entered on a phase II trial. Even with multi-stage designs, limited accrual makes it impractical to conduct an independent trial for each tumour type. The alternative method of pooling all tumour types does not permit identification of drugs whose effectiveness is tumour-specific.

Herson (1979*b*) has begun extending the predictive probability multi-stage design to the several-disease problem in which a phase II trial is conducted for a treatment applied to *d* tumour types, with each patient having exactly one tumour type. In addition to specifying prior information on the response proportion for each tumour type, investigators may specify prior information on the degree of tumour non-specificity in response to the new treatment between each pair of tumour types (for example to what extent will leukaemias respond in the same way as lymphomas, Ewing's sarcomas in the same way as osteosarcomas, etc.). This prior information is corrected by incoming data as the trial progresses. The technique allows for a sharing of accruing response data between tumour types and can result in more efficient trials in the face of tumour-type heterogeneity and limited accrual. More work in this area is needed.

SOURCES OF BIAS

For the estimate of θ to be useful in inferring probability of response in future patients and in deciding on the advisability of further research, it is important that systematic errors in response measurement, known as bias, are not introduced by investigators in the conduct of the trial or in the reporting of results. Several sources of bias will now be described. Some of these have been discussed elsewhere by Herson (1980).

Selection bias based on patient characteristics

If investigators have the opportunity to decide whether or not to enter a patient on a particular phase II trial, they may consciously or subconsciously select certain types of patients for certain agents and other types for other agents. Indeed, if interim results on response are freely disseminated, investigators might enter only very advanced patients on a trial whose early results show poor response.

One approach to this problem is to 'blind' interim results from clinicians. The ethics of this approach are questionable and the policy does not allow for collective decision-making regarding the course of the trial or in the planning of future trials. A better approach would be to motivate clinicians to strictly follow the treatment priority list for each malignancy.

'Wait and see' bias

'Wait and see' bias may occur when investigators have the opportunity to begin treatment and observe patient response before deciding whether or not to register the patient on the trial. This phenomenon may result in an over-optimistic estimate of response proportion. This source of bias would occur mainly in multi-institution trials, and a requirement that patients be registered on the trial within 3 days of treatment start should reduce this source of bias.

Selective reporting of results

A 'selective reporting' bias is introduced when investigators issue reports of results ignoring the existence of patients who died shortly after the start of treatment, refused further treatment early in the trial, had inadequate trials due to severe toxic effects, or who went off-study due to major protocol violations. Reports based on selective subsamples of this type provide a misleading impression of treatment effectiveness and feasibility. Investigators must adopt a policy of reporting on every patient entered in the trial in their final report. There is general agreement on a conservative position of classifying patients who are lost to the study before response could be observed as non-responders, rather than ignoring their existence (Peto, Pike, Armitage, Breslow, Cox, Howard, Mantel, McPherson, Peto, and Smith 1976; Cornfield 1971).

'Good news travels first'

Some investigators have conjectured the 'good news travels first' theory whereby an investigator might be likely to report a response to the co-ordinating centre sooner than a non-response. I have no evidence that this occurs in practice. Investigators should establish and enforce rules for timely reporting.

REPORTING OF RESULTS

Most reports of phase II trials in the literature do not present adequate information for the reader to evaluate either the new treatment or the trial.

The following would constitute a minimal subset of data to be included in a report of a phase II trial:

(i) the priority list in effect for this malignancy at the time the trial was conducted;

(ii) explanation of how patients were recruited;

(iii) whether investigators were blinded from interim results;

(iv) time requirements for registering patients and reporting results;

(v) design used;

(vi) sample size—how determined, false-positive and false-negative probabilities, and degree of precision attained;

(vii) patient list—for each patient: response status, and patient characteristics of possible prognostic significance, for example age, number of previous relapses, prior therapy, stage, histology, etc.;

(viii) toxicity—type, time of onset, severity, duration.

The patient list is important because, although all patients in the trial have a common malignancy, considerable heterogeneity exists. Clinical judgement is a vital ingredient in treatment evaluation. This judgement can be properly exercised only with knowledge of the types of patients treated.

SUMMARY AND CONCLUSIONS

I have attempted to introduce some of the statistical issues involved in designing, carrying out, reporting, and interpreting phase II clinical trials. With the response proportion as the measure of effectiveness, the decisions to be made regarding further testing of a new chemotherapeutic agent may be formulated as a statistical hypothesis test. Sample size is determined to control false-positive and false-negative-error probabilities, and precision in estimation of the response proportion. The commencement of trials for which potential patient accrual appears insufficient was discouraged. In a summary of the 'state of the art' of multi-stage designs, nine approaches were presented and contrasted. When several approaches were compared for two-stage designs with a threshold response proportion of 0.20 they were found to be similar in full sample size requirements and criteria for early termination. Warning was given regarding potential sources of bias and misinterpretation, and guidelines were presented for proper reporting of results.

If this paper has a 'bottom line', it should be that it is vital that a trained biostatistician be involved in the phase II trial from the commencement of protocol planning to the writing of the final report. Considerable further development of statistical methods for phase II trials is needed. Progress has been slow in this area largely because the biostatistician, although actively involved as an investigator in phase III trials, has often been absent hitherto as a collaborator on phase II trials. I hope this paper will help give biostatisticians their proper role in phase II trials.

ACKNOWLEDGEMENT

This paper was written while the author was with the M.D. Anderson Hospital, Houston, Texas. The preparation of this paper was supported in part by research grants CA11430 and CA6294 from the National Cancer Institute (USA) and an International Cancer Research Technology Transfer (ICRETT) travel grant from the International Union Against Cancer.

REFERENCES

Armitage, P. (1975). *Sequential medical trials*, 2nd ed. John Wiley and Sons, New York.
—— McPherson, C. K., and Rowe, B. C. (1969). Repeated significance tests on accumulating data. *R. statist. Soc. Series A* **132**, 235–44.

Atkinson, E. N., Brown, B. W., and Herson, J. (1981). KSTAGE—an interactive computer program for designing phase II clinical trials using predictive probability. *Comput. biomed. Res.* **15**, 220–7.

Box, G. E. P. and Tiao, G. E. (1973). *Bayesian inference in statistical analysis.* Addison-Wesley, Reading, Massachusetts.

Byar, D. P., Simon, R. M., Friedewald, W. T., Schlesselman, J. J., De Mets, D. T., Ellenberg, J. H., Gail, M. H., and Ware, J. H. (1976). Randomized clinical trials: perspectives on some recent ideas. *New Engl. J. Med.* **295**, 74–80.

Colton, T. (1963). A model for selecting one of two medical treatments. *J. Am. med. Ass.* **58**, 388–401.

—— (1974). *Statistics in medicine.* Little Brown, Boston.

Cornfield, J. (1971). The University Group Diabetes Program: a further statistical analysis of the mortality findings. *J. Am. med. Ass.* **217**, 1676–87.

Elashoff, R. M. and Beal, S. (1976). Two stage screening designs applied to chemical-screening problems with binary data. *A. Rev. Biophys. Bioeng.* **5**, 561–87.

Fleming, T. R. (1982). One sample multiple testing procedure for phase II clinical trials. *Biometrics* **38**, 143–151.

Gehan, E. A. (1961). The determination of the number of patients required in a follow-up trial of a new chemotherapeutic agent. *J. chron. Dis.* **13**, 346–53.

George, S. L. (1980). Sequential clinical trials in cancer research. *Cancer Treat. Rep.* **64**, 393–7.

Herson, J. (1979a). Phase II clinical trials for several diseases with limited patient entry. Paper contributed to the *1979 Eastern Regional Statistical Meetings*, New Orleans, Louisiana.

—— (1979b). Predictive probability early termination plans for phase II clinical trials. *Biometrics* **35**, 775–83.

—— (1980). Patient registration in a cooperative oncology group. *Control. clin. Trials* **1**, 101–10.

—— (1983). The practical side of multistage clinical trials for screening new agents. *Cancer Treat. Rep.* **67**, 71–5.

Lee, Y. J., Staquet, M., Simon, R., Catane, R., and Muggia, F. D. (1979). Two stage plans for patient accrual in phase II cancer clinical trials. *Cancer Treat. Rep.* **63**, 1721–6.

Muggia, F. M., Rozencweig, M., Staquet, M. J., and McGuire, W. P. (1980). Methodology of phase II clinical trials in cancer. In *Recent Results in Cancer Research* (eds. S. K. Carter and Y. Sakurai) Vol. 70, pp. 53–60. Springer-Verlag, Berlin.

Peto, R., Pike, M. C., Armitage, P., Breslow, N. E., Cox, D. R., Howard, S. V., Mantel, N., McPherson, K., Peto, J., and Smith, P. G. (1976). Design and analysis of randomized clinical trials requiring prolonged observation of each patient. I. Introduction and design. *Br. J. Cancer* **34**, 585–612.

Pocock, S. J. (1977). Group sequential methods in the design and analysis of clinical trials. *Biometrika* **64**, 191–9.

—— (1978). Size of cancer clinical trials and stopping rules. *Br. J. Cancer* **38**, 757–66.

Schultz, J. R., Nichol, F. R., Elfring, G. L., and Weed, S. D. (1973). Multiple stage procedures for drug screening. *Biometrics* **29**, 293–300.

Sylvester, R. J. and Staquet, M. M. (1977). An application of decision theory of phase II clinical trials in cancer. In *Recent advances in cancer treatment* (eds. H. J. Tagnon and M. J. Staquet). Raven Press, New York.

—— and —— (1980). Design of phase II clinical trials in cancer using decision theory. *Cancer Treat. Rep.* **64**, 519–24.

Wald, A. (1947). *Sequential analysis.* John Wiley and Sons, New York.

Williams, C. J. and Carter, S. K. (1978). Management of trials in the development of cancer chemotherapy. *Br. J. Cancer* **37**, 434–47.

WHO (1979). *WHO handbook for reporting results of cancer treatment.* WHO offset publication no. 48. WHO, Geneva.

Part VI
Design of phase III trials

16 Designs for phase III trials

Maurice Staquet and Otilia Dalesio

INTRODUCTION

Phase III trials are the last step in the planned evaluation of new treatment modalities. They have one of the following purposes (Simon 1982*a*):

(1) to determine the effectiveness of a treatment relative to the natural history of the disease. In this instance, the trial has a no-treatment or a placebo arm;

(2) to determine the effectiveness of the new treatment with regards to the best current standard therapy;

(3) to determine if a new treatment is as effective as a standard therapy but is associated with less severe toxicity.

These studies are disease-oriented studies aiming to either corroborate previous positive findings (confirmatory trials) or to modify an established regimen (explanatory trials) (Carter 1980*a*). The confirmatory trial in a large number of patients is an essential part of the evaluation of a new treatment since the reproducibility of the observed results needs to be established before the use of the treatment in a given population of patients can be recommended. Its function is to reduce the delta error (the proportion of all trials reported as positive which are false positives), especially if the sample sizes of the earlier trials were small (Staquet, Rozencweig, Von·Hoff, and Muggia 1979; Simon 1982*b*).

The explanatory study is an attempt to modify an established treatment. Typically, the goal may be to prove an equivalence in effectiveness between two treatment modalities, one being less toxic or more convenient than the other. This type of trial also requires a large number of patients in order to substantiate a conclusion that the two treatments are practically equivalent with respect to response or survival time. It also contributes to the reduction of the epsilon error (Staquet *et al.* 1979).

CONTROLS

The evaluation of a new treatment modality in a phase III trial is performed by comparison with a group of similar patients treated with a control therapy. One of the major controversies in clinical trials today is related to the selection of a control group to use as the base against which the new treatment is to be evaluated. This issue has been addressed in a number of papers which will not be reviewed here (Ingelfinger 1972; Chalmers, Block, and Lee 1972; Gehan and Freireich 1974; Byar, Simon, Friedewald, Schlesselman, DeMets, Ellenberg, Gail, and Ware 1976; Byar 1980). Allocation of treatments by a random process is generally considered as the method of choice for phase III trials. This procedure guarantees the validity of the statistical comparisons between outcomes and assures, on the average, an equal distribution of the known and unknown prognostic factors between the treatment arms. Unfortunately, random allocation does not assure that for a given trial all the prognostic factors will be equally distributed and therefore that the groups of patients will differ only by treatment. As a matter of fact, the probability that several prognostic factors are all evenly distributed between two groups of patients is low for small size trials. Imbalances between known prognostic factors which occur by chance must be corrected a posteriori.

Investigators have often been tempted to use historical controls, but the only case where there is general agreement that historical controls may indeed be used is when a new treatment is overwhelmingly effective in comparison with historical data. In such an instance, the control group is implicit in so far as it is common knowledge that the disease status cannot be improved with other existing therapies. Even then, the discovery of an outstanding treatment does not necessarily pre-empt further phase III comparative trials. This is exemplified in Hodgkin's Disease where MOPP was found highly effective by means of a non-randomized trial, but was subsequently compared with other chemotherapy regimens in phase III randomized trials (DeVita and Hellman 1982).

TYPES OF TREATMENTS INVESTIGATED IN PHASE III TRIALS

Single modality treatment

Comparative trials of surgical procedures and of radiation therapy are rare. These modalities are more generally tested when used in combination. In addition to the comparison of combination chemotherapies (simultaneous, cyclic, or sequential), comparisons of single experimental drug regimens against established chemotherapy regimens in advanced disease are common (Staquet 1978).

Combined modality treatment

The combined modality approach consists of using, for the treatment of early (that is adjuvant therapy—see below) or of advanced disease, a sequence of two or more of the following therapies: surgery, radiotherapy, chemotherapy, immunotherapy, and endocrine therapy.

Some of the problems related to the design and analysis of such types of studies have been delineated by Schwartz and Lellouch (1967). In particular, the relative timing of each of the modalities to be administered must be considered with respect to the final analysis. For instance in the comparison of pre-operative radiotherapy or not, eligible patients are randomized to one of these two options. Clearly a patient randomized to no pre-operative radiotherapy could be operated immediately, or after a period equivalent to the time needed to administer radiation therapy to the other group. The statistical results will be interpreted differently according to the design chosen.

Adjuvant therapy

Adjuvant therapy is a treatment modality given to patients treated by a potentially curative primary therapy, but for whom there is a substantial risk of recurrence. The primary therapy is usually surgery, but may also include radiation therapy, chemotherapy, or a combination of these. Adjuvant therapy consists in most instances of chemotherapy, but the other modalities are sometimes applied (Glatstein 1981; Ultmann and Karnofsky 1979).

The concept of adjuvant therapy is based on the observation that micrometastases can in some cases be totally eradicated in experimental models after removal of the primary tumour. Such a result has been documented in a number of human tumours (DeVita 1982). Guidelines for the indication of adjuvant therapy have been described by Bonadonna, Tancini, Rossi, and Gasparini (1978). In essence, adjuvant therapy is to be administered at full dose in subgroups of patients with a high risk of relapse, as soon as possible after completion of primary treatment.

The delineation of a high-risk group requires the access to large data bases and the use of sophisticated statistical methods of prediction. Even in this case, the high-risk group will contain a number of patients who have been cured by the primary treatment and for whom adjuvant therapy is unnecessary. Possible strategies to balance between morbidity and benefit have been proposed by Ultmann and Karnofsky (1979).

The design of comparative adjuvant trials, or of trials with a maintenance programme, is characterized by several specific features which are related to the standardization of the primary therapy, the timing of the randomization procedure, and the comparison of survival times.

The standardization of the primary treatment is essential to permit valid comparisons between the different adjuvant treatments (Durant, Bartolucci, and Birch 1981). Indeed, it is desirable that the various adjuvant therapies being tested be administered to groups of patients which are similar with respect to their probability and number of micrometastases. The only way to produce such comparable groups is to use the same primary treatment in all the patients and to investigate the completeness of the remission or response with the same thoroughness in all the subjects. The same need for comparability of the groups requires that the process of randomization between the arms of the adjuvant study be performed *after* the primary intervention is completed, even if it is standardized. This procedure is required to avoid unconscious variation in the primary therapy which can result from the knowledge of the subsequent treatment that the patient will receive if randomization is performed before the primary therapy. Whenever possible, it is also desirable that all patients receive the same salvage therapy (that is the treatment given after relapse) in order to simplify interpretation of survival comparisons.

Another characteristic of adjuvant therapy trials is the necessity for large sample sizes and long-term follow-up of the same frequency and nature in both arms of the study. Large sample sizes are needed because the power of statistical comparisons of survival and disease-free interval depend on the number of deaths or recurrences in each sample rather than on the total number of patients studied.

UNEQUAL ALLOCATION OF PATIENTS TO TREATMENT GROUPS

Usually, the same number of patients are assigned to the various treatment arms, because statistical considerations show that this is the most efficient design with regards to the power of the statistical tests.

Pocock (1979) has indicated that a slight imbalance, that is a ratio of 2 to 1 or less of treatment to control, entails a small loss of power and could therefore be used in some cases. Investigators may request, for instance, assignment of more patients to a new promising treatment than to a standard well-known therapy (Peto, Pike, Armitage, Breslow, Cox, Howard, Mantel, McPherson, Peto, and Smith 1976). However, such an option is not unanimously accepted (Friedman, Furberg, and DeMets 1981). These authors state that equal allocation is more consistent with the fact that there is no preconceived idea as to which treatment is better.

TYPES OF DESIGNS FOR PHASE III TRIALS

Unstratified design

In this design, patients are randomly assigned to treatment arms as they become sequentially available. As the size of the trial increases, the number of patients assigned to the various arms becomes approximately equal, but at any point in time, and especially for trials with small sample sizes, an imbalance between the number of patients on each arm could occur by chance. Since, for the sake of statistical power, it is desirable to have treatment arms of approximately equal size, the randomization is often 'blocked' or 'restricted'. A block is a sequence of *n* patients in which each treatment is allocated an equal number of times. For instance, successive blocks of six patients can be formed, in which three patients will receive treatment A and the three others treatment

B. For a sample size of say 49 subjects, at most 25 but at least 24 will have received treatment A (eight blocks of six plus one or zero).

The appropriate way to perform a blocked randomization is to select the arrangement of treatments within each block at random among all the possible sequences. For instance, for a block of four patients, there are six possible treatment sequences: AABB, BBAA, ABAB, BABA, ABBA, and BAAB. The order in which each of the six possible sequences will be used for the next 24 patients is decided by a random process. Each sequence could be numbered one to six and a die cast to determine the order of use of the sequences. In general for the case of two treatments, one would use blocks of size four, six, or eight depending on the predicted total sample size (the number of distinct treatment sequences for a block of size six is 20 and 70 for a block of size eight).

The major drawback to blocked randomization, when the treatments are not blinded, is that the investigator may figure out the block size and thus will know exactly what treatment will be assigned to the last patient(s) of the block and, therefore, can select the patients for a given treatment. This is especially true for single-centre studies where only one or two physicians are entering the patients in the trial. Several methods to limit this type of bias are discussed by Simon (1979a) and Pocock (1979). The simplest one is to vary the dimension of the blocks and to keep the investigators unaware of their sizes.

Stratified designs

When the factors influencing the response to treatment are known, they must be taken into account when evaluating the meaning of the observed difference between outcomes.

The ideal way to account for the possible influence of the prognostic factors is to distribute them equally between the treatment groups. In such a scheme, the random assignment of the treatments is performed within each stratum of patients. A stratum of patients is a mutually exclusive grouping of subjects according to factors known to influence the end-points of the trial. For example, if it is known that prior therapy and sex are important prognostic factors, patients can be grouped in four categories: males with and without prior treatment, females with and without prior treatment. In each of these four strata, randomization between treatments must then be carried out using blocked randomization.

It is obvious that stratification by more than two factors, or more than two levels for each of the two factors rapidly leads to impractical designs because the number of strata becomes too large. In this case, an imbalance between treatment numbers can easily arise by chance. To illustrate this idea, let us suppose that we stratify by two prognostic factors for two treatments using blocks of six patients. The four blocks of six allocations selected at random among the 20 possible are displayed in Table 16.1 (upper part). Of note is that within each stratum the number of subjects receiving A is the same as the number receiving B, provided the randomization is not stopped before the end. Suppose for the sake of demonstration that we examine the data after 10 patients have been entered. Since, in general, the number of patients without prior therapy will be low, it is conceivable that by chance four males and four females with prior therapy and one male and one female without prior therapy were randomized. By counting the number of treatments administered it can be seen (Table 16.1, lower part) that three A's were given against seven B's. The two patients without prior therapy have both received treatment B as well as

Table 16.1. *Random allocation of two treatments (A and B) to patients in four strata: status of the trial after the first 10 entries*

Males (M)		Females (F)	
No prior treatment	Yes prior treatment	No prior treatment	Yes prior treatment
B*	B*	B*	B*
A	A*	B	B*
B	A*	A	B*
A	B*	B	A*
A	A	A	A
B	B	A	A

	A	B	Total
M prior treatment	2	2	4
M no prior treatment	0	1	1
F prior treatment	1	3	4
F no prior treatment	0	1	1
Total	3	7	10

* Patients entered in the trial at the time of this analysis.

four of the five females. In practice much larger numbers of patients would usually be involved, but appreciable imbalances can still arise if block sizes are large or there are many strata even if proper rules for blocked randomization were used.

This tendency for imbalance will decrease by increasing the number of patients entered or decreasing the block size provided the number of prognostic factors is kept low. On the contrary, increasing the number of strata will increase the probability of an unequal number of patients on each treatment.

For instance, a multi-centre trial with 20 institutions for a disease with three important prognostic factors (each with two levels) would need

$20 \times 2 \times 2 \times 2 = 160$ strata. With medium sample sizes, it is certain that some strata will be empty or severely unbalanced since a minimum of 320 patients is needed to assign two patients per stratum. Excessive stratification in itself is useless as demonstrated by Pocock and Simon (1975), Zelen (1975), and Simon (1979a), because, in the long run, it amounts to no stratification and unblocked randomization. Moreover, randomization within a large number of strata is conducive to administrative errors because of its complexity.

An extreme view on stratification is expressed by Peto *et al.* (1976) who argue that prior stratification is unnecessary providing that an adjusted statistical analysis is undertaken. Still, as indicated by Brown (1980a), the trial will be more convincing, at least subjectively, if it can be shown that the most important prognostic variables were taken into account before randomization. This will also guard against the possibility of an unequal distribution of prognostic factors in any single trial, and does not rely on 'expectation' to achieve this goal (Green and Byar 1978).

Adaptive stratified designs

When a large number of strata exist, an effective way to avoid a severe imbalance in the number of patients on each treatment for any given factor has been proposed by Taves (1974). The 'minimization' method, further developed by Pocock and Simon (1975), Freedman and White (1976), and White and Freedman (1978) does not attempt to assign an equal number of treatments to each possible combination of the prognostic factors, but tends to equalize treatment numbers within each level of each prognostic variable separately.

A simple example with three treatments will illustrate the procedure. The two-treatment case will be illustrated by Lagakos and Pocock (1983) in the next chapter using a slightly different method. Suppose that treatments A, B, and C are being compared in patients who need to be stratified by institution (numbered 1 to 10), prior therapy (yes or no), and stage (I, II, III, and IV). Complete stratification for all the factors would require random allocation of the three treatments to 80 mutually exclusive strata $(10 \times 2 \times 4)$. With a moderate sample size, it can be expected that there will be many empty and partially-filled strata in the trial (80 strata with three treatments requires a minimum of 240 patients to fill all the strata if a minimal block size of three is chosen) and that a treatment imbalance is likely to occur at the end of the trial. The 'minimization' technique of randomization is illustrated here by selecting an arbitrary point in time during the trial. Suppose that a patient becomes available for randomization and that he is from institution 1, with no prior therapy and in stage I. An examination of the treatments already allocated in these three specific strata is performed (Table 16.2, upper part: 'before'). To determine which treatment will be assigned to the patient, it must be found what total imbalance between treatments would result with each of the three possible treatment allocations. Suppose that treatment A is given, then the numbers in the first column of Table 16.2 (upper part, 'before') are increased by one. The result is shown in Table 16.2, option 1. The total amount of imbalance is calculated by adding the ranges[16.1] (the difference between the largest and the smallest number) for all strata. So, for option 1 and institution 1, the range is $10-6$; for option 1 and no prior therapy, it is $2-1$ and for option 1 and stage I it is $7-4$. The sum of imbalances is equal, therefore, to $(10-6)+(2-1)+(7-4)=8$ for option 1. The same computation is repeated, supposing treatment B or C is given (Table 16.2, options 2 and 3). It can be seen that option 3, assigning treatment C, produces the minimum of imbalance within the three strata, and therefore treatment C is selected for the incoming patient. In case of equality between imbalances, the treatment is chosen by simple randomization.

Table 16.2. *Treatment numbers for various prognostic factors before and after assignment of the next patient to each possible treatment*

	Treatment		
	A	B	C
Before			
Institution 1	8	10	6
No prior treatment	1	1	1
Stage I	6	4	5
Option 1: assigning treatment A			
Institution 1	9	10	6
No prior treatment	2	1	1
Stage I	7	4	5
Imbalance $=(10-6)+(2-1)+(7-4)=8$			
Option 2: assigning treatment B			
Institution 1	8	11	6
No prior treatment	1	2	1
Stage I	6	5	5
Imbalance $=(11-6)+(2-1)+(6-5)=7$			
Option 3: assigning treatment C			
Institution 1	8	10	7
No prior treatment	1	1	2
Stage I	6	4	6
Imbalance $=(10-7)+(2-1)+(6-4)=6$			

It should be noted that the figures for each treatment cannot be added up to yield the number of patients with these characteristics already entered on this treatment. For instance, a previously treated patient in institution 1 with stage I disease and who has received treatment A is counted twice, once in the row 'institution', and once in the row 'stage I'.

[16.1] Other measures of imbalance have been suggested, such as the sum of the variances for all strata as illustrated by Lagakos and Pocock (1983) in the next chapter.

Such a 'minimization' procedure is not without inconvenience since the next treatment can often be predicted, if the investigators have a knowledge of data similar to those displayed in Table 16.2 (upper part, 'before'). This is generally not the case in multi-centre trials with central co-ordination where the physician has no access to information outside his own institution before the end of the trial.

A slight modification of this 'minimization' method has been proposed by Begg and Iglewicz (1980) for the comparison of two treatments and prognostic factors having only two levels. Another approach, especially valuable when there is a strong interaction between prognostic factors, has been studied by Nordle and Brantmark (1977). It can be observed that in these dynamic randomization methods, the patients are not assigned to treatment groups by a random process. So, in order to fulfil the requirement of random allocation, it must be assumed that the order of arrival of the patients in the trial is random.

Factorial designs

The factorial arrangement of treatments is a useful tool in clinical research whenever two or more treatments need to be investigated simultaneously.

The simplest factorial design, called a 2×2 factorial, involves the simultaneous study of two different treatments. Such a design was used in an EORTC adjuvant study in epidermoid carcinoma of the lung where 600 patients were allocated to four groups after primary treatment (Table 16.3): no adjuvant treatment (N), chemotherapy alone (C), immunotherapy alone (I), and chemotherapy and immunotherapy (C + I). This design allows the data to be used 'twice', once for assessing the efficacy of the chemotherapy and once for that of immunotherapy. To assess the effectiveness of chemotherapy, one will compare the two treatment groups C and C + I together with the two other groups, N and I together, stratifying retrospectively for the presence or absence of I. Likewise, the effect of I can be investigated by comparing the patients receiving I and C + I to the subjects treated by N and C, stratifying retrospectively for the presence or absence of C. The advantage of such a design is that the evaluation of the 'main effects' (that is C and I) can be performed at the same level of statistical power using half of the patients that would be needed as compared with two separate studies comparing I with N and C with N and one-third less patients than in a three-arm trial (I versus C versus N). In addition C can be compared with I and C + I can be compared with N, although the power of these comparisons will be less than for comparing the main effects.

A potential problem in the factorial design is the presence of an interaction[16.2] between the treatments. If, for instance, the effect of I is lower

---

[16.2] An interaction between A and B means that the effect of A is not the same in the absence as it is in the presence of B and vice versa. This differential effect can be either in the same or in the opposite direction.

Table 16.3. *Patient allocation to a factorial arrangement of two treatments in an EORTC adjuvant study (protocol 08741) of epidermoid carcinoma of the lung*

| | | Chemotherapy | | |
		No	Yes	Total
Immunotherapy	No	150	150	300
	Yes	150	150	300
Total		300	300	600

when chemotherapy is given concomittantly than when it is given alone, then using the grouping of patients indicated above will result in computing an average effect of I which does not necessarily reflect the true potential of I in not otherwise treated patients.

Peto (1978), however, has indicated that the problem is not serious if the effect of one treatment goes in the same direction in the two groups defined by the other treatments.

Cross-over designs

In this design, each patient serves as his own control in so far as each of the treatments being investigated is given to all the subjects in sequence. In the two-period cross-over design, treatment A followed by B is administered to half of the patients and B followed by A to the other half, each subject being assigned at random to one of the two options AB or BA. Of note is that the two periods must be equal in length for all subjects. A mathematical treatment of the problem is given by Brown (1980*b*) and is presented in non-mathematical terms by Hills and Armitage (1979).

The advantage of such a scheme is an increase in precision and therefore a decrease in the sample size needed. However, the assumption of no carry-over effect and no time (period) effect from period one to period two must be made in order to validate the comparison between the two treatments. That is to say at the beginning of the second period, the patients must be in a state comparable with that at the beginning of the first period (Brown 1980*a*). Such an assumption is generally not valid for patients with cancer. Hills and Armitage (1979) have pinpointed a number of reasons for period–treatment interaction. These are the change in pathological state from period one to two, the possible persistence of the initial treatment effect during period two (including the long half-life of the drugs), and the possible relationship between treatment effects and level of response. Also in many instances of cancer trials, the second treatment is given at the time of disease progression, thus rendering the two periods unequal in length. For these reasons, the design and the analysis of cross-over studies in cancer phase II and III trials is tricky and needs careful consideration.

Multi-centre design with institutional option

When institutions disagree on which of three or more treatments should be studied, the investigators are sometimes allowed to select the arms of the trial to which they will participate. For instance, in a design involving the comparison of two new treatments (A and B) and a standard therapy (C), each institution may decide to use the three arms or to restrict its study to A versus C or to B versus C. The rationale of such a scheme stems from the fact that the two separate studies will have a common arm (C). Schoenfeld and Gelber (1979) have developed methods for analysing such studies and have shown that, in the case of three treatment arms, the total sample size must be increased by a factor of at least 2.6 compared with the classical three-arm design without option in order to achieve the same precision.

In addition, Makuch and Simon (1978) have shown that multi-centre designs with institutional options suffer from basic defects. Indeed, besides the low power of the tests used to compare the two control groups, it is not possible to separate the institution effect from the treatment effect.

The possibility of including non-randomizing centres in a multi-centre randomized trial has been studied by Machin (1978). In this design, the centres can either randomize between the control and the new treatment or opt for a single arm of the study. It was shown that little can be gained from such a strategy. By and large, designs with institutional options are to be widely discouraged because the assumptions required are too strong and the increase in sample size too large in addition to the high risk of spurious results.

Multi-stage designs

Two-stage clinical trials are often designed when two different treatments are applied sequentially. This is the case for example when the first treatment is intended to achieve a complete remission (CR) (induction–consolidation) whereas the second treatment is applied to patients in complete response to help maintain this condition as long as possible (maintenance). Thus if two induction regimens, A and B, and two maintenance treatments, C and D, are to be compared, patients will be randomized first between A and B and then those who achieve a CR will be re-randomized between C and D, thus forming a four-arm trial (AC, AD, BC, BD).

Sometimes, because of low sample sizes, the four arms are 'collapsed' into two arms when studying C and D under the assumption that the patients in complete remission are identical with respect to their true disease status, irrespective of the first treatment. This assumption is questionable (Simon 1979*b*) (Durant, Bartolucci, and Birch 1981) since it implies that all patients achieving complete response have an identical neoplastic cell burden. An analysis of the four arms separately (Simon 1979*b*) or stratification for induction regimens (Durant *et al.* 1981) is necessary in this situation.

Another aspect of the two-stage design has been discussed by Simon (1982*b*). In this approach, the evaluation of a new treatment is performed in two steps, the second stage being a confirmation study for therapy found promising in the first stage. Such a design will keep the delta error (Staquet *et al.* 1979) low, even with small sample size for the first stage. Such a scheme could be useful considering the possibility that investigators will be more willing to participate to a deliberately designed two-stage study rather than to simply repeat an earlier positive trial.

CONCLUSIONS

The choice of a design for a phase III trial is an important decision with regards to the final analysis of the study. The adoption of a poor or inadequate design is often recognized too late in the course of the study, for example at the time of the first interim statistical analysis, and leads to unreliable final conclusions.

The use of a proper treatment allocation technique is essential in phase III trials to increase the probability of a valid conclusion. Any procedure which does not assume that the treatment for each patient is allocated by a random procedure must be rejected. In multi-centre trials, a centralized randomization is helpful to fulfil this requirement. In single centres, it is recommended that the investigator rely on the statistician or an independent investigator to randomize the patients on his behalf.

Most investigators recognize intuitively that randomization is warranted to make the treatment groups comparable, but very few realize that the very concept of randomization is central to the statistical analyses performed on phase III trial data. To elaborate on this, it is useful to distinguish between 'random sampling' of patients from a specified population and 'random assignment' of treatments to the patients in the sample.

In the field of clinical trials, random sampling is almost never possible. In fact, the population of interest to the clinician is likely to be inaccessible and the investigator must take whatever patients are available in the participating institutions, that is a highly selected, non-representative, non-random sample of the diseased population of interest. Thus the automatic inference from sample to population is usually not valid.

Random assignment of treatments to available patients is the kind of randomization most clinicians rely upon in phase III trials. This latter procedure is essential to perform valid statistical tests; but the generalization of the conclusions to a larger population has no statistical basis if a random sample has not been drawn. Indeed, nothing in statistical theory allows one to infer from a sample to a population which is defined a posteriori when the trial is completed. However such a generalization is needed because the very purpose of a trial is to find a better treatment for the patients of tomorrow. The process is then purely judgemental and the result of the statistical analysis is one of the elements to consider. In general, the examination of all aspects of a trial, logistic, medical, and statistical, will reveal the necessity of carrying out confirmatory phase III studies to validate positive early results.

ACKNOWLEDGEMENT

This article was written while the first author was a Guest Worker in the Clinical and Diagnostic Trials Section, Biometry Branch, National Cancer Institute, Bethesda, USA. Although the opinions here are those of the authors, appreciation is expressed for stimulating discussions with the staff of the Section, as well as with members of the EORTC Data Center.

REFERENCES

Begg, C. B. and Iglewicz, B. (1980). A treatment allocation procedure for sequential clinical trials. *Biometrics* **36**, 81–90.

Bonadonna, G., Tancini, G., Rossi, A., and Gasparini, M. (1978). Chemotherapy in prevention of the recurrence of resectable cancer. *A. Rev. Med.* **29**, 149–75.

Brown, B. W. (1980*a*). Statistical controversies in the design of clinical trials. Some personal views. *Control. clin. Trials* **1**, 13–27.

—— (1980*b*). The crossover experiment for clinical trials. *Biometrics* **36**, 69–79.

Byar, D. P. (1980). Why data bases should not replace randomized clinical trials. *Biometrics* **36**, 337–42.

—— Simon, R. M., Friedewald, W. T., Schlesselman, J. J., DeMets, D. L., Ellenberg, J. H., Gail, M. H., and Ware, J. H. (1976). Randomized clinical trials: perspectives on some recent ideas. *New Engl. J. Med.* **295**, 74–80.

Carter, S. K. (1980*a*). Clinical considerations in the design of clinical trials. *Cancer Treat. Rep.* **64**, 367–71.

—— (1980*b*). Surgery plus adjuvant chemotherapy. A review of therapeutic implications. I. Breast cancer. *Cancer Chemother. Pharmac.* **4**, 147–63.

Chalmers, T. C., Block, J. B., and Lee, S. (1972). Controlled studies in clinical cancer research. *New Engl. J. Med.* **287**, 75–8.

Ciampi, A. and Till, J. E. (1980). Null results in clinical trials: the need for a decision theory approach. *Br. J. Cancer* **41**, 618–29.

DeVita, V. T. (1982). Principles of chemotherapy. In *Cancer: principles and practice of oncology* (eds. V. T. DeVita, S. Hellman, and S. A. Rosenberg) pp. 132–55. J. B. Lippincott, Hagerstown.

—— and Hellman, S. (1982). Hodgkin's disease and the non-Hodgkin's lymphoma. In *Cancer: principles and practice of oncology* (eds. V. T. DeVita, S. Hellman, and S. A. Rosenberg) pp. 1331–401. J. B. Lippincott, Hagerstown.

Durant, J. R., Bartolucci, A. A., and Birch, R. (1981). Importance of stratification in later stages of clinical trials. *Control. clin. Trials* **2**, 319–25.

Efron, B. (1971). Forcing a sequential experiment to be balanced. *Biometrika* **58**, 403–17.

Freedman, L. S. and White, S. J. (1976). On the use of Pocock and Simon's method for balancing treatment numbers over prognostic factors in the controlled clinical trial. *Biometrics* **32**, 691–4.

Friedman, L. M., Furberg, C. D., and DeMets, D. L. (1981). *Fundamentals of clinical trials*, p. 41. John Wright–PSG, Bristol.

Gehan, E. A. and Freireich, E. J. (1974). Non-randomized controls in cancer clinical trials. *New Engl. J. Med.* **290**, 198–203.

Glatstein, E. (1981). Radiation therapy as an adjuvant in cancer treatment. In *Adjuvant therapy of cancer III* (eds. S. E. Salmon and S. E. Jones) pp. 45–52. Grune and Stratton, New York.

Green, S. B. and Byar, D. P. (1978). The effect of stratified randomization on size and power of statistical tests in clinical trials. *J. chron. Dis.* **31**, 445–54.

Hills, M. and Armitage, P. (1979). The two-period cross-over clinical trial. *Br. J. clin. Pharmac.* **8**, 7–20.

Ingelfinger, F. J. (1972). The randomized clinical trial. *New Engl. J. Med.* **287**, 100–1.

Lagakos, S. W. and Pocock, S. J. (1983). Randomization and stratification in cancer clinical trials: An international survey. In *Cancer clinical trials: methods and practice* (eds. M. Buyse, M. Staquet, and R. Sylvester) pp. 276–86. Oxford University Press, Oxford.

Machin, D. (1978). On the possibility of incorporating patients from non-randomizing centres into a randomized clinical trial. *J. chron. Dis.* **32**, 347–53.

Makuch, R. W. and Simon, R. (1978). Note on the design of multi-institution three-treatment studies. *Cancer clin. Trials* **1**, 301–4.

Nordle, Ö. and Brantmark, B. (1977). A self-adjusting randomization plan for allocation of patients into two treatment groups. *Clin. Pharmac. Ther.* **22**, 825–30.

Peto, R. (1978). Clinical trial methodology. *Biomedicine* Special Issue **28**, 24–36.

—— Pike, M. C., Armitage, P., Breslow, N. E., Cox, D. R., Howard, S. V., Mantel, N., McPherson, K., Peto, J., and Smith, P. G. (1976). Design and analysis of randomized clinical trials requiring prolonged observation of each patient. i. Introduction and design. *Br. J. Cancer* **34**, 585–612.

Pocock, S. J. (1979). Allocation of patients to treatment in clinical trials. *Biometrics* **35**, 183–97.

—— Simon, R. (1975). Sequential treatment assignment with balancing for prognostic factors in the controlled clinical trials. *Biometrics* **31**, 103–15.

Schoenfeld, D. A. and Gelber, R. D. (1979). Designing and analyzing clinical trials which allow institutions to randomize patients to a subset of the treatments under study. *Biometrics* **35**, 825–9.

Schwartz, D. and Lellouch, J. (1967). Explanatory and pragmatic attitudes in therapeutic trials. *J. chron. Dis.* **20**, 637–48.

Simon, R. (1979a). Restricted randomization designs in clinical trials. *Biometrics* **35**, 503–12.

—— (1979b). Heterogeneity and standardization in clinical trials. In *Controversies in cancer. Design of trials and treatment* (eds. H. J. Tagnon and M. J. Staquet) pp. 37–49. Masson, New York.

—— (1982a). Design and conduct of clinical trials. In *Cancer. Principles and Practice of Oncology* (eds. V. T. DeVita, S. Hellman, S. A. Rosenberg) pp. 198–225. J. B. Lippincott, Hagerstown.

—— (1982b). Randomized clinical trials and research strategy. *Cancer Treat. Rep.* **66**, 1083–7.

Staquet, M. (1978). *Randomized trials in cancer. A critical review by sites.* Raven Press, New York.

——Rozencweig, M., Von Hoff, D. D., and Muggia, F. M. (1979). The delta and epsilon errors in the assessment of cancer clinical trials. *Cancer Treat. Rep.* **63**, 1917–21.

Taves, D. R. (1974). Minimization: a new method of assigning patients to treatment and control groups. *Clin. Pharmacol. Ther.* **15,** 443–53.

Ultmann, J. E. and Karnofsky, J. R. (1979). Adjuvant therapy: principles and state of the art. In *Adjuvant therapy of cancer II* (eds. S. E. Jones and S. E. Salmon) pp. 637–59. Grune and Stratton, New York.

White, S. J. and Freedman, L. S. (1978). Allocation of patients to treatment groups in a controlled clinical study. *Br. J. Cancer* **37,** 849–57.

Zelen, M. (1975). Importance of prognostic factors in planning therapeutic trials. In *Cancer therapy: prognostic factors and criteria of response* (ed. M. Staquet) pp. 1–35. Raven Press, New York.

17 Randomization and stratification in cancer clinical trials: an international survey

Stephen W. Lagakos and Stuart J. Pocock

INTRODUCTION

The use of randomization to allocate treatments to patients in cancer clinical trials is widely accepted as the best and, by some, the only way of achieving scientifically valid results. Randomization avoids selection biases and tends to make the treatment groups comparable in all respects (see Byar 1976; Byar, Simon, Friedewald, *et al.* 1979; Zelen 1974).

The simplest type of randomization independently assigns each treatment to each patient with equal probability. In a trial comparing two treatments this amounts to tossing a coin for each patient. Although this type of randomization *tends* to lead to balance between the treatment groups, both with respect to total numbers assigned and prognostic factors, it assures only that balance is achieved on the average. Thus, particularly in small trials, imbalances can occur between the numbers of subjects assigned to the various treatment groups, or with respect to one or more baseline patient characteristics (see for example Pocock 1979). Consequently, a number of alternative methods of randomization have been proposed which force various kinds of balance. An extensive discussion of most of these methods can be found in Pocock (1979).

Some methods are static in the sense that a specific allocation plan is set out in advance of the trial. The most common static method is called random permuted blocks. Suppose there are T treatments and K is a positive integer, often taken to be two. Then, for each block of $k = KT$ successive patients, a random ordering of K assignments to each treatment is produced. The mechanics for implementing this are quite simple (Zelen 1974), and the procedure guarantees that the number of subjects assigned to each treatment is balanced after every k enter. Extension of the method to balance assignments with respect to prognostic factor(s) is achieved by having a separate set of permuted blocks for each level of the factor(s).

Other randomization methods are dynamic, and utilize the actual treatment assignments and/or the baseline characteristics of previously enrolled patients in the determination of a treatment for a new patient. One such method is the biased coin technique (Efron 1971), in which the chances of assigning a new patient to a given treatment are inversely related to the proportion of previous patients that have been assigned to this treatment. Other dynamic methods which attempt to balance one or more baseline characteristics have been proposed by Pocock and Simon (1975) and by Begg and Iglewicz (1980). Extensions and variations of the Pocock–Simon approach have been developed by Freedman and White (1976) and White and Freedman (1978) and will be described in greater detail in the Section dealing with current methods of randomization.

In addition to the issue of static versus dynamic allocation, randomization methods also differ with respect to the degree of chance involved in each treatment assignment. Some are essentially deterministic, while others involve varying elements of chance.

There is no single method of randomization that is universally acknowledged as best for all situations. Virtually everyone feels that perfect balance is ideal. However, the implementation of more elaborate randomization methods is usually associated with additional complexities, and these can increase the chances of something 'going wrong'. As a result, it is often preferable to use a simpler method which is easier to carry out. The trade-off between statistical efficiency and practical applicability depends on numerous factors associated with the institutions participating in the trial, and few hard-and-fast results exist for selecting the 'best' randomization method for a given trial.

The purpose of this chapter is to describe current approaches to randomization by reporting the results of a survey of 15 major cancer centres in Europe and the United States. We describe the *mechanics* involved in the patient registration/randomization procedure—that is the actual steps taken between the time a patient is deemed appropriate for a particular trial and when he or she receives a treatment assignment. We then discuss the statistical methods used by the centres. Finally, we make recommendations on how randomization should be carried out in cancer trials. Since no single approach is best for every trial, our recommendations attempt to strike a balance between statistical efficiency and practical feasibility.

THE SURVEY

The survey was undertaken to learn how cancer research centres actually randomized patients into clinical trials. We surveyed a number of established centres with which we had had previous personal contact. All these centres have a broad experience at co-ordinating cancer clinical trials. Table 17.1 lists the 15 centres included in the survey.

The centres offer broad geographical coverage in Europe and North America. Eight had over 30 active clinical trials and three had less than 10 active trials. Each centre was involved in at least one multi-institutional trial, although in three the majority of trials were confined to their own hospital.

Table 17.1. *Centres included in randomization survey*

Organization	Location	Contact
Institut Gustave Roussy	Paris	R. Flamant
Cancer Research Centre of the USSR Academy of Medical Sciences	Moscow	A. Klimenkov
European Organization for Research on Treatment of Cancer	Brussels	R. Sylvester
Medical Research Council Cancer Trials Unit	Cambridge	L. Freedman
Christie Hospital	Manchester	M. Palmer
Oxford Clinical Trials Centre	Oxford	R. Peto
Scottish Breast Group	Edinburgh	R. Prescott
Childrens Cancer Study Group	Los Angeles	H. Sather
Memorial Sloan Kettering Cancer Center	New York	D. Braun
Northern California Oncology Group	San Francisco	B. Brown
Biometry Branch of National Cancer Institute	Bethesda	D. Byar
Mayo Clinic	Rochester	T. Fleming
University of Texas System Cancer Center	Houston	E. Gehan
Cancer and Leukemia Group B	New York	O. Glidewell
Eastern Cooperative Oncology Group	Boston	K. Stanley

Our method of enquiry was for one or both of us to visit each centre or otherwise interview the person(s) primarily responsible for the system of patient registration and randomization that was used. We had a formal questionnaire which we used as a guide to obtain details on the methods used to randomize patients, their rationale, practicality, and effectiveness.

MECHANICS OF RANDOMIZATION

When a patient is deemed appropriate for a particular clinical trial, a first step is often to obtain *informed consent*. This is a legal requirement in the US, although not in the seven European centres. Two of the European centres indicated that each participating hospital decided on whether and how to handle informed consent.

In 12 of the 15 centres, the primary method of obtaining a randomized treatment assignment was by *centralized registration by telephone*. The patient's attending physician or nurse would telephone the centre's randomization office, provide certain information about the patient and themselves, and then receive a treatment assignment over the phone. In the other three centres, the primary method of obtaining a treatment assignment was by the *sealed envelope* technique. Here a collection of sealed envelopes is maintained at each institution participating in the trial. When a patient is ready to be randomized, the next available envelope is opened, disclosing treatment assignment.

As regards *documentation*, it was standard practice for the centres to maintain a randomization *log sheet* containing patient name, institution, stratifying factors, and treatment assignments. For trials using sealed envelopes, receipt of this information relied on investigators notifying the centre. Some centres also recorded the physician's name, the name of the person phoning, and the patient's birthday (the latter as a means of distinguishing patients having the same name). Only four of the 12 centres that routinely used centralized telephone registration sent a written *confirmation* of each randomization to the patient's institution. One centre required that institutions follow-up each randomization by sending a written confirmation to the centre.

Eight of the 12 centres using a centralized telephone registration carried out some degree of *eligibility checking* during the telephone call in an attempt to avoid randomizing patients who were not in the target population. In some centres it was customary to review all patient eligibility requirements that were specified in the protocol, but in most centres only a limited number of key eligibility requirements were checked. In trials using sealed envelopes there is no real scope for eligibility checks.

One centre made use of a *computer* during the telephone registration. Information was keyed into the computer by the person at the registration office, and the resulting treatment assignment was passed on to the institution before the call ended.

We asked each centre about problems that occurred with the registration of patients. One potential problem with centralized telephone registration is off-hours calls. Most centres made no provision for off-hours randomizations. One centre permitted the participating institution to make a random treatment assignment when the central office could not be reached. The centre that utilized a computer during the telephone registration had a prepared randomization list in the event that the computer was temporarily not working. In some centres that preferred centralized telephone registration, envelopes were used in a few trials or for a few institutions in a given trial because of language or distance problems. One difficulty cited with the envelope technique was the time delays before the centre was notified of randomization and the corresponding inability to monitor the trial.

All centres reported that *ineligible patients* were occasionally randomized into studies, but most felt that this occurred relatively rarely. One centre documented all such occurrences and found that about 6 per cent of their randomized patients were ineligible (this centre also carried out some eligibility checking during registration). This information formed a part of the annual report of the centre.

Most centres indicated that *non-randomized* patients could not be entered into their randomized studies, although two centres indicated that a few non-randomized patients had entered studies which used sealed envelopes.

In general, all centres felt that their primary system of registering and randomizing patients was manageable and effective. Several centres were contemplating a few changes, but most seemed minor. When asked why they used the systems they did, most centres cited practicality as the primary consideration.

CURRENT METHODS OF RANDOMIZATION

In all but two of the centres the standard method of randomizing patients was by *random permuted blocks within strata.* As stated above, patient types are classified into several strata based on the levels of two or more prognostic factors. A separate list of random treatment assignments is then prepared for each stratum, with the constraint that each list has equal numbers on each treatment after every so many (say k) patients. For example, for a trial comparing two treatments (say A and B) in which it is desired to balance with respect to institution and gender, two randomization lists are prepared for each institution, one per sex. If k, the so-called block size, is six, each list consists of a sequence of random permutations of three As and three Bs: for example A,B,B,A,A,B; B,A,B,A,A,B; B,B,A,B,A,A, etc.

Although the use of random permuted blocks within strata was standard in 13 of the centres, there was considerable variability in the specifics of how it was used. Consider firstly the number and types of stratification factors. Some form of *institutional balance* was standard in all but one of the centres. Two of the European centres generally did not stratify by anything other than institution, and two others had at least one trial without additional stratification. The American centres generally used more stratification than the European centres, although no centre tended to use more than five patient factors.

Two of the centres that used random permuted blocks within strata did not use institution as a stratification factor in the usual way, but instead balanced treatments within institution dynamically; whenever the treatment difference in the next patient's institution exceeds a certain number, usually two or three, the treatment assignment specified by the randomization list is ignored, and the patient is assigned to the treatment with the smallest number of patients at that institution. The rationale for this way of balancing seemed to be that there were sufficiently many institutions that the usual method would produce too many strata.

The most common choice for block size (k) was twice the number of treatments. Thus, in a two-arm study a block size of four was typically used. One centre used a block size equal to the number of treatment groups. Some trials used larger block sizes, but none exceeded 10.

Some centres using permuted blocks within strata sometimes achieved an additional degree of balance by imposing constraints between randomization lists. For example, one centre used a system in which each treatment would be the first assignment in the same number of randomization lists.

Four centres were using *dynamic* allocation procedures in which the $(n+1)^{st}$ patient's treatment assignment can depend on his and the previous n patients stratification factors. One centre used a form of *minimization* based on *Efron's biased coin* design almost exclusively (Efron 1980). Another centre used a deterministic type of minimization in 80 per cent of their trials (White and Freedman 1978), and two other centres used minimization in a single trial.

Since practicality is a primary concern in selecting a randomization method, we feel it instructive to illustrate the details of how minimization was used by one centre in a two-arm trial for head and neck cancer. In this trial it was desired to balance treatments across 15 institutions, seven disease sites, and nodal involvement (yes or no). Use of conventional methods would therefore require $15 \times 7 \times 2 = 210$ strata, which is clearly impractical. Minimization attempts to achieve balance by balancing the treatments within the $15 + 7 + 2 = 24$ levels of the three stratification factors. Specifically, one keeps a tally of the number of patients on each treatment within each of these 24 levels. Then, when the next patient is to be entered, the three levels corresponding to him or her are used to determine the treatment assignment. For example, suppose the patient is from the Royal Marsden Hospital, has oropharynx cancer, and no nodal involvement, and suppose that until now the numbers of patients on each treatment arm for each of these levels are as follows:

	Misonidazole	*Placebo*
Royal Marsden	13	14
Oropharynx cancer	25	23
No nodal involvement	80	80
Sum = 118	117

That is, of the patients already in the trial, $27 (= 13 + 14)$ are from Royal Marsden, $48 (= 25 + 23)$ have oropharynx cancer, and $160 (= 80 + 80)$ have no nodal involvement. One then totals these three categories and assigns the treatment with the smaller total (in this case placebo). If the totals were equal, treatment is assigned at random. Hence, to implement this method, a total of 24 tally sheets must be kept, and for each new patient three of these are used to determine the treatment assignment and subsequently updated. Other forms of minimization are similar, but combine the three levels somewhat differently or introduce a degree of randomness in the treatment assignment.

We asked each centre whether any unequal or blinded randomization designs were used. Seven centres had tried designs where unequal numbers of patients were intentionally assigned to the treatment groups, although this was not a common practice. Three centres had undertaken double-blind studies. Two of these had 'blinded' and coded drug packages sent in advance to each centre, and the appropriate code was given over the phone for each patient. In the third centre the institution pharmacist phoned the centre to obtain the treatment assignment and then gave this, in blinded form, to the patient's physician.

RECOMMENDATIONS

Having reviewed how various cancer centres handle patient registration and randomization, we will make some general recommendations. It should be noted that the following are our views and not necessarily shared by each centre.

Telephone randomization

For multi-institutional trials the most reliable means of randomizing patients is to have the institution telephone a central office each time they enter a patient. The alternative of using sealed envelopes at each institution does not allow central monitoring of the randomization procedure or eligibility checking and carries a greater risk of things going wrong. If central telephone randomization is not feasible, for example in some international trials, then telex or telegram may provide an acceptable alternative. However, in some circumstances, it may be necessary to use sealed envelopes. It is then important to monitor patient entry retrospectively to check the scheme was followed. For single-centre trials one should aim for the same formal approach via a randomization office, except personal contact may replace the telephone call.

Eligibility checks

Some centres formally checked that each patient was eligible for the trial immediately before treatment was assigned. We endorse this approach as an effective method of reducing the number of patients who are mistakenly put into a trial. While one can try to preserve a trial's validity by retrospectively eliminating ineligible cases, suspicions may arise if it is done too often or arbitrarily. More importantly, the inclusion of ineligible patients in a study may mean that they fail to receive the best treatment for their disease.

Confirmation of randomization

In multi-institutional trials, it is advisable to follow-up telephone randomization by a written confirmation of patient entry and treatment assignment. This was done in only a few centres and one wonders what drop-outs might occur in other centres due to lack of confirmation. Confirmation notices can also include an opportune reminder of certain aspects of the protocol such as when patient data is to be submitted.

The sequence of events

The one essential aspect of randomization is that the investigator cannot anticipate in advance which treatment any given patient will receive. Thus, before treatment assignment is given one must ensure that both investigator and patient are willing to accept randomization. The validity and credibility of a trial can be seriously compromised when there are investigators or patients who refuse the treatments they were assigned.

Statistical methods for randomization

The simplest method is to prepare a single randomization list in advance, using either a table of random numbers or a computer. This is the equivalent of tossing a coin and has the advantages of simplicity, unpredictability, and hence reliability. Its disadvantage is that one has no guarantee that the treatment groups will be equal in size and similar in type of patient, although in large trials serious imbalances are unlikely to occur. However, it is standard practice to impose some form of restriction on randomization to ensure reasonable balance and the remainder of this paper discusses the various options.

Random permuted blocks

One can arrange each randomization list so that it has equal treatment numbers every so many patients by using random permuted blocks. The number of patients per block will depend on the extent of stratification (see below) but should preferably not be so small as to enable investigators to predict the next assignment, nor so large as to allow serious inequality mid-block. The choice of block size to be twice the number of treatments, as used by most centres, seems to us a sensible one.

Institution balance

In multi-centre trials it is desirable to have approximately equal patient numbers on each treatment within each institution. In the previous Section about current methods of randomization we described three possible approaches: the choice will depend on the extent of other stratification.

Stratification

In principle it is useful to take account of patient factors affecting response by trying to arrange comparable treatment groups (Feinstein and Landis 1976). The standard approach is to choose a few such factors, divide patients accordingly into different strata and use the method of random permuted blocks within each stratum. The problem is to know which patient factors to stratify by and how many such factors it is feasible to include.

Which patient factors?

One should only stratify by factors which are known, or thought very likely, to affect response. Clinicians often favour rather 'technical' factors, such as oestrogen receptors or histological classification, whereas it often turns out that more 'patient oriented' factors, such as weight loss or performance status, have a greater bearing on patient response. For instance, in studies of advanced disease one should consider stratifying by performance status (Zelen 1973). The arbitrary stratification by factors which are of clinical interest but of unknown effect on response should be avoided. Such factors can be included satisfactorily in the analysis of results but need not affect trial design.

Also, one should only stratify by factors which are reliably reported at the time of randomization. For instance, tumour pathology may be unsuitable if local hospital pathologists are inconsistent or if one has to wait for centralized diagnosis to be done.

How many factors?

If institution is one of the stratifying factors in a permuted block design, then one can usually include only one or two other factors in the determination of strata. Otherwise the number of strata becomes too large and this could actually reduce the chances of balance with respect to any individual factor (Pocock 1979). If institutions are balanced dynamically (see the previous section about current methods of randomization), then additional factors might be used.

Minimization

As explained in the section on current methods of randomization, one or two centres have decided to use minimization methods for treatment allocation. The advantage is that balance can be assured across more patient factors, but a certain amount of additional effort is needed as each patient is randomized. The method seems workable in those centres that have tried it, but others might find it more awkward to use. Further experiences may identify more clearly the role of minimization. The method should be particularly valuable in trials of limited size in which several factors are known to affect response.

Is imbalance a problem?

It is statistically efficient for treatment groups to be as similar as possible with respect to prognostic factors. Imbalances can be adjusted for retrospectively, (for example by analysis of covariance methods), and the loss of efficiency relative to a balanced study is usually small, provided the appropriate model is used for adjustment. Thus, on scientific basis alone, imbalance is not usually of serious consequence. Rather, the main problem is a certain loss of credibility associated with non-comparable treatment groups. Clinicians and other consumers of the results of a trial are likely to be sceptical of findings in which the unadjusted treatment comparisons are different from the adjusted comparisons. This scepticism is often well founded. When adjustment is necessary, the choice of statistical models is more important than when it is not, and different statistical models can lead to different 'adjusted' results. Thus, it becomes important to ensure that the correct statistical model is used for adjustment.

Is stratification worthwhile?

Many trials would be well balanced even if no stratification were used. Thus, stratification is like an insurance policy to guarantee this balance. The greatest advantage over non-stratified randomization is the safeguard against the unlikely event of a sizeable difference in the number of patients on each treatment in one or more patient factors. The larger a trial becomes the less important is stratification since the chances of imbalance are progressively reduced. However, even in the largest of trials, if interim analyses are required one should contemplate stratification. In any sized trial, it is advisable to stratify or otherwise balance for institution.

One's decision, as to whether to stratify or not, must be a compromise between the ideal of achieving perfect balance and the feasibility of day-to-day running of a randomization centre. One should not attempt stratification if it cannot be carried out reliably. For example, it is not often feasible to stratify if sealed envelopes are used. With a central phone registration, however, stratification usually does not complicate the randomization procedure.

Reliability and simplicity

One essential in any randomization procedure is that it should work in practice for every patient entered. Hence, one should avoid undue complexity in the cause of exact scientific design. One should aim for a system which is effective in ensuring that the protocol is followed, with appropriate methods to achieve good balance which can be implemented by the resources available at the randomization centre.

ACKNOWLEDGEMENTS

This work was undertaken as part of the UICC project on controlled therapeutic trials, and has been reported in the *British Journal of Cancer*,

September 1982. We are very grateful to the members of the cancer centres participating in our survey, to Laurence Freedman for the example in the section on current methods of randomization, and to Marc Buyse and Richard Sylvester for beneficial suggestions.

REFERENCES

Begg, C. B. and Iglewicz, B. (1980). A treatment allocation procedure for sequential clinical trials. *Biometrics* **36**, 81–90.

Byar, D. P. (1979). The necessity and justification of randomized clinical trials. In *Controversies in cancer: design of trials and treatment* (eds. H. J. Tagnon and M. J. Staquet) pp. 75–82. Masson, New York.

—— Simon, R. M., Friedewald, W. T., *et al.* (1976). Randomized clinical trials: perspectives on some recent ideas. *N. Engl. J. Med.* **295**, 74–80.

Efron, B. (1971). Forcing a sequential experiment to be balanced. *Biometrika* **58**, 403–17.

—— (1980). Randomizing and balancing a complicated sequential experiment. In: *Biostatistics casebook* (eds. R. G. Miller, B. Efron, B. W. Brown, Jr, and L. E. Moses) pp. 19–23. Wiley, New York.

Feinstein, A. R. and Landis, J. R. (1976). The role of prognostic stratification in preventing the bias permitted by random allocation of treatment. *J. chron. Dis.* **29**, 277–84.

Freedman, L. A. and White, S. J. (1976). On the use of Pocock and Simon's method for balancing treatment numbers over prognostic factors in the controlled clinical trial. *Biometrics* **32**, 691–4.

Pocock, S. J. (1979). Allocation of patients to treatment in clinical trials. *Biometrics* **35**, 183–97.

—— and Simon, R. (1975). Sequential treatment assignment with balancing for prognostic factors in the controlled clinical trial. *Biometrics* **31**, 103–15.

White, S. J. and Freedman, L. S. (1978). Allocation of patients to treatment groups in a controlled clinical study. *Br. J. Cancer* **37**, 849–57.

Zelen, M. (1973). Keynote address on biostatistics and data retrieval. *Cancer Chemother. Rep.* **4**, 31–42.

—— (1974). The randomization and stratification of patients to clinical trials. *J. chron. Dis.* **27**, 365–75.

18 The required size and length of a phase III clinical trial

Stephen L. George

INTRODUCTION

Most clinical trials are quite simple in their experimental design. The standard procedure is to allocate eligible patients at random to one of the available treatments, perhaps balancing the randomization separately within two or more 'strata', or groupings, of patients based on some measure of disease severity or prognosis. Summary measures of outcome are then compared among treatments.

It is the purpose of this paper to review the general principles involved in the determination of the required size and length of such a clinical trial, to provide tables suitable for practical application, and to discuss the effect on size and length of study of such complicating factors as censoring, loss to follow-up, unbalanced randomization, and stratification by risk groups. Calculation formulae are given so that cases not covered by the tables can be handled if desired but detailed derivations are omitted and the text may be read without following the mathematics. A fairly detailed set of recent references is provided for those who wish to pursue the subject further.

BACKGROUND AND GENERAL PRINCIPLES

In a review of 71 'negative' randomized clinical trials reported in the medical literature in the 1960s and 1970s, Freiman, Chalmers, Smith, and Kuebler (1978) discovered that most of the trials included too few patients to provide much assurance that a clinically meaningful difference would not be missed. Similarly, Pocock (1978), in a review of 40 randomized clinical trials in cancer, uncovered some serious problems in planning, ranging from extreme optimism in anticipated results (yielding very small numbers of patients) to lack of projections of adequate patient accrual. Peto (1982) argues that larger (and simpler) cancer trials are urgently needed. Thus, despite the widespread use of clinical trials as a therapeutic research tool, there remains a need for a greater appreciation of fundamental design issues. One of the most fundamental of these issues is the determination of how many patients are needed and how long the trial must last to achieve the desired objectives.

The problem of determining the required sample size in a statistical study is, of course, not a new one. In general terms, the most common procedures involve the determination of some minimum sample size such that the statistical testing procedure is sufficiently sensitive to detect differences of interest and that the estimation of these differences is sufficiently precise. These notions are made more concrete in the following paragraphs.

Perhaps the most conventional approach to the problem is that of hypothesis testing. In this approach, one first specifies the null hypothesis of no difference among the various treatments under study and fixes the rate α, the type I error rate, at which this hypothesis will be erroneously rejected when it is in fact correct. For two treatments it is necessary to distinguish between one-sided tests, in which only one direction of difference is being tested, and two-sided tests, in which deviations in either direction are being tested. Then, for some specified hypothetical deviation from the null hypothesis, one determines the sample size N necessary to achieve a specified probability, $1 - \beta$, of correctly rejecting the null hypothesis when in fact the deviation holds. The quantity β is referred to as the type II error rate and $1 - \beta$ is the power of the test at the specified alternative hypothesis. The power of the test is the most natural index of the sensitivity of the test procedure. Although there is no necessity to do so, it is fairly common practice to set β four or five times as large as α. For example (α, β) pairs of $(0.01, 0.05)$ and $(0.05, 0.20)$ are common.

Thus one can, in principle, determine the sample size from the quantities α, β and Δ (where Δ is used here as a generic index of deviation from the null hypothesis), plus knowledge of the probability distribution of the test statistic, Y, used to test the null hypothesis. An excellent general review of these areas is provided by Lachin (1981) and the references therein. In the absence of any complicating factors, such as censoring, loss to follow-up or drop-outs, tables for the required number of patients are provided in various references (for example Cochran and Cox 1957) for the more common testing situations. The solutions for the normal distribution are of primary importance since most of the test statistics or some simple transformation will be approximately normally distributed except for very small sample sizes.

A second approach to the determination of N is to specify the required precision in the estimation of treatment effects (or in the differences of these effects). This approach may be used in addition to the hypothesis testing approach or instead of it. It is an obvious choice for those situations in which tests of hypothesis are not of primary importance. Also, some statisticians object on general principles to the design of clinical trials based on arbitrary tests of hypotheses and prefer, instead, some estimation approach.

In the estimation approach, one specifies that the standard error of the difference of the treatment effects is to be less than some value ε. Thus, one can determine N for a given ε given knowledge of the standard deviation. Although this general approach is independent of any hypothesis testing considerations, the two approaches (testing and estimation) can obviously be linked by an appropriate choice of ε. Also, as mentioned earlier, there is no reason why one could not design a study to satisfy both types of criteria simultaneously.

Both the testing and estimation approaches as defined above result in a requirement of a fixed number of patients on the various treatments. This 'fixed-sample' design is the most common one used in the design of clinical trials but, in practice, ethical and practical considerations require periodical assessment of the results during the course of the trial. This practice will affect the size and length considerations and lead to sequential or semi-sequential designs, a topic which is discussed in Chapter 19 of this book. Therefore, the results given in this chapter should be taken as approximate guidelines in the design of a trial, not as rigid requirements.

COMPARING SUCCESS RATES

One of the most common and simple outcome variables in a clinical trial is the 'success rate'. That is, each subject is classified as a success (response to therapy, survival to a fixed time T, etc.) or as a failure (non-response, death before T, etc.) so that each observation is simply a binary variable. The general problem is to estimate and compare the success rates in different treatment groups. This section provides the necessary background to determine the numbers of patients required in this setting. Fleiss (1981) gives a clear elementary description of the mathematics involved. The case of paired observations is not covered here but is discussed by Lachin (1981).

Comparing two success rates

Suppose we wish to compare the unknown success rates, θ_i $(i = 1, 2)$, in two treatment groups based on n independent observations from each treatment. If we wish to test equality at a two-sided significance level α with power $1 - \beta$ at a specified alternative (θ_1, θ_2), where $\theta_1 \neq \theta_2$, then a commonly used approximation to the required n is:

$$n = \left[\frac{(z_{\alpha/2} + z_\beta)^2}{2(\arcsin\sqrt{\theta_1} - \arcsin\sqrt{\theta_2})^2} \right] \tag{18.1}$$

where here, and in the following, $[x]$ is the smallest integer greater than or equal to x, z_x is the $100(1-x)$ percentile of the standard normal distribution and the arcsin is given in radians. For a one-sided test, simply replace $\alpha/2$ by α. This expression is based on the variance stabilizing transformation $\arcsin\sqrt{\hat\theta}$, where $\hat\theta = x/n$, the observed proportion of successes (Cochran and Cox 1957; Cohen 1977; Feigl 1978). Tables of n based on equation (18.1) are given in Cochran and Cox (1957) and isographs are given in Feigl (1978). Note that all (α, β) pairs yielding the same $z_{\alpha/2} + z_\beta$ result in the same required n. For example, the n required for $(\alpha = 0.05, \beta = 0.10)$ is nearly identical to $(\alpha = 0.01, \beta = 0.25)$. Nelson (1980) gives a graphical aid to determine such pairs.

However, as recently shown by Casagrande, Pike, and Smith (1978) and Hasemann (1978), the values of n obtained from eqn (18.1) are too low in comparison with the n required for an exact test. An improved approximation formula is given by Casagrande *et al.* (1978) as:

$$n^* = \left[\frac{\{\sqrt{A} + \sqrt{(A+4\delta)}\}^2}{4\delta^2} \right] \tag{18.2}$$

where $\sqrt{A} = z_{\alpha/2}\sqrt{2\bar{\theta}(1-\bar{\theta})} + z_\beta\sqrt{\{\theta_1(1-\theta_1) + \theta_2(1-\theta_2)\}}$, $\delta = \theta_1 - \theta_2$ and $\bar{\theta} = (\theta_1 + \theta_2)/2$. Isographs of n^* are given by Aleong and Bartlett (1979) and detailed tables are available in Fleiss (1981). Table 18.1 gives n^* for selected cases of practical importance.

Details of the exact approach to this problem are given in several papers (Gail and Gart 1973; Garside and Mack 1976; Hasemann 1978). The primary difficulty with the exact approach is computational complexity. This difficulty would be even more acute in the K-sample case, which is discussed in the next section.

In certain situations one may wish to select unequal numbers of patients to place on the two treatments (Walter 1977; Brittain and Schlesselman 1982). For example, if one of the two treatments is a 'control' treatment for which prior information is available, it may be more desirable to place more patients on the 'new' treatment in order to estimate its effect with more precision. In this case, we select one group of size n_1 and the other of size $n_2 = rn_1$ where $r > 0$. That is, the two group sizes are in the ratio $r:1$.

The generalization of eqn (18.2) to cover unbalanced treatment assignment is easily shown to be (see Fleiss, Tytun, and Ury 1980):

$$n_1 = \left[\frac{\{\sqrt{A'} + \sqrt{\{A' + 2(r+1)\delta\}}\}^2}{4r\delta^2} \right] \tag{18.3}$$

where

$$\sqrt{A'} = z_{\alpha/2}\sqrt{(r+1)\bar{\theta}(1-\bar{\theta})} + z_\beta\sqrt{\{r\theta_1(1-\theta_1) + \theta_2(1-\theta_2)\}}.$$

The size of the second sample is, or course, just r times n_1. Another approximation yielding similar results is given in Ury and Fleiss (1980).

The total population required in the unbalanced case ($r \neq 1$) is always larger than that required in the balanced case ($r = 1$). Similarly, for the same total number of patients, the maximum power is obtained by equal allocation of the patients to the two treatments. Some idea of this effect is given by the 'relative efficiency' of an unbalanced allocation, the ratio of the total number of patients required in the balanced case to the unbalanced case expressed as a percentage. This is given by the ratio of $2n^*$ to $n_1 + n_2$. A much simpler approximation for the relative efficiency is given by:

$$\frac{4r}{(r+1)^2} \times 100\%. \tag{18.4}$$

Table 18.1. Number of patients required on each of two treatments to compare success rates

θ_1 (Smaller success rate)	$\delta = \theta_2 - \theta_1 =$ Larger minus smaller success rate						
	0.05	0.10	0.15	0.20	0.25	0.30	0.35
0.10	580 (725)	176 (219)	92 (113)	58 (72)	41 (51)	31 (38)	25 (30)
	787 (957)	237 (286)	121 (146)	77 (92)	54 (65)	41 (49)	32 (38)
	917 (1061)	275 (317)	141 (162)	89 (102)	63 (72)	47 (54)	37 (43)
0.20	901 (1134)	251 (313)	122 (151)	74 (91)	50 (62)	37 (45)	28 (35)
	1233 (1504)	339 (412)	163 (198)	98 (118)	66 (80)	48 (58)	37 (44)
	1439 (1668)	395 (457)	190 (219)	114 (131)	77 (89)	56 (65)	43 (49)
0.30	1124 (1416)	300 (376)	141 (176)	83 (103)	55 (68)	40 (49)	30 (37)
	1541 (1882)	408 (496)	190 (230)	111 (134)	73 (88)	52 (63)	39 (47)
	1800 (2088)	476 (550)	221 (255)	129 (149)	85 (98)	61 (70)	45 (52)
0.40	1248 (1573)	325 (408)	149 (186)	86 (107)	56 (70)	40 (49)	29 (36)
	1713 (2092)	442 (538)	202 (244)	115 (140)	75 (90)	52 (63)	38 (46)
	2001 (2322)	516 (597)	235 (271)	134 (155)	87 (100)	61 (70)	45 (51)
0.50	1273 (1605)	325 (408)	147 (183)	83 (103)	53 (66)	37 (45)	27 (33)
	1747 (2134)	442 (538)	198 (240)	111 (134)	71 (85)	48 (58)	35 (41)
	2041 (2369)	516 (597)	230 (266)	129 (149)	82 (94)	56 (65)	41 (46)

Table 18.1 *(continued)*

θ_1	$\delta = \theta_2 - \theta_1$				
	0.40	0.50	0.60	0.70	0.80
0.10	29 (25) 26 (31) 30 (34)	14 (17) 18 (21) 21 (24)	11 (13) 13 (15) 16 (18)	8 (10) 10 (11) 12 (13)	6 (7) 7 (9) 9 (10)
0.20	23 (28) 29 (35) 34 (39)	15 (19) 19 (23) 23 (26)	11 (13) 13 (16) 16 (18)	8 (10) 10 (11) 12 (13)	— — —
0.30	23 (29) 30 (36) 35 (40)	15 (19) 19 (23) 23 (26)	11 (13) 13 (15) 16 (18)	— — —	— — —
0.40	23 (28) 29 (35) 34 (39)	14 (17) 18 (21) 21 (24)	— — —	— — —	— — —
0.50	20 (25) 26 (31) 30 (34)	— — —	— — —	— — —	— — —

Upper figure: $\alpha = 0.05$, $\beta = 0.20$.
Middle figure: $\alpha = 0.05$, $\beta = 0.10$.
Lower figure: $\alpha = 0.01$, $\beta = 0.20$.
Entries without parentheses are for one-sided tests. Numbers in parentheses are for two-sided tests.

Equation 18.4 is based on the same approximations that led to n. One point to notice from this is that relatively little efficiency is lost even for fairly severe imbalance. For example, if $r = 2$, the relative efficiency is approximately 89 per cent and for $r = 3$, the relative efficiency is approximately 75 per cent. Thus, one should not be overly concerned about the loss of efficiency in setting up an imbalanced treatment assignment scheme, particularly if there is some reason to be more precise about the effect of one of the treatments than the other one.

The inverse problem of calculating the power obtainable for a given sample size can be approached by solving eqn (18.3) for z_β. The power $1 - \beta$ is then easily calculated or read from ordinary tables of the standard normal distribution. However, since these equations must be solved iteratively, a simpler approach is to use the approximate equality (Fleiss *et al.* 1980):

$$z_\beta = \frac{\{r\delta^2 N/(r+1) - (r+1)\delta\}^{1/2} - z_{\alpha/2}\{(r+1)\bar\theta(1-\bar\theta)\}^{1/2}}{\{r\theta_1(1-\theta_1) + \theta_2(1-\theta_2)\}^{1/2}} \tag{18.5}$$

where N is the total sample size available.

Comparing more than two success rates

In order to compare the success rates in K populations, where $K > 2$, it is necessary to specify the deviation from the null hypothesis that it is desired to detect. The simplest way to do this is to specify the maximum response rate and the minimum response rate, and to assume the remaining $K - 2$ rates are exactly midway between extremes. This is the so-called 'least favourable' configuration since any other configuration would lead to higher power.

In this case, the required number of patients on each treatment, based on the arcsin transformation, can be shown to be:

$$n = \left[\frac{\lambda^2}{2(\arcsin\sqrt{\theta_1} - \arcsin\sqrt{\theta_0})^2} \right] \tag{18.6}$$

where θ_1 is the maximum θ, θ_0 is the minimum θ and λ^2 is the non-centrality parameter from a chi-squared distribution with $K - 1$ degrees of freedom for the specified α and β. There are computer programs available to calculate λ^2 as well as tables from which it can be obtained (for example Hayman, Govindarajula, and Leone 1970).

Alternatively, since eqn (18.6) is simply a multiple of eqn (18.1) for the two-sided case, one can obtain the required n by knowledge of this multiplication factor and the values of n for $K = 2$. By analogy with the case $K = 2$, we can use eqn (18.2) rather than eqn (18.1) in this approach. Thus, the approximate number of patients required in the case $K > 2$ can be obtained from Table 18.1 and the multiplication factors as given in Table 18.2. Note that the total number of patients required to compare K groups simultaneously is always greater than K times the number of patients needed in each group for a

Table 18.2. *Factors for determining the number of patients required to compare K > 2 success rates*

K = number of rates to be compared			
3	4	5	6
1.23	1.39	1.52	1.63
1.20	1.35	1.47	1.57
1.19	1.32	1.43	1.53

Upper figure: $\alpha = 0.05$, $\beta = 0.20$.
Middle figure: $\alpha = 0.05$, $\beta = 0.10$.
Lower figure: $\alpha = 0.01$, $\beta = 0.20$.
Least favourable configuration assumed.

comparison of two groups. The multiplication factor increases as a function of K.

It is important to emphasize that the factors given in Table 18.2 are for the least favourable configuration of the parameters. If there is reason to assume that this is not the case then considerably fewer patients may be required. For example, if all except one of the unknown success rates are equal, then the factors in Table 18.2 may themselves be multiplied by a factor of $[2(1 - 1/K)]^{-1}$. For example, if $K = 3$, the number of patients required when two of the three rates are equal is only three-quarters of the number required in the least favourable configuration. Further, in the extreme case, of the *most* favourable configuration (that is one-half of the success rates equal to θ_0 and the other half equal to θ_1), the savings is even more dramatic with a multiplication factor of approximately $2/K$ (exactly $2/K$ if K is even). While it is unlikely, in the absence of any prior knowledge, that one would be willing to assume the most favourable distribution for the success rates, the rather extreme conservatism of the factors in Table 18.2 should be kept in mind.

The power and sample sizes for approximate chi-square tests are discussed in Guenther (1977) and may be applied in the current setting. The related topic of testing for homogeneity in $R \times C$ trials is discussed by Lachin (1977). This latter topic is of interest when one is comparing K treatments with more than two outcomes.

Comparing a single success rate with a standard rate

Tests of hypotheses of the form $\theta \geq \theta_0$ versus $\theta < \theta_0$, where θ_0 is some standard (fixed) rate with which we wish to compare the rate θ, are based on a single sample of size N. The arcsin transformation approach yields an N of exactly one-half of n as given by eqn (18.1), with α in place of $\alpha/2$ since this is a one-sided test. Since n gives the number in each sample, the number of patients required in a single sample is exactly one-quarter of the total number required when comparing a single rate with a control population (rather than some fixed arbitrary standard). However, this dramatic saving in the number of patients required must be interpreted properly. For example, it does *not* provide a justification for use of historical controls. For a comparison with an historical control group, a minimum requirement would be to use the number of patients in the historical group as given (n_1) and find the number (n_2) of patients needed on the current treatment group by arguments similar to those leading to eqn (18.3). This approach would require more patients than the one-quarter factor mentioned above.

A better approach would be to take into account the fact that the results from the historical control group are fixed. This is the approach taken by Makuch and Simon (1980), who give the appropriate equation for n_2 and provide some limited tables for this situation. One important point here is that a solution is not always possible when the historical group is small.

Testing the equivalence of two proportions

Recent progress in the treatment of certain diseases (for example Hodgkin's Disease) has led investigators to design new treatment regimens which reduce the acute or chronic toxicity of some standard treatment while maintaining adequate disease control. One would like to reduce the unwanted side-effects without reducing effectiveness but, unfortunately, there is no way to be certain that the new treatment is really identical in effectiveness to the standard treatment.

In this setting, Makuch and Simon (1978) propose that enough patients be entered so that the confidence interval on the difference in success rates is nearly certain to be less than some specified length. If 'equivalence' of the two treatments is taken to mean simply that the success rate on the new treatment is very close (not necessarily identical) to that of the standard treatment, this approach is appropriate. The related approach of testing a non-null hypothesis is examined by Dunnett and Gent (1977) and Blackweder (1982).

Simple formulae for the required number of patients similar in form, but different in interpretation, to formulae for the usual significance testing approach are given in Makuch and Simon (1978). For most cases in which this approach would be adopted in practice (that is reasonably large success rates), smaller numbers of patients are required than for the significance testing approach. The important point is to avoid interpreting a simple lack of statistical significance as evidence of equivalence unless sufficient numbers of patients have been studied.

Cross-over designs

In some clinical settings (for example clinical pharmacology) it is possible to allow each patient to be treated serially with two or more treatments, which are applied in random order. For two treatments, this design is called a two-treatment two-period cross-over design and has been compared with other simple designs in reviews by Brown (1980) and Hills and Armitage (1979).

The relative advantages are largely dependent on the lack of a carry-over effect (that is a residual effect of a treatment in the first period on response in the second period). If there is no carry-over effect the efficiency of a cross-over design to a completely random design achieving the same precision can be quite large (how large depends on the intra-subject correlation; see Brown (1980) for details). On the other hand, if we cannot assume that the carry-over effect is negligible and must test for this possibility (Grizzle 1965), then the cross-over design can require considerably more patients than a completely random design.

COMPARING SURVIVAL DISTRIBUTIONS

Many clinical trials have as a major objective the comparison of two or more treatment groups with respect to the distributions of the times to some critical event, usually referred to as survival time. This time can be the time to recurrence of disease, the time to death, or any other clearly defined measure of time. For simplicity, the problem of determining the number of patients can be formulated and solved as in the previous section by defining 'success' as survival to some arbitrary time t. However, this approach is clearly inefficient in that it takes no account of the actual failure times before or after t. Also, this approach does not usually correspond to the analyses actually planned. A more realistic approach must take account of the facts that patients enter the study serially and that the complete survival times for all patients are not known at the time of analysis (George and Desu 1974; Pasternack and Gilbert 1971; Lustbader and Litwin 1981).

In this section, the following model is assumed:

(1) patients enter the study randomly according to a Poisson process with intensity γ (that is an average of γ patients per unit time);

(2) each patient, on entry, is assigned to one of K treatments with probability π_i $(i=1, \ldots, K)$. Usually, $\pi_i = K^{-1}$ (that is equal probabilities of assignment);

(3) the survival time of a patient assigned to treatment i has an exponential distribution with mean λ_i^{-1} (this assumption is not as restrictive as it first appears and will be discussed further below);

(4) entry continues to chronological (study) time T, after which patients are followed for an additional time τ.

The statistical hypothesis to be tested is that all of the λ_i are equal. The problems to be solved are: how many patients need to be entered and how long do they need to be followed in order to obtain a power of $1-\beta$? Thus, the notions of size and length are inextricably linked in a clinical trial designed to compare survival distributions. In our formulation, since the entry rate γ is considered fixed, these problems reduce to finding an appropriate entry time T and follow-up time τ such that a power of $1 - \beta$ is obtained at $T + \tau$. Without further assumptions, there is no unique solution to this problem. The general problem of selecting T and τ is deferred to the next section. In this section we derive the number of patients needed when all patients are followed until failure (that is no censoring) and describe the effect of censoring on these derivations.

Comparing two survival distributions

Suppose we wish to compare the unknown hazard rates λ_i ($i = 1, 2$) in two treatment groups based on n independent observations from each group. If we wish to test equality at a two-sided significance level α with power $1 - \beta$ at some specified alternative $\Delta = \lambda_1/\lambda_2$, then the required number of patients in each group, all followed until failure, is:

$$n = [2(z_{\alpha/2} + z_\beta)^2/(ln\ \Delta)^2].$$ (18.7)

This expression is based on the approximate normality of the distribution of $ln\ \bar{x}_i$ where $\bar{x}_i$ is the mean of the observations from the ith treatment group ($i = 1, 2$). Equation (18.7) yields values of n very close to those required by the exact approach based on the distribution of $\bar{x}_2/\bar{x}_1$ (George and Desu 1974; Lesser and Cento 1981). A one-sided test is obtained by replacing $\alpha/2$ by α. Note that the required n does not depend on knowledge of the individual λs but only on their ratio Δ.

Table 18.3 gives n for commonly used (α, β) pairs, both one- and two-sided, and Δ from 1.1 to 4.0. Any Δ larger than 2.0 is unrealistic for most clinical trials. The entries in this table are actually calculated using the exact approach but differ from eqn (18.7) by at most two only in the cases with the largest n (that is for $\Delta = 1.1$). Nomograms are provided by Schoenfeld and Richter (1982).

The expected length of study may be calculated from Table 18.3. Since the average number of patients entered per year is γ, the expected entry time T to enter $2n$ patients is simply $2n/\gamma$ years. After the patients are entered, the expected follow-up time τ can also be calculated but, unlike the case for the required number of patients, is a function of the individual λ_is and not merely their ratio Δ.

If an unequal number of patients is to be entered, n_1 on treatment one, and $n_2 = rn_1$ on treatment two, the number of patients required is obtained by a simple modification of eqn (18.7) as in the previous section. The number required on treatment one is:

$$n_1 = \left[\frac{(r + 1)(z_{\alpha/2} + z_\beta)^2}{r(ln\ \Delta)^2} \right]$$ (18.8)

Table 18.3. *Number of patients required on each of two treatment groups to compare survival distributions*

	Δ = Ratio of medians (or hazard rates); larger to smaller						
	1.1	1.2	1.3	1.4	1.5	1.6	1.7
	1364	373	181	110	76	57	45
One-tailed	1888	516	250	152	105	78	62
	2212	605	293	178	123	92	72
	1731	473	230	140	96	72	57
Two-tailed	2316	633	306	187	129	96	76
	2574	704	340	207	143	107	84
	1.8	1.9	2.0	2.5	3.0	3.5	4.0
	37	31	27	16	11	9	7
One-tailed	50	42	37	21	15	12	10
	59	50	43	25	18	14	11
	46	39	34	20	14	11	9
Two-tailed	62	52	45	26	18	14	12
	69	58	50	29	20	16	13

Upper figure: $\alpha = 0.05$, $\beta = 0.20$.
Middle figure: $\alpha = 0.05$, $\beta = 0.10$.
Lower figure: $\alpha = 0.01$, $\beta = 0.20$.

and the number required on treatment two is simply rn_1. Comments on the relative efficiency yielded by different choices of r would be similar to those in the previous section. The relative efficiency eqn (18.4) also holds in this case.

Comparing more than two survival distributions

The number of patients required for comparing $K > 2$ survival distributions may be derived in a similar manner to that of comparing K response rates. Based on the approximate normality of $ln \ \bar{x}_i$ ($i = 1, \ldots, K$), the required number of patients in each group is given by:

$$n = \left[\frac{2\lambda^2}{(ln \ \Delta)^2} \right]$$
(18.9)

where λ^2 refers to the non-centrality parameter of a chi-square distribution with $K - 1$ degrees of freedom, and Δ is the ratio of the maximum and minimum hazard rates. The factors given in Table 18.2 for the K-sample comparison of survival distributions, and the comments concerning the least favourable configuration of the alternatives also hold.

To find the number of patients required in a K-sample comparison, the two-sample population requirement (two-tailed) is read from Table 18.3 (with $\Delta = \lambda_{max}/\lambda_{min}$) and multiplied by the appropriate factor in Table 18.2. For specifications not covered in the tables, eqn (18.9) must be calculated.

Comparing a single survival distribution with a standard distribution

Tests of hypotheses of the form $\lambda \leq \lambda_0$ versus $\lambda > \lambda_0$, where λ_0^{-1} is the mean of the survival distribution achieved by some standard treatment, are based on a single sample of size N. This situation is similar to that discussed with respect to success rates and the same comments with respect to historical controls hold here also. If the comparison is truly between the current sample and some fixed (hypothetical) standard distribution, then the required number of patients is exactly one-half of eqn (18.7), with α replacing $\alpha/2$ since this is a one-sided test. The required N can be obtained easily from Table 18.3 by dividing the one-sided entries by one half.

The effect of censoring

The above derivations assume that all patients are followed until failure. In practice it is rare to wait until all patients have failed before making the desired comparisons. Tests are usually made at various times during the study when many patients are still alive (or censored, in statistical terminology) and the effect of censoring on the power of tests must be clearly understood.

Under the assumptions of this section, it is well known that the distribution of the total observed survival time divided by the number of failures is such that the earlier expressions are still valid, but with n representing the required number of failures, not the number of entries. For example, in the case of two treatment groups, the power $(1 - \beta)$ can be obtained by solving eqn (18.8) for z_β:

$$z_\beta = z_{1 - \alpha/2} + \left(\frac{d_1 d_2}{d_1 + d_2}\right)^{1/2} (ln\ \Delta) \qquad (18.10)$$

where d_1 and d_2 are the number of failures in the two treatment groups. The number of patients entered on the two treatments does not appear in eqn (18.10). That is, for the comparison of treatments with respect to survival the number of patients entered is unimportant. The ability to detect treatment differences is a function of the number of failures only. However, this result is dependent on the proportional hazards model. Otherwise, as shown by Benedetti, Liu, Sather, Seinfeld, and Epton (1982), the number of patients entered can be important as well as the number of failures.

Robustness of calculations based on the exponential assumption

The assumptions made in deriving the above are quite general with the exception of the assumption of an exponential survival in each treatment group. This assumption implies that the risk of failure in each interval of time is constant. Since this assumption is unrealistic in many clinical trials, it is natural to investigate the robustness (that is insensitivity to deviations from assumptions) of the calculations based on it. The most commonly used test to compare two survival curves is the logrank test (Peto, Pike, Armitage, Breslow, Cox, Howard, Mantel, McPherson, Peto, and Smith 1976), which is itself a member of a more general class of rank tests (Tarone and Ware 1977). These are general non-parametric tests which do not assume any specific distributional form for the survival times. If the ratio of the hazard functions is constant (that is independent of time) then it can be shown (Schoenfeld 1981) that the number of patients on treatment one required by these tests is:

$$n_1 = \left[\frac{(r+1)\ (z_{\alpha/2} + z_\beta)^2}{rd(\ln \Delta)^2} \right] \tag{18.11}$$

where $\Delta = \lambda_1(t)/\lambda_2(t)$ is independent of t and d is the combined probability of failure (a function of the censoring mechanisms). Freedman (1982) gives a similar formula and related sample size tables. Equation (18.11) is equal to (18.8) except for the divisor d. Thus, Table 18.3 may be used by simply dividing the entries by d, which, as an approximation, can be set equal to the overall proportion of failures expected at the time of analysis. If $d = 1$ (that is no censoring) the results are identical. Similar results apply in the case of $K(>2)$ treatments but the details have not been published.

Thus, in the very important case of proportional hazards and the use of general rank tests, the derivation of the required number of patients via an exponential distribution may be used directly. Since these tests are so heavily used in the analysis of survival data from clinical trials, this result is of considerable practical importance. Of course, if there is strong reason to suspect the proportional hazards model, other approaches should be investigated following the general principles outlined here. Details are omitted since they would depend on the model chosen.

LENGTH OF SURVIVAL STUDIES

In the previous section the required number of patients was derived and it was noted that, for the important case of proportional hazards, this number refers to the number of failures, not the number entered. In this section, guidelines are given for choosing an appropriate entry period (T) and follow-up period (τ) such that the requisite number of failures is obtained at $T + \tau$. The average yearly entry rate to the trial (γ) is assumed to be constant. For simplicity, we assume no loss to follow-up (this assumption can be easily dropped as indicated below).

A unique solution to the choice of an optimum T and τ requires that some criteria of optimality be set. For example, if it is desired to minimize the total study length $(T+\tau)$, then it is shown in George and Desu (1974) that the optimum choice is $\tau=0$. That is, patients are entered continuously until the required number of failures occurs. If γ is large relative to the λ_i, application of this procedure may lead to an excessive number of patients entered in the trial since it maximizes the expected number of patients entered on-study.

A different criterion would be to minimize the number of patients entered. In the absence of loss to follow-up, this requires entry equal to the number of failures needed. The follow-up time τ is then as long as necessary for all patients to fail. This approach maximizes the expected total study length $T+\tau$.

Some compromise between these two extremes seems warranted. Some general decision theoretical approach could be used but would require assigning a cost or loss function to the incommensurables 'patient entry' and 'length of study'. Except for purely administrative or economic purposes, this does not seem practical in most applications.

A pragmatic approach is to select T and τ such that the expected number of patient-years at risk is large enough for the required number of failures to be obtained. That is, require $T+\tau$ to be such that (for the case of two treatments):

$$\frac{\gamma T}{2} \sum_{i=1}^{2} \left\{ 1 - \left(\frac{\exp(-\lambda_i \tau) - \exp(-\lambda_i(T+\tau))}{\lambda_i T} \right) \right\} \lambda_i^{-1} \cong n \sum_{i=1}^{2} \lambda_i^{-1} \quad (18.12)$$

Details on the derivation of the above are given in George and Desu (1974). Equation (18.12) may be solved iteratively for T if τ is given. For $\tau=0$, Table 18.4 gives the required minimum length of study for a comparison of two treatments as a function of the yearly entry rate and the hazard ratio Δ. The minimum median survival is taken to be 1 year so the entries may be changed easily (by multiplying by the true median time) for other situations.

By solving eqn (18.12) for non-zero τ it may be seen that, although the required $T+\tau$ is somewhat larger than that given in Table 18.4, the excess is quite small even for fairly large τ, while the savings in patient entry is dramatic. Accordingly, one compromise would be to specify the maximum proportionate increase (p) in patients actually entered over the required number of failures. Then we set the entry period equal to a maximum of $2n(1+p)/\gamma$ and solve for τ. Rubinstein, Gail, and Santner (1981) give a more complete exposition of the issues involved and provide several useful tables and figures based on a somewhat different approach.

SOME COMPLICATING FACTORS

The previous sections cover the situations generally encountered in designing

Table 18.4. *Required duration of study (in years) to compare two survival distributions (continuous entry)*

Ratio of hazards (Δ)	Yearly entry rate (γ)						
	20	40	60	80	100	150	200
	138.0	69.0	47.0	35.0	29.0	19.0	15.0
1.10	190.0	96.0	64.0	49.0	39.0	26.0	20.0
	240.0	121.0	81.0	61.0	49.0	33.0	25.0
	26.0	14.0	9.9	7.9	6.6	4.9	4.0
1.25	36.0	19.0	13.0	10.0	8.5	6.2	5.0
	45.0	23.0	16.0	12.0	10.0	7.4	5.9
	9.5	5.6	4.2	3.5	3.0	2.3	2.0
1.50	12.0	7.1	5.2	4.3	3.7	2.8	2.4
	15.0	8.4	6.2	5.0	4.3	3.3	2.7
	4.6	3.0	2.3	2.0	1.7	1.3	1.2
2.00	5.7	3.6	2.8	2.4	2.1	1.6	1.4
	6.8	4.2	3.3	2.7	2.4	1.9	1.6

Assumes one-sided test, $\alpha = 0.05$.
Upper figure: $\beta = 0.20$.
Middle figure: $\beta = 0.10$.
Lower figure: $\beta = 0.05$.
The smaller median survival is 1 year. For different medians, the entries can be modified accordingly by multiplication.
Entries over 10 years were rounded to the nearest year.

the size and length of clinical trials. In this section some potential complicating factors are considered with respect to their effect on size and length calculations. These are the effect of patients who are lost to follow-up or who drop out in long-term therapy trials, the effect of stratification by important risk groups, the effect of using historical information, and the effect of adjustment for covariates.

Loss to follow-up

In any clinical trial involving follow-up it is almost inevitable that some patients will be lost from the study before the final outcome is observed. The simplest approach to handling this problem is to increase the required number of patients by a factor equal to $(1-r)^{-1}$ where r is the anticipated loss rate. When survival is being studied, a better approach is that of Rubenstein *et al.* (1981), who extend the methods of George and Desu (1974) to cover loss to follow-up and provide tables for various cases likely to be encountered in practice.

Drop-out (non-adherence to treatment)

In a long-term therapy for some chronic disease one problem is the patient who stops the assigned therapy prior to the time at which full benefit could be expected to accrue. Such patients are not the same as those who are lost to follow-up since they may still be followed to the final outcome even though they do not adhere to the treatment. Halperin, Rogot, Gurian, and Ederer (1968) give tables of the number of patients required in this setting when one treatment is a control group (that is no drop-outs by definition) and the other is a treatment group for which the drop-out rate may be estimated beforehand. No loss to follow-up or censoring is allowed, but the simple approximation mentioned earlier may be used to handle losses. Similarly, Schork and Remington (1967) consider a similar case in which patients may change from one treatment to the other during the course of a trial. Formulae, but no tables, are given. In general terms, the drop-out problem may be handled via internal time-dependent covariates (Kalbfleish and Prentice 1980), but no results seem to have been published with respect to the necessary number of patients required using this approach. Other approaches are given by Palta and McHugh (1979; 1980) and Wu, Fisher, and DeMets (1980).

Stratification by risk groups

In many trials there are factors that are known (or suspected) to yield differing prognoses. In this case it is common to define certain risk groups (or strata) based on these factors and to assign the treatments randomly within each group in such a way that there is a balance among treatments within each stratum. Treatment effects are expected to vary by risk group or there would be no reason to do the stratification. It is important to keep in mind that the primary purpose of the stratification is to ensure a balance that may not occur if the assignment is completely random. It is not intended to compare the treatments in a definitive way in each stratum. Some writers (Peto *et al.* 1976) have argued that stratification is unnecessary and perhaps counter-productive from a statistical viewpoint, since the variables used in the stratification can be taken into account in the analysis, but this argument is not universally accepted. Stratification has a strong appeal to clinicians and is certainly widely used in practice. Green and Byar (1978) discuss the effect of ignoring important risk groups on the size and power of tests.

Ordinarily, the assumption is made that the difference in treatment effects (in some scale) is constant across strata although, of course, the effect of individual treatments may vary widely from stratum to stratum. This is the key assumption that permits a single pooled estimate of treatment differences to be made by weighting each stratum inversely proportional to the variance of the treatment difference. If, in addition, the variance of the difference does not depend on the magnitude of the difference, then the number of patients required is exactly the same as would be required in the absence of stratification and without any stratum effect. Tables 18.1 and 18.3 may be used without modification. If we require separate results in each stratum, which is almost never the case, the above gives the number required in each stratum.

The reason that the above result is so simple is that we assumed that the variance of the outcome variable is not dependent on the stratum mean. This is approximately correct for some transformations but there are cases in which this is not a reasonable assumption. For example, if we assume that the relative odds for success on two treatments is constant across strata (Gail 1973), then the number of patients required on each treatment is:

$$\left[\frac{(z_{\alpha/2} + z_\beta)^2}{\delta^2 \Sigma w_j \sigma_j^{-2}} \right] \tag{18.13}$$

where w_j is the proportion of patients in the jth stratum, δ is the log odds and σ_j^2 is proportional to the approximate variance of the sample log odds in the jth stratum. In order to compute eqn (18.13) knowledge of σ_j^2 is required. Note that w_j, the proportion of patients falling in the jth stratum, can be set by the design of the trial to decrease the required number of patients. Gail (1973) provides further information and a table to facilitate calculations. As a general guide, if the success rates in all strata are in the range of 25 per cent to 75 per cent, then we would not be too far off to calculate the average success rate and use Table 18.1 as if there were no strata. If some strata have large or small success rates this simple approach is inappropriate and eqn (18.13) must be used.

The key assumption in the above is that the difference in treatment effects, as measured by δ_j, is the same in all strata. If this is not the case, then there are real difficulties in planning the trial since the lack of homogeneity cannot generally be known beforehand. One way out of this difficulty is to design the study so that a sufficient number of patients is entered in order to test for homogeneity as well as equality. The test of homogeneity could be based on $\Sigma(\hat{\delta}_j - \hat{\delta})^2/\sigma_j^2$ which, under the hypothesis of equal treatment differences in each stratum, has approximately a χ^2 distribution with degrees of freedom equal to one less than the number of strata. Unfortunately, this adds another level of complexity that is not warranted unless one has strong reason to suspect the homogeneity assumption.

For survival studies, the complicating factors of censoring and slow accrual must also be considered. Bernstein and Lagakos (1978) give the necessary theory and a computer program to calculate the required size of study (in this case specified as required entry rate) in the case of uniform entry, exponential survival, and specified follow-up. Expected survival in each stratum must be specified.

Using historical information

One of the major improvements brought about by the use of clinical trials, as a device to compare competing treatments, is the principle that the comparisons of most validity are those made among treatments applied concurrently. Comparisons made with historical results are correctly given much less weight. However, there are situations, for instance when there are results from a previous trial in the same organization, in which it may be appropriate to combine the historical data with the current data to improve the treatment comparisons. The general issue of when such a combination is appropriate is beyond the scope of this paper. Our concern here is to assess the effect of the use of historical information on the size of the current trial.

One approach is that taken by Pocock (1976), who extends some suggestions of Meier (1975). The model assumes that we are to compare treatments one and two in a concurrent trial and have historical information on treatment one. The number of patients (n_1) required on treatment one in the randomized study is:

$$n_1 = n_2 - \frac{n_h}{(1 + \sigma_\delta^2 n_h / \sigma^2)}$$

where n_2 = the number of patients assigned to treatment two, n_h = the number of patients on the historical treatment one, σ^2 = the variance of the outcome (assumed equal in all three treatment groups), and σ_δ^2 is the prior variance of the bias (difference in outcome between the two treatment one groups). The key points are: (1) In general, fewer than one-half of the new patients need to be assigned to treatment one; (2) if σ_δ^2 is small relative to σ^2, then the historical results count equally with the current results; (3) if σ_δ^2 is large, then approximately equal assignment is required.

All of these results are more intuitive than practical since σ_δ^2 is a subjectively assigned quantity and would likely not be used in the analysis. However, the qualitative results are informative. If large differences are found in results between the two treatment one groups, usually one would not use the historical results at all.

Adjustment for covariates

In some clinical trials, a major purpose may be the estimation and testing of the parameters in some multivariate regression model. For example, it may be desirable to identify prognostic factors that are significantly related to response or survival. This is done commonly through models such as the linear logistic regression model:

$$\log[\theta/(1-\theta)] = \beta_0 + \boldsymbol{\beta}'\mathbf{x}, \tag{18.14}$$

where θ is the probability of success, $\mathbf{x}$ is a vector of covariates, β_0 is a constant, and $\boldsymbol{\beta}$ is a vector of unknown parameters. The proportional hazards regression model of Cox (1972) is also used:

$$\lambda(t) = \lambda_0(t)\exp\{\boldsymbol{\beta}'\mathbf{x}\} \tag{18.15}$$

where $\lambda_0(t)$ is an arbitrary unspecified baseline hazard function.

In general, the number of patients required to test hypotheses concerning $\boldsymbol{\beta}$ depends on both β_0 and the distribution of $\mathbf{x}$. Very little work has been done on this general problem. One notable exception is the work of Whittemore (1981), which provides some approximate formulae and tables for some special cases based on the approximate normality of the maximum likelihood estimators.

CONCLUDING REMARKS

The previous sections of this paper assume that it is possible to enter and treat a fixed number of patients. However, the ethical requirements in clinical trials have led to considerable developments in the area of sequential statistical procedures applied to such trials (Armitage 1975). A sequential design is distinguished from fixed-sample designs primarily by allowing the number of patients required to depend on the results of the trial. In general terms, a decision is made to continue or stop the trial after each observation. Recent modifications of the general approach have allowed the same principles to be applied to survival studies in which the events do not necessarily occur in sequential order (Jones and Whitehead 1979; Tsiatis 1981). Sequential procedures are a natural development of taking observations in groups or stages and a substantial literature on the subject has developed during the last 35 years (see George (1980) for a brief history).

In the context of the current paper, the important point is that, on average, sequential procedures can lead to a substantial savings in the number of patients required in a trial although this saving cannot be guaranteed. Fully sequential procedures are not usually very practical for large scale trials, so that use of a two-stage or multi-stage design may be appropriate (Pocock 1977). These designs can also reduce the required number of patients dramatically (Colton and McPherson 1976; Nagelkerke, Hart, and Strackee 1981) and generally correspond more closely to the practical imperatives of clinical trials. The related topic of adaptive treatment assignments, designed to maximize the number of patients entered on the best treatment, is reviewed by Simon (1977).

In all the material above, both fixed-sample and sequential, the usual hypothesis-testing framework is applied. A quite different approach is provided by selection designs (Gibbons, Olkin, and Sobel 1977) in which it is generally desired merely to select the best of K treatments with some reasonable probability (P) when the treatments differ by some specified amount. Ramberg (1972) gives some approximations to the required sample sizes in this case.

Finally, with the current widespread access to computing facilities, there is no need to depend on published tables of sample size or power when planning a clinical trial. All of the procedures outlined here can be easily programmed. An excellent interactive package (STPLAN) covering most the standard situations, is described by Brown and Herson (1981). Another program, covering stratified survival studies is given in Bernstein and Lagakos (1978). These routines are written in ISO FORTRAN and are easily converted to most computer systems.

ACKNOWLEDGEMENTS

This paper was prepared in part with the support of grants CA20180 and CA21765 from the National Cancer Institute.

REFERENCES

For the most part, the references in this chapter are to publications within the last ten years. References to earlier work are contained in these papers for those seeking a more complete historical account.

Aleong, J. and Bartlett, D. E. (1979). Improved graphs for calculating sample sizes when comparing two independent binomial distributions. *Biometrics* **35**, 875–82.

Armitage, P. (1975). *Sequential medical trials*, 2nd edn. Blackwell Scientific Publications, Oxford.

Benedetti, J. K., Liu, P., Sather, H. N., Seinfeld, J., and Epton, M. A. (1982). Effective sample size for tests of censored survival data. *Biometrika* **69**, 343–9.

Bernstein, D. and Lagakos, S. W. (1978). Sample size and power determination for stratified clinical trials, *J. statist. Comput. Simulat.* **8**, 65–73.

Blackwelder, W. C. (1982). 'Proving the null hypothesis' in clinical trials. *Controlled Clinical Trials* **3**, 345–53.

Brittain, E. and Schlesselman, J. J. (1982). Optimal allocation for the comparison of proportions. *Biometrics* **38**, 1003–9.

Brown, B. W. (1980). The crossover experiment for clinical trials. *Biometrics* **36**, 69–80.

Brown, B. W. and Herson, J. (1981). STPLAN: an interactive study planning package. *Am. Statist.* **35**, 164.

Casagrande, J. T., Pike, M. C., and Smith, P. G. (1978). An improved approximate formula for calculating sample sizes for comparing two binomial distributions. *Biometrics* **34**, 483–6.

Cochran, W. G. and Cox, G. M. (1957). *Experimental designs*, 2nd edn. John Wiley and Sons, New York.

Cohen, J. (1977). *Statistical power analysis for the behavioral sciences*, revised edition. Academic Press, New York.

Colton, T. and McPherson, K. (1976). Two-stage plans compared with fixed sample size and Wald SPRT plans. *J. Am. statist. Assn.* **71**, 80–6.

Cox, D. R. (1972). Regression models and life tables. *Jl R. statist. Soc. Series B* **34**, 187–202.

Dunnett, C. W. and Gent, M. (1977). Significance testing to establish equivalence between treatments, with special reference to data in the form of 2×2 tables. *Biometrics* **33**, 593–602.

Feigl, P. (1978). A graphical aid for determining sample size when comparing two independent proportions. *Biometrics* **34**, 111–22.

Fleiss, J. L. (1981). *Statistical methods for rates and proportions*, 2nd edn. John Wiley, New York.

—— Tytun, A., and Ury, H. K. (1980). A simple approximation for calculating sample sizes for comparing independent proportions. *Biometrics* **36**, 343–6.

Freedman, L. S. (1982). Tables of the number of patients required in clinical trials using the logrank test. *Statistics in Medicine* **1**, 121–9.

Freiman, J. A., Chalmers, T. C., Smith, Jr, H., and Kuebler, R. R. (1978). The importance of beta, the type II error, and sample size in the design and interpretation of the randomized controlled clinical trial. *New Eng. J. Med.* **299**, 690–4.

Gail, M. (1973). The determination of sample sizes for trials involving several independent 2×2 tables. *J. chron. Dis.* **26**, 669–73.

—— and Gart, J. J. (1973). The determination of sample sizes for use with the exact conditional test in 2×2 comparative trials. *Biometrics* **29**, 441–8.

Garside, G. R. and Mack, C. (1976). Actual type 1 error probabilities for various tests in the homogeneity case of the 2×2 contintency table. *Am. Statist.* **30**, 18–21.

George, S. L. (1980). Sequential clinical trials in cancer research. *Cancer Treat. Rep.* **64**, 393–7.

—— and Desu, M. M. (1974). Planning the size and duration of a clinical trial studying the time to some critical event. *J. chron. Dis.* **27**, 15–24.

Gibbons, J. D., Olkin, I., and Sobel, M. (1977). *Selecting and ordering populations: a new statistical methodology*. John Wiley and Sons, New York.

Green, S. B. and Byar, D. P. (1978). The effect of stratified randomization on size and power of statistical tests in clinical trials. *J. chron. Dis.* **31**, 445–54.

Grizzle, J. (1965). The two-period change-over design and its use in clinical trials. *Biometrics* **21**, 467–80.

Guenther, W. C. (1977). Power and sample size for approximate chi-square tests. *Am. Statist.* **31**, 83–5.

Halperin, M., Rogot, E., Gurian, J., and Ederer, F. (1968). Sample sizes for medical trials with special reference to long-term therapy. *J. chron. Dis.* **21**, 13–24.

Haseman, J. K. (1978). Exact samples sizes for use with the Fisher–Irwin test for 2×2 tables. *Biometrics* **34**, 106–09.

Hayman, G. E., Govindarajula, Z., and Leone, F. C. (1970). Tables of the cumulative non-central chi-square distribution. In *Selected tables in mathematical statistics* (eds. H. L. Harter and D. B. Owen) Vol. 1. Markham Publishing Co., Chicago.

Hills, M. and Armitage, P. (1979). The two-period cross-over clinical trial. *Br. J. clin. Pharmac.* **8**, 7–20.

Jones, D. and Whitehead, J. (1979). Sequential forms of the log rank and modified Wilcoxon tests for censored data. *Biometrika* **66**, 105–14.

Kalbfleish, J. D. and Prentice, R. L. (1980). *The statistical analysis of failure time data*. John Wiley and Sons, New York.

Lachin, J. M. (1977). Sample size determinations for r × c comparative trials. *Biometrics* **33**, 315–24.

—— (1981). Introduction to sample size determination and power analysis for clinical trials. *Control. clin. Trials* **2**, 93–113.

Lesser, M. L. and Cento, S. J. (1981). Tables of power for the F-test for comparing two exponential survival distributions. *J. Chron. Dis.* **34**, 533–44.

Lustbader, E. D. and Litwin, S. (1981). Design of censored survival studies. *Biometrics* **37**, 697–704.

Mace, A. E. (1964). *Sample size determination*. Reinhold Publishing Co., New York. (Reprinted 1973, R. E. Krieger Publishing Co., New York.

Makuch, R. and Simon, R. (1978). Sample size requirements for evaluating a conservative therapy. *Cancer treat. Rep.* **62**, 1037–40.

—— and —— (1980). Sample size considerations for non-randomized comparative studies. *J. chron. Dis.* **33**, 175–81.

Meier, P. (1975). Statistics and medical experimentation. *Biometrics* **31**, 511–29.

Nagelkerke, N. J. D., Hart, A. A. M., and Strackee, J. (1981). Sample size in sequential survival clinical trials. *Biometrical Journal* **23**, 709–14.

Nelson, L. S. (1980). Sample sizes for comparing two proportions. *J. quality technol.* **12**, 114–15.

Palta, M. and McHugh, R. (1979). Adjusting for losses to follow-up in sample size determination for cohort studies. *J. chron. Dis.* **32**, 315–26.

—— and —— (1980). Planning the size of a cohort study in the presence of both losses to follow-up and non-compliance. *J. chron. Dis.* **33**, 501–12.

Pasternack, B. S. and Gilbert, H. S. (1971). Planning the duration of long-term survival time studies designed for accrual by cohorts. *J. chron. Dis.* **24**, 681–700.

Peto, R. (1982). Size of the therapeutic benefit that can be expected in a trial, and its implications in the design and organization of the trial. In *Evaluation of methods of treatment and diagnostic procedures in cancer* (eds. R. Flamant and C. Fohanno) pp. 49–65. UICC, Geneva.

—— Pike, M. C., Armitage, P., Breslow, N. E., Cox, D. R., Howard, S. V., Mantel, N., McPherson, K., Peto, T., and Smith, P. G. (1976). Design and analysis of randomized clinical trials requiring prolonged observation of each patient. I. Introduction and design. *Br. Cancer* **34**, 585–612.

Pocock, S. J. (1976). The combination of randomized and historical controls in clinical trials. *J. chron. Dis.* **29**, 175–88.

—— (1977). Group sequential methods in the design and analysis of clinical trials. *Biometrika* **64**, 191–9.

—— (1978). Size of cancer trials and stopping rules. *Br. J. Cancer* **38**, 757–66.

Ramberg, J. S. (1972). Selection sample size approximations. *Ann. math. Statist.* **43**, 1977–80.

Rubinstein, L. V., Gail, M. H., and Santner, T. J. (1981). Planning the duration of a compatative clinical trial with loss to follow-up and a period of continued observation. *J. chron. Dis.* **34**, 469–79.

Schoenfeld, D. (1981). The asymptotic properties of nonparametric tests for comparing survival distributions. *Biometrika* **68**, 316–19.

Schoenfeld, D. A. and Richter, J. R. (1982). Nomograms for calculating the number of patients needed for a clinical trial with survival as an end point. *Biometrics* **38**, 163–70.

Schork, M. A. and Remington, R. D. (1967). The determination of sample size in treatment—control comparisons for chronic disease studies in which drop-out or non-adherence is a problem. *J. chron. Dis.* **20**, 233–9.

Simon, R. (1977). Adaptive treatment assignment methods and clinical trials. *Biometrics* **33**, 743–9.

Tarone, R. E. and Ware, J. (1977). On distribution-free tests for equality of survival distributions. *Biometrika* **64**, 156–60.

Tsiatis, A. A. (1981). The asymptotic joint distribution of the efficient scores test for the proportional hazards model calculated over time. *Biometrika* **68**, 311–15.

Ury, H. K. and Fleiss, J. L. (1980). On approximate sample sizes for comparing two independent proportions with the use of Yates' correction. *Biometrics* **36**, 347–51.

Walter, S. D. (1977). Determination of significant relative risks and optimal sampling procedures in prospective and retrospective comparative studies of various sizes. *Am. J. Epidemiol.* **105**, 387–97.

Whittemore, A. S. (1981). Sample size for logistic regression with small reponse probability. *J. Am. statist. Ass.* **76,** 27–32.

Wu, M., Fisher, M., DeMets, D. (1980). Sample sizes for long-term medical trial with time-dependent dropout and event rates. *Control. clin. Trials* **1,** 111–23.

19 Alternative designs: sequential, multi-stage, decision theory and adaptive designs

Boris Iglewicz

INTRODUCTION

Of the large number of phase III oncology trials performed each year, very few designs, if any, depart from the classical (Neyman–Pearson) hypothesis-testing formulation with random allocation of treatments to patients using fixed-sample size. That is, the trials are designed with a preassigned significance level and require a sufficient number of observations in order to detect, with reasonable probability, a specified treatment difference. The statistical theory of such standard designs is well developed and relatively straightforward to use. In addition, practitioners have developed familiarity and expertise in designing and analysing such phase III trials through the learning process of extensive previous utilization.

A number of alternative designs have been discussed in the statistical literature. These include a formulation based on decision theory models, the use of sequential stopping rules, and adaptive treatment assignment plans which recommend allocating treatments to future patients based on inform-ation attained from previous patients. Numerous theoretical publications based on each of the above types of alternative designs have appeared in the literature. Despite this very active theoretical activity, alternative designs have seldom been used in practice. A discussion of many of the practical reasons for this lack of usage can be found in Bailar (1976) and Simon (1977). These review papers did not seem to slow the level of theoretical research on alternative designs nor reduce the resistance of most practitioners.

The alternative designs are based on a modification of one or more important features of a well-designed phase III clinical trial. All well-designed phase III clinical trials must contain a rule for terminating the experiment, a method for allocating treatments to patients, and a rule for deciding between treatments. There are clearly many reasonable approaches for deciding when to terminate an experiment. In addition, many possible methods can be formulated for allocating treatments to patients or for making a decision. A number of such modifications have been extensively investigated.

The sample size of a clinical trial may be fixed in advance or be a random variable. Such plans are called *fixed sample* or *sequential* plans, respectively.

Note that the termination rule of a sequential trial is a function of the previous responses while that of a fixed-sample plan is independent of such responses. Sequential plans can be further subdivided into *one-patient* (or pair of patients) *at-a-time designs* or *multi-stage designs*. In the one-patient-at-a-time design the decision to terminate or continue the trial is made either continuously or each time a patient responds, while in multi-stage designs such decisions are made in stages with each stage consisting of the responses from a group of patients. In general, the stages subdivide the trial period with, say, a 1 year two-stage trial possibly consisting of two half-year stages. In order to differentiate between one-patient-at-a-time and multi-stage plans, the former will be called sequential plans. In addition, because of major practical and theoretical differences between sequential and multi-stage designs, they will be discussed in separate sections.

Another design consideration is the method for allocating treatments to patients. Such allocations are usually performed randomly. Alternative *adaptive* schemes have been developed which allocate treatments based on information from previous patients. A very important purpose of adaptive allocation is to balance the patients on the trial over the important prognostic factors. This type of adaptive balancing has been discussed in Chapters 16 and 17. Here consideration will be given to adaptive schemes which are designed to place more patients, on the average, on the superior treatment. Such schemes have been extensively studied and this research will be summarized.

Although the classical Neyman–Pearson approach has been used universally for comparing treatments, it has been severely criticized by a number of notable statisticians. They argue that trials should not be designed to control the size of the type I and type II errors, but rather to minimize the total ethical cost of the losses incurred by patients receiving the inferior, rather than the superior, treatment. Such *decision theoretical* formulations lead to different types of decision rules which usually require a larger number of patients for an optimally designed trial. It is useful to have some familiarity with decision theoretical models as they provide a very different and interesting approach to clinical trial design.

It should be noted that theoretical models for clinical trials may combine a number of the features discussed above. Thus, one may consider an adaptive sequential, decision theory model or a multi-stage adaptive procedure. Clearly, many combinations are possible and the statistical literature contains selections from each.

This chapter contains a review of the common alternative designs which may be used in oncology trials on humans. Each major design type will be illustrated with a practical example and its basic properties will be summarized. Also included will be a critical review of each type of alternative design, giving both the advantages and disadvantages of practical usage and providing a relatively extensive bibliography for further reading. It should be noted that many of these designs have not been used in practice. Some rationale for this lack of usage will be provided through comparisons between these alternative designs and comparable ones based on Neyman–Pearson hypothesis tests. I shall consider single, multi-stage, and sequential designs which use either a classical or decision theory formulation. Adaptive designs will also be discussed. The purpose in each case is to provide sufficient familiarity for the non-statistician, and a brief introduction and relatively extensive bibliography for the statistically more sophisticated reader.

SEQUENTIAL DESIGNS

Sequential analysis was developed during the Second World War as a technique for reducing the sample sizes required for quality control inspection plans. Rather than the data being analysed based on a fixed sample size, the accumulating data are continuously re-analysed as they become available in an effort to reach an early conclusion. During this period, Abraham Wald and his colleagues developed the sequential probability ratio test (SPRT) and obtained many of its properties. This work is summarized in Wald (1947) where a very easy to use sequential test procedure is discussed and approximate formulae for the expected sample size and power are given.

Following the publication of Wald's pioneering book, biostatisticians immediately recognized the potential of this new tool for making early decisions and began the task of developing sequential methods useful for clinical trials. The appearance of the 1960 edition of Armitage's *Sequential Medical Trials* helped popularize this new approach and provided useful tables for sequential trial implementation. This led to the use of sequential techniques on a fair number of medical trials which include Anderson and Hutchison (1969), Brown, Mohamed, Montgomery, Armitage, and Lawrence (1960), Carroll, Mowbray, and Davies (1970), Cattaneo, Luccelli, Bona, and Maccacaro (1966), Grenville-Mathers and Trenchard (1964), Watkinson (1958), Russel, Frain-Bell, Riddell, Stevenson, Djavahiszwili, and Morrison (1960), Smith (1958), and Smith and Devey (1968). Additional sequential trials are discussed in Armitage (1975) and Wetherill (1975).

A detailed example will be given now in order to illustrate the implementation of a sequential plan and as a basis for further discussion. Consider the trial conducted by Anderson and Hutchison (1969) for comparing two chemotherapy regimens for cancer of the lung. A control regimen of nitrogen mustard was compared with a mixed regimen starting with 5-fluorouracil and then methotrexate, and finally ethyl hydrazide of pedophyllic acid as the disease progressed. This alternative treatment regimen was labelled chronofusor. Treatments were assigned by a scheme which consisted basically of random pairing of adjacent patients. A binary measure was used with survival of 6 or more months classified as a success. From a strictly practical point of view it would have been better to consider survival times, rather than survival at 6 months. Such an alternative approach can be implemented easily by assuming exponential survival and using a sequential method discussed in Armitage's book.

Let us denote success and failure by S and F, respectively. Then the following four responses are possible for each pair of patients:

S–F
S–S
F–F
F–S

Of the possible responses only F–S and S–F are used in the sequential trial and the information from the other responses is ignored in the decision process. For this reason, the measure used to compare treatments is the proportion of untied pairs yielding the preference A. That is, if π_1 and π_2 are the success rates of treatment A and B, respectively, then

$$\theta = \frac{\pi_1(1-\pi_2)}{\pi_1(1-\pi_2)+\pi_2(1-\pi_1)}$$

is the proportion of untied pairs yielding preference A. Armitage (1975, Table 4.1) tabulated values of θ for selected pairs of π_1 and π_2. Notice that the null hypothesis $\pi_1 = \pi_2$ corresponds to $\theta = 0.5$, while $\pi_1 > \pi_2$ corresponds to $\theta > 0.5$ and $\pi_1 < \pi_2$ is equivalent to $\theta < 0.5$.

Returning to our example, it is necessary first to specify values for π_1 and π_2. Anderson and Hutchison (1969) felt that nitrogen mustard is expected to yield a $\pi_2 = 0.2$ success rate. Because of the resources at hand, π_1 was chosen to be 0.5. This leads to $\theta = 0.8$. In addition, a two-sided test was used because it was not clear which, if either, of the two treatment regimens would prove to be superior. The authors also chose $\alpha = \beta = 0.05$ which resulted in testing H_0: $\theta = 0.5$ with a power equal to 0.95 of detecting $\theta = 0.8$.

It is possible now to choose between a number of types of sequential plans. Among these are the open and restricted plans which can be implemented easily by using the appropriate tables from Armitage (1975). While both types of trials will eventually terminate, restricted plans contain an upper sample-size limit while open plans do not. The difference between an open and a restricted plan should become clearer from the boundaries illustrated in Fig. 19.1, from which it can be noticed that the use of an open plan may on occasion require far more observations than initially anticipated.

Using a two-sided open plan with significance level $\alpha = \beta = 0.05$, Anderson and Hutchison obtained a continuation region which is reproduced in Fig. 19.1a (Armitage 1975, Table 3.1). From this figure one notices that the trial continues as long as one stays within either of the two pairs of parallel lines, while termination occurs with the acceptance of the alternative hypothesis if the outside upper or lower lines are either reached or passed. The trial also terminates with the acceptance of the null hypothesis when the right-hand inner lines are either reached or passed.

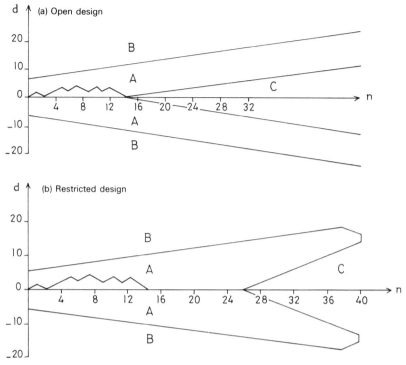

Fig. 19.1. Two-sided open and restricted plans for the Anderson and Hutchinson (1969) data (From Armitage 1975). n, number of preference pairs; d, number of positive preferences minus the number of negative preferences; A, region of trial continuation; B, region of accepting the alternative hypothesis; C, region of accepting the null hypothesis.

The survival data will now be sequentially listed in the form (chronofusor, nitrogen mustard) and with the S–F and F–S pairs being denoted by + and −, respectively. An S denotes survival of at least 6 months while an F indicates a survival of less than 6 months. The condensed data required to make a decision are listed below:

(S, F)+	(F, S)−	(S, S)
(F, S)−	(S, S)	(F, F)
(S, F)+	(S, F)+	(S, F)+
(F, F)	(F, F)	(F, S)−
(S, S)	(F, F)	(S, F)+
(S, F)+	(F, S)−	(F, S)−
(S, F)+	(F, F)	(F, S)−
(F, F)	(F, S)−	

These data are charted in Fig. 19.1 with a horizontal followed by an upward step for each + and a horizontal and downward step for each − Since the first pair of observations is a '+', the first point is placed by moving one unit horizontally and one upward unit. The second pair, a '−', leads to one more unit of horizontal movement followed by one downward unit. The process is continued until a boundary is reached or passed at which point the trial is terminated and the appropriate hypothesis accepted.

Notice that only 14 preference pairs were used to make a decision for the open plan, compared with 30 preference pairs required for an equivalent fixed sample trial (Armitage 1975, Table 3.1). Thus, the use of sequential analysis can, in this case, be termed a great success, as the required number of patients was drastically reduced. The potential for such drastic sample-size reductions is advanced as the major reason for favouring sequential designs.

Notice also that the equivalent restricted plan, illustrated in Fig. 19.1b, did not terminate after 14 preference pairs. This is a common characteristic of sequential trials where a specific response pattern may lead to a termination with one plan but not with another, even though both plans have the same α and β values.

Although the above trial terminated rapidly using the open plan, similar such trials may require additional observations to terminate. An important measure of sequential trial performance is the expected sample size, often called the *average sample number* (ASN). Fortunately ASN comparisons can be made easily for restricted plans by using the entries of Tables 3.1 and 3.7 of Armitage (1975).

Consider again the Anderson and Hutchison (1969) trial with H_0: $\theta=0.5$, $\alpha=\beta=0.05$ and an alternative θ value of 0.8. An equivalent fixed sample size trial would require 30 preference pairs. For the restricted sequential design, the ASN is a function of θ with ASN equal to 29.2, 30, 27.6, and 18.7 for $\theta=0.50$, 0.60, 0.70, and 0.80, respectively. Notice that $\theta=0.50$ corresponds to $\pi_1=\pi_2$. Thus, the ASN values are close to the ones required for an equivalent fixed sample-size trial when θ is close to $\frac{1}{2}$ and decrease considerably as θ approaches θ_1 (the alternative hypothesis value). As most oncology trials seem to have θ in the neighbourhood of $\frac{1}{2}$, such sequential trials would require an ASN similar to that of equivalent fixed plans. On the other hand, if it is strongly felt that θ is considerably larger than $\frac{1}{2}$, then ethical considerations would lead to the favouring of a sequential trial with the potential of a speedy decision in favour of the innovative treatment.

While the above ASN comparisons were made for binary responses, similar results were observed when sequential designs were investigated with other types of response measures. One such comparison for open and restricted sequential *t* tests was made by Suich and Iglewicz (1970). They include values for the sample-size standard deviation and show that such standard deviation values are approximately one-half the size for the restricted, as compared with the open plans. Thus, restricted plans have two practical advantages over open plans. They contain an upper bound on the required number of observations which helps greatly in designing a sequential plan based on the resources at hand. Such plans also have much lower sample-size variability which is an important practical consideration in estimating the approximate trial duration.

A number of discussion papers on the practical aspects of using sequential analysis in clinical trials have appeared. One very interesting discussion occurred between Mainland (1967; 1968) and Colton (1968). In this discussion, Mainland criticizes sequential techniques for reducing the chance for proper blinding, for increasing the possibility of wrong decisions due to clerical errors in charting, for creating a difficult practical dilemma if the trial terminates very rapidly, for example after five pairs of patients. Colton's rebuttal maintains that charting can detect practical problems, for instance improper randomization, at an early stage, that blinding can be maintained, and that early termination of many sequential trials is of great advantage. Their discussion stimulates thought on many of the practical considerations involved in using sequential methods in clinical trials.

Other interesting discussions of the practical aspects of using sequential designs can be found in Bross (1958), Cornfield (1966), and Armitage (1963). Cornfield argues against sequential methods by explaining that the only conclusions one can draw from observations should depend on the observations and not on the technique used to terminate the trial. For an alternative view see Armitage (1963).

A number of papers have appeared dealing with specific aspects of sequential designs. Anderson (1964) considered the incorporation of information contained in delayed observations, Siegmund (1978) discusses methods of confidence interval estimation following the use of sequential tests, and Lim and Fung (1980) consider the robustness of sequential procedures. Notice that the latter consideration is very important because an outlier, occurring early in a sequential trial, may lead to an early wrong decision.

Sequential procedures have also been investigated on response variables useful in oncology trials. Some examples are papers by Breslow and Haug (1972) who consider the sequential comparison of exponential survival curves, Whitehead (1978) who investigates sequential 2×2 tables, Jones and Whitehead (1979) who discuss sequential logrank tests for censored data, and Sigmund (1980) who considers sequential χ^2 and F tests. The above papers are just a small sample of the many theoretical sequential articles which have appeared in the statistical literature.

The practical difficulties encountered in implementing sequential oncology trials should not be overlooked. One difficulty is caused by the considerable duration between initiation of treatment and the observation of response. This may bias unduly the decision of a sequential trial in the direction of the rapid respondents whose responses may not be representative of the true effectiveness of the treatments used in the trial. The need for pairing also causes difficulties because of the large proportion of pairs which lead to no treatment preference. This makes it difficult to estimate the upper bound of the trial duration, even when a restricted plan is used.

The main advantage claimed by advocates of sequential procedures is the possibility of early trial termination. This is most likely to occur when there is a considerable treatment difference, which is precisely the situation when ethical considerations warrant early trial termination. Unfortunately, such large treatment differences occur rather infrequently in oncology trials, so that it is questionable whether there are actual advantages in implementing sequential oncology trials.

MULTI-STAGE DESIGNS

Oncology trials are often of long duration and, as a consequence, considerable time elapses between the first responses and the termination of the trial. During this lengthy trial period, interim analyses are often made and reports written. Such interim investigations may lead to a modification of the trial protocol or even to an early trial termination. Since a fair number of patients are gathered between interim reports, it would seem natural to use a formal multi-stage decision rule designed to protect the overall significance level.

The protection of the overall significance level is a very important consideration when performing an interim analysis. The use of repeated significance tests during the performance of such analyses may greatly distort the overall significance level and make it far more likely for a significant result to be reported. Armitage (1975, p. 29) summarizes the effect of using repeated t tests following each pair of responses. Using a nominal significance level of 0.05 he finds that the use of 20 pairs (19 such repeated tests) leads to an overall significance level of 0.26 versus a nominal value of 0.05.

One approach is to use repeated significance tests on accumulating data, but to use a lower nominal significance level at each stage. This approach has been considered by a number of authors and will be discussed in more detail. Such an approach leads to the correct overall significance level, the potential for early trial termination, but also the possibility of requiring a somewhat larger sample size than needed for a corresponding fixed sample-size plan.

Multi-stage trials are not new and have been used in quality control for many years, see, for example Dodge and Romig (1959). A heightened interest has recently been shown in the development of multi-stage procedures useful in clinical trials. Among the recent papers on this topic are articles by Haybittle (1971), Elfring and Schultz (1973), Canner (1976), Pocock (1977), Madsen and Hewett (1978), O'Brien and Fleming (1979), Demets and Ware (1980), and Pasternak and Shore (1980). Of these papers, the one by Pocock (1977) discusses a relatively simple and practical procedure for normally distributed response data with known variance. This procedure is further shown to be a good approximation for a number of other types of responses and, for this reason, provides a simple multi-stage procedure for performing many types of two-sided tests.

Let us review the Pocock multi-stage group sequential procedure in more detail. He assumes that the responses are normally and independently distributed with means μ_A and μ_B, respectively, and known common variance σ^2. He further assumes that the study consists of at most, N stages and that at each stage a group of n patients per treatment is studied. Of interest is testing $H_0: \mu_A = \mu_B$ versus $H_1: \mu_A \neq \mu_B$ at significance level α. Using these assumptions, the difference between the sample means for the jth group,

$$\bar{X}_{Aj} - \bar{X}_{Bj},$$

is normally distributed with mean $\delta = \mu_A - \mu_B$ and variance $(2\sigma^2)/n$. Following the accumulation of responses from i such groups, the statistic

$$\bar{Z} = \sqrt{\frac{ni}{2\sigma^2}} \left[\sum_{j=1}^{i} (\bar{X}_{Aj} - \bar{X}_{Bj})/i \right]$$

is, under the null hypothesis, distributed as standard normal.

The above test statistic can be employed for group testing if caution is used regarding the significance level at each stage. The significance level used for each stage will be called the *nominal significance level* which will depend on the maximum number of stages N and the overall significance level α. For example, if an overall significance level of $\alpha = 0.05$ is desired and $N = 5$, then the nominal significance level (α') is found from Pocock (1977) to equal 0.0158. Thus, the critical value is 2.413 and rejection of the null hypothesis, $H_0: \mu_A = \mu_B$, at the end of any stage occurs if $|\bar{Z}| > 2.413$.

Consider a hypothetical trial designed to compare the effects of two treatments on tumour growth. Assume that the trial duration is planned to be at the most 20 months and interim reports are expected at the end of each 4-month period. This leads to $N = 20/4 = 5$. The hypotheses to be tested are $H_0: \mu_A = \mu_B$ versus $H_1: \mu_A \neq \mu_B$ and assume that the overall level of significance is set at $\alpha = 0.05$. If observations on 21 patients are expected to be available at the end of each stage, then the power equals 0.90 of detecting a treatment difference of $\delta = 0.5\sigma$.

While the maximum number of patients per treatment of this five-stage design equals $5 \times 21 = 105$, the actual number of required patients is often far less than 105. For example, the expected number of patients when $\delta = 0.5\sigma$ equals 58 which is less than the 84 required for an equivalent fixed-sample-size plan. Thus, the use of this five-stage procedure can, at its worst, lead to a penalty of requiring 25 per cent more patients than the corresponding fixed-sample plan, but this multi-stage plan also has the potential for a substantial reduction in the required number of patients.

In general, an increase in the maximum number of stages (N) results in a decrease in the required number of patients per stage, an increase in the maximum number of patients required for the trial ($2nN$) and a decrease in the expected number of patients under the alternative hypothesis. For instance, if $N = 20$ in the above example, then nN changes to 120 and the average number of patients per treatment under the alternative hypothesis becomes 56. There was clearly little gained in going from $N = 5$ to $N = 20$. In general, there seems to be hardly any advantage in using more than five stages and multi-stage procedures with $N = 2$ to 5 should serve most purposes.

Pocock's group sequential plan is relatively insensitive to its use with other types of response variables. It can be used for the unknown σ^2 case by estimating σ^2 with the accumulated data. Exponential responses can be used by taking the logarithms of the ratio of sample means while binary responses follow directly by choosing $\delta = \pi_A - \pi_B$ and estimating $\sigma^2 = \pi_0(1 - \pi_0)$, where $\pi_0 = (\pi_A + \pi_B)/2$. Let r_A and r_B be the number of responses on treatment A and B, respectively, following the conclusion of the kth stage. The objective, then, is to make the appropriate substitution into $\bar{Z}$ by letting $\hat{\pi}_A = r_A/(nk)$, $\hat{\pi}_B = r_B/(nk)$ and $\hat{\sigma}^2 = \hat{\pi}_0(1 - \hat{\pi}_0)$. Substituting into $\bar{Z}$ results in

$$\frac{(\sqrt{2})[r_A(nk - r_B) - r_B(nk - r_A)]}{[nk(r_A + r_B)(2nk - r_A - r_B)]^{\frac{1}{2}}}$$

which is approximately standard normal under the null hypothesis H_0: $\pi_A = \pi_B$. The above test statistic is used as a replacement for $\bar{Z}$ in the binary case.

Some caution should be used in applying the above approximate binary multi-stage procedure. Basically, the approximation is quite good when $N \geq 5$ and $n \geq 10$, while $n = 50$ is required for $N = 2$ and α very close to 0.05. Even in this latter case, the use of $n = 25$ would lead to a reasonable value of α. A rule of thumb is to refrain from using this binary approximation directly for $nN < 50$. Even in such a situation the procedure can be safely used by choosing slightly smaller α' values.

The Pocock model can be modified by choosing unequal values for the α's. O'Brien and Fleming (1979) consider the use of monotonically increasing α's by choosing the critical values at stage k proportional to $1/\sqrt{k}$. This approach leads to a slight increase in the maximum sample size ($2nN$), as compared with an equivalent fixed-sample plan and still allows for the possibility of early trial termination. The drawback of the O'Brien and Fleming procedure lies in the increase of the expected sample size under the alternative hypothesis. Such a modified Pocock plan basically leads to expected sample sizes far closer to those used for an equivalent fixed-sample plan over a wide range of values of δ. This unequal nominal significance-level approach thus leads to a multi-stage design which is adjusted for the effects of repeated significance testing and has a maximum sample size close to the value required for an equivalent fixed-sample plan.

The Pocock multi-stage plan can also be compared with an equivalent restricted sequential procedure. Basically multi-stage plans lead to a reduction in the maximum number of patients required for the trial while, at the same time, requiring a somewhat larger expected number of patients under the alternative hypothesis. From a practical standpoint, the group sequential plan has the advantage of not requiring continual monitoring and computation, of being less sensitive to outlying observations, and of making it easier to design the plan in order to properly control randomization and blinding.

Demets and Ware (1980) consider one sided multi-stage plans and compare the use of a one-sided Pocock procedure with one using a sequential probability ratio type of decision boundary. The latter is called the constant likelihood ratio approach. Both methods use the same test statistic, but the latter requires a larger maximum sample size and a far smaller expected sample size under the null hypothesis. The expected sample sizes under the alternative hypothesis are about the same for both plans. An example is given where the Pocock model requires a maximum of $2nN = 950$ patients and an expected number of patients under the null and alternative hypothesis of 902 and 415, respectively. The corresponding values for the constant likelihood ratio procedure are 1060, 534, and 414, respectively. This example illustrates the advantage of using the constant likelihood approach for a one-sided multi-stage test, especially when it is quite likely that δ is near zero. It should be noted that the Pocock two-sided plan can be similarly modified by the inclusion of an inner boundary which would lead to an earlier trial termination when $\delta = 0$.

These multi-stage techniques are quite general and can be adapted to many possible applications. One such use is discussed by Pasternak and Shore (1980) who consider the use of the Pocock model in survival analysis. They discuss the application of the Mantel–Haenszel technique in a multi-stage experiment with mice, and provide a detailed discussion of the practical consequences. One problem with the use of multi-stage procedures in survival analysis is the long delay between commencement of treatment and the observation of the response. As a consequence, the early termination of a trial will lead to the accrual of many additional responses which could result in a different final conclusion. This slight risk should not deter practitioners from using such multi-stage procedures as the most reasonable policy was used to terminate the trial.

In summary, multi-stage procedures seem to be a very good compromise between sequential and fixed sample-size methods. Such plans have most of the advantages of fixed-sample procedures and also allow for proper interim analysis with the possibility of early trial termination. At the same time it should be noted that a number of adjustments in the formulae need to be made when using such simple multi-stage designs in actual oncology trials, because practical oncology trials can seldom be implemented with equal numbers of patients for each group or for each treatment within group. The equal sample-size plans could still be used as reasonable approximations as long as the sample sizes do not differ drastically.

DECISION THEORY APPROACH

The classical approach to the design of a well-controlled clinical trial consists of choosing a decision rule with preassigned probability of a type I error and which, in some sense, maximizes the power of the test. A very different approach to clinical trials was advanced simultaneously by Anscombe (1963), in a lengthy review of Armitage's 1960 edition of *Sequential Medical Trials* and by Colton (1963). Also worthy of note is Armitage's (1963) response to Anscombe's paper. The decision theoretical approach was already recommended for other applications by a number of statisticians, including Raiffa and Schlaifer (1961), Maurice (1959), and Bross (1950).

Since the decision theory model differs greatly from the classical approach, we will consider the Colton (1963) paper in some depth. For the Colton model it is assumed that two treatments are to be compared and the responses are normally distributed. Let us denote by $X \sim N(\mu, \sigma^2)$ that the random variable X is normally distributed with mean μ and variance σ^2. Independent observations from $2n$ patients, n from each treatment, are observed and the responses are assumed to be distributed as $Z_{ij} \sim N(\mu_i, \sigma^2)$; $i = 1, 2$; $j = 1, 2, \ldots, n$. The difference between the treatment means $\delta = \mu_2 - \mu_1$ is used as the measure of treatment quality. In practice, δ might be the difference between the mean duration of remission or between the mean response rates. To simplify future discussions, let us assume that positive values of δ are preferred, or equivalently that large values of μ are desirable.

Unlike the classical approach, the decision theoretical model measures losses for each treated patient. The Colton model assumes the loss to be proportional to the absolute value of δ. In order to measure the overall loss one needs to know the total number of patients who receive either treatment. This number N is called the *finite patient horizon*. Thus, the Colton model assumes that there will be $2n$ patients on the trial, n on each treatment, and the remaining $N-2n$ patients are to receive the treatment chosen as superior.

An interpretation of the finite patient horizon is that it measures the number of patients who are to receive either of the above treatments, that is, until a treatment superior to both becomes ready for use. The finite patient horizon is clearly a difficult value to estimate, although past experience may be of some help.

In order to obtain the optimum sample size it is assumed that prior information on δ is available. Such prior information is needed because the amount of loss per patient is a function of δ and, as a consequence, some knowledge of the distribution of δ is required in order to obtain the expected loss (risk), which is to be minimized through the proper choice of sample size. Colton assumed that $\delta \sim N(0, \sigma_0^2)$. The decision rule is based on the difference between sample means with a decision in favour of treatment two if

$$\bar{X}_2 - \bar{X}_1 > 0,$$

and treatment one otherwise. The optimum risk and sample size can now be obtained by minimizing the overall expected loss given by

$$C|\delta|(n+(N-2n)P_I),$$

where C is a proportionality constant and P_I is the probability of making the wrong decision and choosing the inferior treatment.

The solution to the above equation leads to a very simple formula for the optimum sample size given by

$$\frac{n}{N} = \frac{1}{3+(9+4R)^{\frac{1}{2}}},$$

where

$$R = (N\sigma_0^2)/(2\sigma^2).$$

The above formula for R was derived from the mathematics used to obtain an optimum solution and there does not seem to be a simple practical explanation of the meaning of this term. A reasonable approximation of R, in a practical setting, also seems very difficult and may be obtained by estimating N as discussed above and σ_0^2 from estimates of δ from prior trials. If the values of N and R can be guessed with reasonable accuracy, then it becomes very easy to determine the optimum sample size and decision rule. For example, if $N = 100\ 000$ and $R = 100$, then $n = 4306$. This means that the optimum use of the Colton model would require $2n = 8612$ patients on the trial; a value which is clearly far too large for most oncology trials. Notice that when $R = 0$, which is equivalent to $\delta_0 = 0$, that $2n = 33\ 333$.

It should be noted that these large sample sizes are very strongly dependent on the Colton model, rather than the decision theory approach. Mendoza and Iglewicz (1978) considered a slightly modified model which leads to a considerable reduction in the optimum sample size. They assume that while the trial is in progress, most patients receiving treatment do not participate in the experiment. These patients may be receiving the inferior treatment and a lengthy trial may lead to considerable ethical losses. Assume that only 5 per cent of the patients during the trial phase particpate in the experiment. Then, using our example and equation 2.5 from Mendoza and Iglewicz (1978), we come to $2n = 1192$. This is still quite a large sample size, but is considerably smaller than the value obtained using Colton's model.

While the Colton design is quite easy to use, it has the drawbacks of requiring knowledge of R and N and of often leading to an optimum sample size which is far larger than is feasible in a practical trial. These drawbacks may not be as critical as initially assumed, since the risk is relatively insensitive to changes in N, R and n. Iglewicz, Huang, and Mendoza (1978) observe that moderate changes in either N, R or n lead to relatively small changes in risk. This means that choosing a smaller sample size than the optimum may be almost as good as choosing the optimum value.

Other theoretical research involving different aspects of the Colton model can be found in Begg and Mehta (1979), Chernoff and Petkau (1981), Colton (1965), Day (1969a, b), Donner (1977), Langenberg and Srinivasan (1981), Mendoza and Iglewicz (1977), and Petkau (1981).

A very interesting extension of the Colton model is given by Cornfield, Halperin, and Greenhouse (1969). They consider a multi-stage version with the number of observations on each treatment at the next stage determined by the results from the previous stages. This model simultaneously incorporates two important considerations of multi-stage clinical trials. It determines the sample size for each stage and, in addition, subdivides this sample between the two treatments in a proportion which is based on the previous responses.

Let us look at the Colton model again, but not from the view of the finite patient horizon or optimum sample size, but rather by considering the recommended decision rule. Consider a simple comparison of the Colton model with binary data and the corresponding classical procedure. Assume that n patients are placed on each treatment and that the number of successes on treatment i is S_i; $i = 1$, 2. Canner (1970) obtained the following decision rule for a symmetrical prior:

$$\text{choose treatment two if } S_2 > S_1$$

$$\text{and choose treatment one otherwise.}$$

The above rule is modified for $S_1 = S_2$ by choosing each treatment with probability $\frac{1}{2}$. If treatment one is considered the standard treatment then the classical approach would recommend treatment two if $S_2 - S_1 > c$, where c is chosen to attain the proper significance level.

Next consider a simple example. Suppose that 50 patients are placed on each treatment and that $\pi = \frac{1}{2}$ and $\pi = \frac{1}{2} + \Delta$ are the success rates on the standard and innovative treatments, respectively. A one-sided test is used to decide between $H_0 : \Delta = 0$ and $H_1 : \Delta > 0$. Often Δ is assumed to be a fairly large value, say $\Delta = 0.2$, in order for the trial to require a moderate sample size with sufficient power to detect $\pi + \Delta$. In reality there are numerous oncology trials performed each year. If a fair number of them had $\Delta = 0.2$, then rapid progress would be made each year and cancer would cease to be a problem. Thus, the true value of Δ must usually be very small and the value of Δ used for a typical alternative hypothesis can be best described as a mathematical nicety which serves the purpose of constructing a practical clinical trial. In this context it is worth noting that most oncology trials consist of a moderate or relatively small number of patients, which makes it impossible to identify small treatment differences; see, for example Pocock, Armitage, and Galton (1978).

The standard one-sided test with $\alpha = 0.05$ for deciding between $H_0 : \Delta = 0$ and $H_1 : \Delta > 0$ has power equal to 0.257 for detecting $\Delta = 0.1$. If the above Canner model was used instead, the power would increase to 0.843. If, on the other hand, $\pi = \frac{1}{2} - \Delta$ for the innovative treatment, then the use of the classical approach leads to the choosing of the alternative hypothesis with probability 0.004 versus a corresponding value of 0.157 when the Canner model is used. Thus, the decision theory approach leads to a higher probability for choosing a superior innovative treatment and, at the same time, a greater chance of choosing an inferior innovative treatment.

An even more important consideration is the effect of using a particular decision policy over an extended period of time. Consider the situation of 20 innovative treatments, 16 of which have success probability π, two have success probability $\pi + \Delta$ and two have success probability $\pi - \Delta$. Assume that we start with a standard treatment having success probability π, which is to be compared with one of the innovative treatments chosen at random and with the successor of the treatment comparison being chosen as the next standard treatment. The object is to determine the proportion of the final standard treatments which have success probabilities π, $\pi + \Delta$ and $\pi - \Delta$, respectively.

Five thousand such 20 trial cases were simulated by using random sampling without replacement, from an urn model with 16 values of π, two of $\pi + \Delta$, and two of $\pi - \Delta$, respectively. The results are given in Table 19.1 where it can be

Table 19.1. *The proportion of times that a 20-trial policy will result in choosing either π, $\pi + \Delta$ or $\pi - \Delta$ as the final treatment based on using the Canner decision theory model and the classical approach*

		Proportion of final treatments	
Δ	π	Decision theory	Classical with $\alpha = 0.05$
0.05	$\frac{1}{2}$	0.735	0.695
	$\frac{1}{2} + \Delta$	0.230	0.291
	$\frac{1}{2} - \Delta$	0.035	0.014
0.10	$\frac{1}{2}$	0.541	0.490
	$\frac{1}{2} + \Delta$	0.447	0.507
	$\frac{1}{2} - \Delta$	0.012	0.003

noticed that the use of the classical model leads to a higher proportion of the final standard treatment being a $\pi + \Delta$ and a smaller proportion a $\pi - \Delta$ as compared with using the Canner model. This result may indicate an important reason why practitioners prefer the classical approach.

It can be argued that this comparison is unfair as a choice of an asymmetrical prior would have changed the conclusions. No attempt was made to perform an exhaustive comparison between the classical and decision theory approaches, although it is felt that this simple illustration provides some reasons for using caution when considering the application of decision theory models.

The use of prior information in designing clinical trials has been recommended for classical comparisons. Staquet, Rozencweig, Von Hoff, and

Muggia (1979) emphasize the importance of using information on prior oncology trial outcomes in planning future trials. They advocate the estimation of the a priori probability that a new treatment is superior to the control and to use this information as a guide in determining an appropriate significance level and sample size.

Although there may be valid reasons for not using decision theory models, such models should not be ignored by practitioners as they can be of help in designing a clinical trial. Some contemplation on the size of the finite patient horizon may aid in a proper sample-size choice. In addition, Schneiderman (1975) advocates that oncology trials be carefully designed and lead to a decision. Also of importance is some contemplation on the effects of the trial on all patients to potentially receive the investigated treatments. In summary, decision theory models can provide the practitioner with a useful insight into the proper design of a clinical trial.

ADAPTIVE TREATMENT ASSIGNMENT PROCEDURES

Since patients usually enter an oncology trial sequentially, the methods of allocating treatments to patients become very important considerations when designing the clinical trial. The standard approach is to allocate patients randomly. An alternative data-dependent allocation procedure was introduced by Zelen (1969). Zelen considers the Colton model with a *play-the-winner* (PW) allocation scheme where a success on a particular treatment leads to assigning that treatment to a future patient, while a failure with a particular treatment leads to assigning the alternative treatment to a future patient. He also considers the modified PW rule for instantaneous responses with the next patient receiving the treatment indicated by the current patient response. The modified PW model was used in most future theoretical work on PW rules and will subsequently be called the PW rule.

Assume that there are n patients to be allocated in a trial and that a PW rule is used. If π_1 and π_2 are the success proportions on treatment one and two, respectively, then the expected number of patients receiving treatment one using PW allocation is given by

$$\frac{n(1-\pi_2)}{(1-\pi_1)+(1-\pi_2)}.$$

Consider $n = 200$, $\pi_1 = 0.7$ and $\pi_2 = 0.5$. Then 125 patients are expected to be placed on treatment one and 75 on treatment two. Zelen shows that the use of PW allocation in Colton's model assigns more of the N patients to the superior treatment as long as $\pi_1 + \pi_2 > 1$.

A considerable number of papers appeared dealing with PW allocation. Among these are articles by Sobel and Weiss (1970; 1971; 1972), Hoel (1972), Fushimi (1973), Hsi and Louis (1975), Nordbrock (1976), and Christie and Iglewicz (1981). These papers consider deterministic allocation schemes which have been criticized on practical grounds. Wei and Durham (1978) consider an urn PW model which incorporates randomness of treatment assignment, but leads to considerable loss of efficiency (see Christie and Iglewicz 1981).

Most PW plans are discussed in a ranking and selection theory framework. This approach is summarized in Gibbons, Olkin, and Sobel (1977). In this framework a parametric difference Δ and probability of correct treatment selection P are chosen and the trial is designed to have a probability of correct selection of at least P, whenever the parametric difference is at least Δ.

Consider one of the more efficient PW procedures in more detail. Nordbrock (1976) uses a PW allocation scheme with termination of the trial whenever either $|S_1 - S_2| = n$ or $|\hat{\pi}_1 - \hat{\pi}_2| > c/(F_1 + F_2)$, where $S_i(F_i)$ are the current number of successes (failures) on treatment i and

$$\hat{\pi}_i = S_i/(S_i + F_i); \quad i = 1, 2.$$

Consider a simple illustration of Nordbrock's method. For $\Delta = 0.2$ and $P = 0.95$ the values of c and n are 4.2 and 11, respectively. Assume that treatment one is randomly chosen to be given to the first patient and a success is observed. Then $S_1 = 1$, $S_2 = 0$ and $|S_1 - S_2| \neq 11$. The next patient again receives treatment one and assume that the response is a failure. Then $\hat{\pi}_1 = \frac{1}{2}$, $\hat{\pi}_2 = 0$ and $|\hat{\pi}_1 - \hat{\pi}_2| = \frac{1}{2} < 4.2/(1 + 0)$. Thus, the next patient is to receive treatment two and the process is continued until either $|S_1 - S_2| = 11$ or $|\hat{\pi}_1 - \hat{\pi}_2| > 4.2/(F_1 + F_2)$.

Nordbrock computes the critical values c and n and summarizes a simulation study comparing his method with some other procedures. PW allocation schemes are often compared with corresponding *vector-at-a-time* (VT) procedures, which are also sequential, but with patients allocated in pairs with one assigned to each treatment. The entries of Table 19.2 use Nordbrock's (1976) results of a comparison between his and the corresponding VT scheme. In this Table, $\Delta = 0.2$, $P = 0.95$, $E(N)$ is the ASN and $E(N_2)$ the average number of patients on the inferior treatment. Notice that Nordbrock's PW scheme is

Table 19.2. *Comparison of Nordbrock's PW rule with VT for P=0.95 and $\Delta=0.2$ with respect to the average sample number, E(N), and the average number of patients on the inferior treatment, E(N$_2$)*

$\pi_0 = \dfrac{\pi_1 + \pi_2}{2}$	Nordbrock		VT $E(N)$
	$E(N_2)$	$E(N)$	
0.3	14.1	32.1	35.2
0.5	16.8	41.0	33.6
0.7	11.7	34.0	35.2
0.8	7.1	23.9	36.9
0.9	2.4	14.4	37.2

considerably better in terms of $E(N)$ and $E(N_2)$, as compared with VT, when $\pi_0 = (\pi_1 + \pi_2)/2$ is large, while it is inferior for π_0 in the neighbourhood of 0.5. This is a common property of PW schemes, that they perform well for some parameter values and relatively poorly for others. Hoel, Sobel, and Weiss (1972) consider a two-stage scheme with the first stage consisting of a short VT trial, used to estimate π_0, and the second stage consisting of whichever method seems better based on this preliminary estimate of π_0.

Many other variants of PW and other types of adaptive schemes are discussed by Hoel, Sobel, and Weiss (1975). Their excellent review chapter can be used as a guide to the more technical aspects of data-dependent allocation schemes.

PW schemes are special cases of the two-armed-bandit problem which has been researched extensively in the theoretical literature. The armed-bandit problem deals with the optimum allocation of a treatment given complete information on previous responses. If only two treatments are to be compared and π_1 and π_2 are the two success probabilities, then the one-armed-bandit problem considers exactly one of (π_1, π_2) known, while the two-armed-bandit problem deals with both π_1 and π_2 being unknown. The one-armed-bandit problem is discussed by Brandt, Johnson, and Karlin (1965), while the two-armed-bandit problem was introduced by Robbins (1952), and considered by Berry (1972; 1978), Fabius and van Zwet (1970), Feldman (1962), and Kelley (1974).

Consider the example discussed by Berry (1978). The object is to allocate one of two treatments to each of 100 patients. Furthermore, it is known that π_1 is equal to either 0.25 or 0.75 and π_2 equals the other value. If, in addition, π_2 is known beforehand to be 0.75, then it will be used on all 100 patients and the expected number of successes will be 75. This is the best that can be done for these values of π_1 and π_2. Assume further that it is not known which treatment has $\pi = 0.75$ and that it is felt that the prior probability that π_1 is superior equals 0.50. Using the PW allocation scheme on the first n patients and the winning treatment on the remaining $100 - n$ patients, Zelen (1969) obtains the optimum value of n as 14, which leads to an expected number of successes of 72.6. Berry (1978) considers the optimum two-armed-bandit solution given by Feldman (1962). This consists of allocating treatment one whenever

$$S_1 - F_1 > S_2 - F_2$$

and treatment two when the inequality is reversed. Either treatment can be used when $S_1 - F_1 = S_2 - F_2$. Here, again, $S_i(F_i)$ is the number of successes (failures) on treatment i. Using the above procedure for all 100 patients, Berry (1978) obtains 74.0 as the expected number of successes. Notice that this is very close to the ideal value of 75.0. Thus, some improvement in the expected number of patients on the superior treatment can be realized by using the optimum two-armed-bandit solutions versus more specialized adaptive procedures, such as PW rules.

Data-dependent schemes were also considered for other types of response variables. Thus, Flehinger and Louis (1971; 1972) present adaptive schemes, with stopping rules based on likelihood ratios, for normally and exponentially distributed responses. One plan, R_γ, depends on a specified constant γ with $0 < \gamma < 1$. A randomized version is also considered where future patients are assigned to the leading treatment with probability $(1 + \gamma)/2$ and to the other treatment with probability $(1 - \gamma)/2$.

Another approach to this problem for normal observations is given by Robbins and Siegmund (1974). They use a sequential probability ratio approach and assignment rule which follows almost equal allocation when the decision function is far from the decision boundaries, and places most patients on one treatment when the function is close to one of the decision boundaries. A simulation study leads to the obvious conclusion that this method is close to equal allocation, with some penalty in expected sample size, when the treatments do not differ and leads to an approximately 50 per cent reduction on the use of the inferior treatment, from pair-wise sampling, when the two treatments differ greatly.

Louis (1975) uses the measure $N + (\gamma - 1)N_2$, where N and N_2 are the number of patients in the trial and on the inferior treatment, respectively. He considers the minimization of the expected value of $N + (\gamma - 1)N_2$ for a number of choices of γ. Clearly, $\gamma = 1$ implies that only sample size is of importance, while a large value of γ is used when reduction of the number of patients on the inferior treatment is of most consequence. He observes that increasing γ increases the expected sample size and decreases the expected number of patients on the inferior treatment.

Hayre (1979) extends the Louis (1975) paper by the consideration of the minimization of a general class of weighted linear combinations of N and N_2. This is considered further in Hayre and Turnbull (1981) who discuss normal observations with σ_1 and σ_2 unknown and extend their results to binary responses and exponential survival curves.

Despite the extensive theoretical research, such adaptive procedures have not been used in practice. Zelen, in a personal communication, mentioned the application of a specialized type of PW rule in a lung cancer trial. This is the only application of such procedures known to the author. Among the advocates for the use of such procedures is Weinstein (1974). Bailar (1976) and Simon (1977) give a number of reasons for the lack of use of adaptive procedures. Key among these are the limitations of the adaptive designs, such as the requirement for rather quick or instantaneous responses, potential problems with blinding, and increased difficulty in the analysis of auxiliary variables. Perhaps the main consideration is that most oncology trials consist of relatively few patients, with only slight treatment differences. In such circumstances it becomes more important to study other aspects, for instance treatment toxicity, other side-effects, and response on different prognostic factors. The application of adaptive procedures may then only muddy the waters. If, on the other hand, a large treatment difference is suspected, then early trial termination may be of a higher consideration and a relatively simple, restricted sequential design can be considered. In summary, adaptive clinical trials have not been used in practice because practitioners sense that they will gain little through their use, despite the natural inclination to place more patients on what seems to be a superior treatment.

SUMMARY

A number of alternative clinical trial designs have been discussed. While these designs have been subdivided into separate units, they are usually combined in the theoretical literature. Thus, one may find a discussion of an adaptive sequential design or of a multi-stage decision theory model. While these alternative designs have been extensively studied in the statistical literature, they have been applied seldom in actual clinical trials. The main reason for such lack of usage is that alternative designs are modelled on the basis of large treatment differences, whereas most oncology trials show only small treatment differences on the major end-points.

The alternative designs still have an important place in clinical trial methodology, as they model a number of interesting situations. They provide some guidance for a number of important questions, such as, whether one should place more patients on one of the two treatments and what policy to use in making such an unequal allocation, on whether to consider the use of a sequential approach which may lead to early trial termination, or on the consequences of measuring risk differently from the method used in classical trials. Some familiarity with these alternative approaches can be considered part of a well-rounded clinical trial background.

The decision theory approach will play an important role in clinical trial theory as it can be used to model very complex designs. The solution to such complex modelling may provide further insight into the practical design and implementation of oncology trials.

Of the alternative designs considered in this chapter, the multi-stage approach is the most likely to be commonly applied in future trials. Multi-stage designs have the advantage of providing a systematical method for proper interim analysis and of allowing for the periodical monitoring of a lengthy trial.

ACKNOWLEDGEMENTS

Thanks are due to Theodore Christie and Patricia Langenberg for very helpful editorial comments. This work was partially supported by the Radiation Therapy Oncology Group Statistical Center, Grant CA 32115, National Cancer Institute.

REFERENCES

Anderson, J. M. and Hutchison, J. (1969). Sequential analysis of constant and prolonged regional chemotherapy for cancer of the lung. *Br. J. Cancer* **23**, 744–50.

Anderson, T. W. (1964). Sequential analysis with delayed observations. *J. Am. statist. Ass.* **59**, 1006–15.

Anscombe, F. J. (1963). Sequential medical trials. *J. Am. statist. Ass.* **58**, 365–83.

Armitage, P. (1963). Sequential medical trials: some comments on F. J. Anscombe's paper. *J. Am. statist. Ass.* **58**, 384–7.

—— (1975). *Sequential medical trials*, 2nd edn. John Wiley and Sons, New York.

Bailar, J. C., III. (1976). Patient assignment algorithms—an overview. In *Proceedings of the 9th International Biometric Conference*, Vol. I, pp. 189–206. Biometric Society, Raleigh, North Carolina.

Begg, C. B. and Mehta, C. R. (1979). Sequential analysis of comparative clinical trials. *Biometrika* **66**, 97–104.

Berry, D. A. (1972). A Bernoulli two-armed bandit. *Ann. math. Statist.* **43**, 871–97.

—— (1978). Modified two-armed bandit strategies for certain clinical trials. *J. Am. statist. Ass.* **73**, 339–45.

Brandt, R. N., Johnson, S. M., and Karlin, S. (1965). On sequential designs for maximizing the sum of *n* observations. *Ann. math. Statist.* **27**, 1060–70.

Breslow, N. and Haug, C. (1972). Sequential comparison of exponential survival curves. *J. Am. statist. Ass.* **67**, 691–7.

Bross, I. (1950). Two choice selection. *J. Am. statist. Ass.* **45**, 530–40.

—— (1958). Sequential clinical trials. *J. chron. Dis.* **8**, 349–65.

Brown, A., Mohamed, S. D., Montgomery, R. D., Armitage, P., and Laurence, D. R. (1960). Value of a large dose of antitoxin in clinical tetanus. *Lancet* **ii**, 227–30.

Canner, P. L. (1970). Selecting one of two treatments when the responses are dichotomous. *J. Am. statist. Ass.* **65**, 293–306.

—— (1976). Repeated analysis of clinical trial data. In *Proceedings of the 9th International Biometrics Conference* Vol. I, pp. 261–75. Biometric Society, Raleigh, North Carolina.

Carroll, B. J., Mowbray, R. M., and Davies, B. (1970). Sequential comparison of L-tryptophan with E.C.T. in Severe Depression. *Lancet* **i**, 967–9.

Cattaneo, A. D., Luccelli, P. E., Bona, N., and Maccacaro, G. A. (1966). Sequential experimentation and multivariate analysis in the evaluation of a treatment for postoperative intestinal symptoms. *Clin. Pharmac. Therap.* **7**, 429–35.

Chernoff, H. and Petkau, A. J. (1981). Sequential medical trials involving paired data. *Biometrika* **68**, 119–32.

Christie, Jr, T. and Iglewicz, B. (1981). Utilization of run lengths in bonus play-the-winner rules for clinical trials. *J. statist. Comput. Simulat.* **12**, 107–19.

Colton, T. (1963). A model for selecting one of two medical treatments. *J. Am. statist. Ass.* **58**, 388–400.

—— (1965). A two-stage model for selecting one of two treatments. *Biometrics* **21**, 169–80.

—— (1968). Statistical ward rounds—7. *Clin. Pharmac. ther.* **9**, 113–19.

Cornfield, J. (1966). Sequential trials, sequential analysis and the likelihood principle. *Am. Statist.* **20**, 18–23.

——Halperin, M., and Greenhouse, S. W. (1969). An adaptive procedure for sequential clinical trials. *J. Am. statist. Ass.* **64**, 759–70.

Day, N. E. (1969a). Two-stage designs for clinical trials. *Biometrics* **25**, 111–18.

—— (1969b). A comparison of some sequential designs. *Biometrika* **56**, 301–11.

Demets, D. L. and Ware, J. H. (1980). Group sequential methods for clinical trials with a one-sided hypothesis. *Biometrika* **67**, 651–60.

Dodge, H. F. and Romig, H. G. (1959). *Sampling inspection tables—single and double sampling*, 2nd edn. John Wiley and Sons, New York.

Donner, A. (1977). The use of auxiliary information in the design of a clinical trial. *Biometrics* **33**, 305–14.

Elfring, G. L. and Schultz, J. R. (1973). Group sequential designs for clinical trials. *Biometrics* **29**, 471–7.

Fabius, J. and van Zwet, W. R. (1970). Some remarks on the two-armed bandit. *Ann. math. Statist.* **41**, 1906–16.

Feldman, D. (1962). Contributions to the two-armed bandit problem. *Ann. math. Statist.* **33**, 847–56.

Flehinger, B. J. and Louis, T. A. (1971). Sequential treatment allocation in clinical trials. *Biometrika* **58**, 419–26.

—— and —— (1972). Sequential medical trials with data dependent treatment allocation. In *Proceedings of the 6th Berkeley symposium on probability and statistics*. Berkley, Los Angeles, California.

Fushimi, M. (1973). An improved version of a Sobel–Weiss play-the-winner procedure for selecting the better of two binomial populations. *Biometrika* **60**, 517–23.

Gibbons, J. D., Olkin, I., and Sobel, M. (1977). *Selecting and ordering populations—a new statistical methodology*. John Wiley and Sons, New York.

Grenville-Mathers, R. and Trenchard, H. J. (1964). Cytotoxic drugs in bronchial carcinoma. *Lancet* **ii**, 1200–1.

Haybittle, J. L. (1971). Repeated assessment of results in clinical trials of cancer treatment. *Br. J. Radiol.* **44**, 793–7.

Hayre, L. S. (1979). Two-population sequential tests with three hypotheses. *Biometrika* **66**, 465–74.

—— and Turnbull, B. W. (1981). A class of simple approximate sequential tests for adaptive comparison of two treatments. *Communications in statistics*, Vol. A10, No. 22, 2339–60.

Hoel, D. G. (1972). An inverse stopping rule for play-the-winner sampling. *J. Am. statist. Ass.* **67**, 148–51.

—— Sobel, M., and Weiss, G. H. (1975). A survey of adaptive sampling for clinical trials. In *Perspectives in Biometry* (ed. R. Elashof) pp. 29–60. Academic Press, New York.

Hsi, B. P. and Louis, T. A. (1975). A modified play-the-winner rule for sequential trials. *J. Am. statist. Ass.* **70**, 644–7.

Iglewicz, B., Huang, D., and Mendoza, G. (1978). Another look at the robustness of Colton's model for comparing two medical treatments. *J. statist. Comput. Simulat.* **7**, 259–67.

Jones, D. and Whitehead, J. (1979). Sequential forms of the log rank and modified Wilcoxon tests for censored data. *Biometrika* **66**, 105–13.

Kelley, T. A. (1974). A note on the Bernoulli two-armed bandit problem. *Ann. Statist.* **2**, 1056–62.

Langenberg, P. and Srinivasan, R. (1981). On the Colton model for clinical trials with delayed observations-normally-distributed responses. *Biometrics* **37**, 143–8.

Lim, T. K. and Fung, K. Y. (1980). Sequential trimmed *t* tests. *Biometrika* **67**, 181–6.

Louis, T. A. (1975). Optimal allocation in sequential tests comparing the means of two gaussian populations. *Biometrika* **62**, 359–69.

Madsen, R. W. and Hewett, J. E. (1978). Multi-stage tests based on sequential ranks. *J. statist. Comput. Simulat.* **7**, 93–105.

Mainland, D. (1967). Statistical ward rounds—4. *Clinical Pharmac. Therap.* **8**, 615–24.

—— (1968). Statistical ward rounds—8. *Clinical Pharmac. Therap.* **9**, 120–8.

Maurice, R. J. (1957). A minimax procedure for choosing between two populations using sequential sampling. *Jl R. statist. Soc.* Series B, **19**, 255–61.

Mendoza, G. and Iglewicz, B. (1977). A three phase sequential model for clinical trials. *Biometrika* **64**, 201–6.

—— and —— (1978). An extension of Colton's model for comparing two medical treatments. *J. Am. statist. Ass.* **73**, 646–9.

Nordbrock, E. (1976). An improved play-the-winner sampling procedure for selecting the better of two binomial populations. *J. Am. statist. Ass.* **71**, 137–9.

O'Brien, P. C. and Fleming, T. R. (1979). A multiple testing procedure for clinical trials. *Biometrics* **35**, 549–56.

Pasternak, B. S. and Shore, R. E. (1980). Group sequential methods for cohort and case-control studies. *J. chron. Dis.* **33**, 365–73.

Petkau, J. A. (1980). Frequentist properties of three stopping rules for comparative clinical trials. *Biometrika* **67**, 690–2.

Pocock, S. J. (1977). Group sequential methods in the design and analysis of clinical trials. *Biometrika* **64**, 191–9.

——, Armitage, P. and Galton, D. A. G. (1978). The size of a cancer clinical trial: an international survey. *UICC tech. rep.* Series **36**, 5–32.

Raiffa, H. and Schlaifer, R. (1961). *Applied statistical decision theory.* Harvard University Graduate School of Business Administration, Boston.

Robbins, H. E. (1952). Some aspects of sequential design of experiments. *Bull. Am. math. Soc.* **55**, 527–35.

Robbins, H. and Siegmund, D. O. (1974). Sequential tests involving two populations. *J. Am. statist. Ass.* **69**, 132–9.

Russel, B., Frain-Bell, W., Riddell, R. W., Stevenson, C. J., Djavahiszwili, N., and Morrison, S. L. (1960). Chronic ringworm infection of the skin and nails treated with griseofulvin. *Lancet* **i**, 1141–7.

Schneiderman, M. A. (1975). How do you know you've done any better? *Cancer* **35**, 64–9.

Siegmund, D. (1978). Estimation following sequential tests. *Biometrika* **65**, 341–9.

Sigmund, D. (1980). Sequential χ^2 and F tests and the related confidence intervals. *Biometrika* **67**, 389–402.

Simon, R. (1977). Adaptive treatment assignment methods and clinical trials. *Biometrics* **33**, 743–9.

Smith, J. M. (1958). Hydrocortisone hemisuccinate by inhalation in children with asthma. *Lancet* **ii**, 1248–50.

—— and Devey, G. F. (1968). Clinical trial on disodium cromoglycate in treatment of asthma in children. *Br. med. J.* **2**, 340–4.

Sobel, M. and Weiss, G. H. (1970). Play-the-winner sampling for selecting the better of two binomial populations. *Biometrika* **58**, 357–65.

—— and Weiss, G. H. (1971). Play-the-winner rule and inverse sampling in selecting the better of two binomial populations. *J. Am. statist. Ass.* **66**, 545–51.

—— and —— (1972). Recent results on using the play-the-winner sampling rule with binomial selection problems. *Proceedings of the 6th Berkeley symposium on probability and statistics.* Berkeley, Los Angeles, California.

Staquet, M. J., Rozencweig, M., Von Hoff, D. D., and Muggia, F. M. (1979). The delta and epsilon errors in the assessment of cancer clinical trials. *Cancer Treat. Rep.* **63**, 1917–21.

Suich, R. and Iglewicz, B. (1970). A truncated sequential t-test. *Technometrics* **12**, 789–98.

Wald, A. (1947). *Sequential analysis.* John Wiley and Sons, New York.

Watkinson, G. (1958). Treatment of ulcerative colitis with lopical hydrocortisone hemisuccinate sodium. A controlled trial employing restricted sequential analysis. *Br. Med. J.* **2,** 1077–82.

Wei, L. J. and Durham, S. (1978). The randomized Play-the-winner rule in medical trials. *J. Am. Statis. Ass.* **73,** 840–3.

Weinstein, M. C. (1974). Allocation of subjects in medical experiments. *New Engl. J. Med.* **291,** 1278–85.

Wetherill, B. G. (1975). *Sequential methods in statistics.* Chapman and Hall, London.

Whitehead, J. (1978). Large sample sequential methods with application to the analysis of 2 × 2 contingency tables. *Biometrika* **65,** 351–6.

Zelen, M. (1969). Play-the-winner rule and the controlled clinical trial. *J. Am. statist. Ass.* **64,** 131–46.

Part VII
Analysis of phase III trials

20 Estimation and comparison of proportions

Alfred A. Bartolucci

INTRODUCTION

Most phase III studies are designed with several end-points in mind, one of which is to compare treatments with respect to rate of response and/or toxicity. The present chapter deals with an overview of some of the more common methodologies used to achieve that specific objective. We avoid excessive mathematical development and list references for those readers who wish to delve further into the theoretical concepts.

Our applications and examples all deal with fixed sample-size trials. That is to say, those trials in which an established number of patients are assigned or randomized to each treatment group and the trial is then analysed when that number is achieved. This is opposed to the sequential medical trial discussed by Anscombe (1963), or the multi-stage clinical trials presented by Colton (1963), Cornfield (1966), Cornfield, Halperin, and Greenhouse (1969), and Zelen (1969). Also, since our examples are based on actual clinical trials, it should be noted that these examples are for demonstration purposes only and are not to be considered as conclusive results. There are many other end-points to these studies, besides rates or proportions of toxicity or response, which are fully analysed elsewhere and give a more definitive overview of the results of these trials.

Although the techniques described herein are based on classical statistical procedures, it is worth noting that the Bayesian approach also has its place in the literature for analysing rates and proportions. For investigation of this approach, the reader is referred to Lindley (1964), Cornfield (1969), and Gunel and Dickey (1974).

ESTIMATION OF PROPORTIONS AND INTERPRETATION OF CONFIDENCE INTERVALS

In a clinical trial interest sometimes focuses on the question of which therapy produces the highest proportion of successes or responses. For example, if patients on a given trial are allocated prospectively in a random manner to one of two treatments A or B and

S_A = observed number of successes or responses on treatment A and

N_A = total number of patients randomized to treatment A,

then the relative frequency or proportion of responses, or response rate, on treatment A is simply

$$\frac{S_A}{N_A} = p_A \qquad (20.1)$$

where p_A is an estimate of the true proportion of successes on treatment A based on the observed data.

Likewise the proportion of responses on treatment B is

$$\frac{S_B}{N_B} = p_B \qquad (20.2)$$

Response can be defined according to the criteria given in a treatment protocol. Rather well-defined response criteria, for example for metastatic breast cancer, are given by Hayward, Carbone, Heuson, Kimaoka, Segaloff, and Rubens (1977). In a Southeastern Cancer Study Group (SECSG) protocol comparing CHOP (Cytoxan, Adriamycin, Vincristine and Prednisone) to BCOP (BCNU, Cytoxan, Vincristine and Prednisone) in diffuse histiocytic non-Hodgkin's lymphoma there were 59 patients randomized and evaluated on CHOP and 53 randomized and evaluated on BCOP. The number of complete responses (CR) on CHOP and BCOP were 33 and 19, respectively. Thus, the proportion of successes on CHOP and BCOP were

$$\frac{33}{59} = 56 \text{ per cent}$$

and

$$\frac{19}{53} = 36 \text{ per cent.}$$

Likewise $26/59 = 44$ per cent of the CHOP patients and $34/53 = 64$ per cent of the patients on BCOP failed to achieve a CR.

The most common way to represent these response results is via the 'fourfold' table or 'two by two' (2×2) contingency table as follows in Table 20.1.

Table 20.1.

Treatment	CR's	NON-CR's	Total
CHOP	33	26	59
BCOP	19	34	53
Total	52	60	112

Proportions are used also to depict the percentage of patients in a given trial or on a particular treatment who have certain characteristics. For example, if

20 of the 59 patients on CHOP are over the age of 50, then clearly $20/59 = 34$ per cent of the patients on CHOP are in the older age group. Likewise in toxicity studies the proportion of patients on CHOP experiencing severe granulocytopenia (a drop to less than 750 absolute segs and bands) is $16/59 = 27$ per cent.

From the above examples we see that 'proportions' are based on all or none variables. Either one shares or has the characteristic or one does not. Likewise, one either achieves a level of response as defined or one does not.

Having calculated the proportion of successes in a sample, we may wish to know what degree of confidence exists that the true proportion of successes lies in some interval. This interval, called a 'confidence interval', has a minimum or lower limit which we label L, and a maximum which we denote as U. L and U are often called the confidence limits.

Thus, considering p_A in eqn (20.1) we can calculate L and U so that we can be 95 per cent confident that the true proportion of successes lies between L and U or we can calculate a 95 per cent confidence interval for this true proportion. That is, 95 per cent of such confidence intervals will contain the *true* proportion of successes. In general, the formulae for L and U are:

$$L = p_A - z_{\gamma/2} \sqrt{p_A(1-p_A)/N_A}$$

and

$$U = p_A + z_{\gamma/2} \sqrt{p_A(1-p_A)/N_A}$$

(20.3)

where $z_{\gamma/2}$ is a statistical notation for a value computed from the normal probability tables for various degrees of confidence $1 - \gamma$ (See Ostle and Mensing (1975, Appendix 3). For a 95 per cent confidence interval $\gamma = 0.05$ and $z_{\gamma/2}$ takes the value 1.96.

If an investigator wishes to have degrees of confidence other than 95 per cent then the value of $z_{\gamma/2}$ in eqn (20.3) will change accordingly. For example, the following table lists common degrees of confidence and their corresponding value for $z_{\gamma/2}$.

Table 20.2.

Degree of confidence (%)	$z_{\gamma/2}$
85	1.44
90	1.645
95	1.96
99	2.575

Clearly if N_A remains constant in eqn (20.3) and $z_{\gamma/2}$ increases then the confidence limits increase or the interval becomes wider. In turn, if $z_{\gamma/2}$ is left constant and the sample size or N_A increases then the limits decrease or the interval becomes narrower. Obviously a larger sample size for any degree of confidence yields a tighter interval.

To demonstrate the use of all these values in (20.3) let us consider our non-Hodgkins lymphoma example and the CHOP regimen as treatment A. Clearly from eqn (20.1) and Table 20.1

$$S_A = 33, \ N_A = 59$$

and

$$p_A = 33/59 = 0.56, \ 1 - p_A = 0.44.$$

Thus a 95 per cent confidence interval for the true proportion of responses on CHOP is

$$(0.56 - 1.96 \ \sqrt{(0.56)(0.44)/59}, \ 0.56 + 1.96 \ \sqrt{(0.56)(0.44)/59})$$
$$= (0.43, \ 0.69).$$

We then have 95 per cent confidence that the true proportion of successes on CHOP lies between 0.43 and 0.69.

A similar interval can be computed for the true proportion of successes on BCOP or treatment B by substituting B for A in eqn (20.3). In this case $S_B = 19$ and $N_B = 53$.

At times when computing L in eqn (20.3) it may happen that $L < 0.0$. In such cases, to ensure that the lower limit of the interval is non-negative we set $L = 0.0$. Likewise if $U > 1.0$ we impose the restriction $U = 1.0$.

The confidence limits formulated in eqn (20.3) for a proportion were based on the use of the normal probability distribution as an approximation to the binomial distribution. For smaller sample sizes, say less than 30, eqn (20.3) may be inappropriate. Other methods for computing L and U are found in Clopper and Pearson (1934), Hald (1952), Calvert (1955), Muench (1960), and Snedecor and Cochran (1967).

In many clinical trials there may be more than two treatments and certainly more than two levels of response (that is response versus no response). We can generalize all our results above to such a case. In an advanced non-small-cell carcinoma of the lung trial patients were randomized to one of three treatments. They were:

(1) CAMF Cyclophosphamide
Adriamycin
Methotrexate with folinic acid
(2) CAP Cyclophosphamide
Adriamycin
Cis-platinum
(3) CA   Cyclophosphamide
Adriamycin.

Patients were appropriately stratified. To discuss stratification or other variables is irrelevant for our purposes at this point. The levels of response considered in the trial were complete response (CR), partial response (PR), stable, and progression. Thus, in this trial we have three treatments and four levels of response. The results for evaluable patients are presented in the following three by four table (3×4 or three rows and four columns—not counting the totals).

Table 20.3.

Treatment	Response				
	CR	PR	Stable	Progression	Total
CAMF	0	13	35	50	98
CAP	3	6	47	57	113
CA	0	4	47	77	128
Total	3	23	129	184	339

The proportion or percentage of patients achieving a particular level of response for a given treatment can also be presented in tabular form as follows in Table 20.4.

Table 20.4.

Treatment	Response (%)			
	CR	PR	Stable	Progression
CAMF	0	13	36	51
CAP	3	5	42	50
CA	0	3	37	60

Clearly on CAMF there were 0 per cent CRs, 13 per cent PRs, 36 per cent stable, and 51 per cent of the patients had tumour progression or died while on protocol. As in our previous 2×2 example one can find a confidence interval for each of these levels of response percentages per treatment group.

Similar tables can be generated for patient characteristics. The following is such a 2×3 table for prior radiation status by treatment group with proportions in parentheses.

Table 20.5.

	CAMF		CAP		CA	
Prior RT	31	(32%)	40	(35%)	43	(34%)
No prior RT	67	(68%)	73	(65%)	85	(66%)
Total	98		113		128	

Construction of such tables is, of course, not limited to looking at response or other characteristics by treatment group. We may wish to consider response by age or performance status, or toxicity level by response or age or performance status, or any combination of variables that may have clinical significance and proper statistical interpretation. Here the question and problem of 'multiple comparisons' must be dealt with and we will address that problem later in the chapter.

The studies we have discussed thus far have been 'prospective' in nature since the experimental units (patients) are assigned to treatment groups and the observations such as responses or proportion of responses are then recorded. These types of studies contrast to studies which are 'retrospective' in nature and one must be careful of the interpretation of these studies. As an example of a retrospective study, suppose that at a specific hospital a group of lung cancer patients were identified and classified as either 'smoker' or 'non-smoker'. Suppose further that a group of control patients were matched appropriately with these lung cancer patients. We then summarize the data as follows in the following 2×2 table.

Table 20.6.

	Smoker	Non-smoker	Total
Lung cancer patients	56	10	66
Matched controls	27	12	39
Total	83	22	105

Clearly we can make statements about the proportion of patients being smokers given that they have lung cancer. However, what can be said about the proportion of people contracting lung cancer given that they are smokers? People were not randomly assigned to a smoking versus a non-smoking programme and then observations made as to their contracting lung cancer. More will be said about interpretation of retrospective results in the next section. For further reference on retrospective studies, see Mantel and Haenszel (1959) and Mantel (1963).

REVIEW OF STATISTICAL TESTS USED TO COMPARE PROPORTIONS

Chi-square test

We see that in Table 20.1 there are 56 per cent CRs on CHOP and 36 per cent CRs on BCOP. A natural question to ask is 'Is there an association between type of treatment and response rate?' The most common statistic used to measure this association is the chi-square (χ^2) statistic computed for Table 20.1 and which is

$$\chi_1^2 = \frac{(33 \cdot 34 - 26 \cdot 19)^2 \cdot 112}{59 \cdot 53 \cdot 60 \cdot 52} = 4.527. \tag{20.4}$$

If a fourfold table takes the general form as in Table 20.7 below,

Table 20.7.

	Success	Failure	Total
Treatment A	S_A	$N_A - S_A = F_A$	N_A
Treatment B	S_B	$N_B - S_B = F_B$	N_B
Total	$S_A + S_B$	$F_A + F_B$	$N_A + N_B = N$

then the general formula for the χ^2 statistic is:

$$\chi_1^2 = \frac{(S_A \cdot F_B - S_B \cdot F_A)^2 \cdot N}{(S_A + S_B) \cdot (F_A + F_B) \cdot N_A \cdot N_B}. \tag{20.5}$$

The subscript 1 on the χ^2 denotes one degree of freedom. To interpret the value of the χ^2, that is $\chi_1^2 = 4.527$ in (20.4), we first have to know the null hypothesis we are testing and the corresponding alternative hypothesis.

One-sided test

Suppose that the null hypothesis is

H: the proportion of CRs on CHOP and on BCOP are equal;

and the alternative hypothesis is:

H̄: the proportion of CRs on CHOP is greater than the proportion of CRs on BCOP.

Here we are interested in the alternative being in one direction, that is the percentage of CHOP CRs being superior to the percentage of BCOP CRs. Since the data in Table 20.1 are consistent with H̄, we would proceed to compute the χ^2 as we did in eqn (20.4). If H̄ were stated in the other direction, that is the BCOP percentage CRs are greater than the CHOP percentage CRs, then Table 20.1 would be inconsistent with H̄ and we would probably conclude that H̄ is not true without further calculation.

Using the χ^2 value, we have guidelines as to the chance of observing the data we did, if in fact, H were true. For the one-sided test if:

$$\begin{aligned}
&\chi_1^2 > 2.69 \text{ the chance is less than } 0.05 \\
&\chi_1^2 > 4.27 \text{ the chance is less than } 0.02 \\
&\chi_1^2 > 5.42 \text{ the chance is less than } 0.01 \\
&\chi_1^2 > 9.55 \text{ the chance is less than } 0.001
\end{aligned} \tag{20.6}$$

Thus, since $\chi_1^2 = 4.527$, in our case we can say that if BCOP and CHOP were equally effective in their ability to achieve CRs, then the chance of observing the data in Table 20.1 is less than 0.02. In fact, the chance or probability of observing Table 20.1 computed from the cumulative chi-square probability tables is 0.017. Thus the difference in response rate is significant at the 0.017 level and we would reject H in favor of $\bar{\text{H}}$.

Two-sided test

If the alternative hypothesis were

$\bar{\text{H}}$: either CHOP is superior to BCOP or BCOP is superior to CHOP with respect to the percentage achieving CR,

then the χ^2 computed in eqn (20.4) would still be significant but at a higher level. The threshold values for the χ_1^2 for the two sided test are:

$$\text{If } \chi_1^2 > 3.84 \text{ the chance is less than } 0.05$$
$$\chi_1^2 > 5.42 \text{ the chance is less than } 0.02 \qquad (20.7)$$
$$\chi_1^2 > 6.63 \text{ the chance is less than } 0.01$$
$$\chi_1^2 > 10.80 \text{ the chance is less than } 0.001.$$

Thus, since $\chi^2 = 4.527$, our response rate difference is significant at least at the 0.05 level. The significance level is, in fact, 0.033. Thus, we would still reject H in favour of $\bar{\text{H}}$.

Using the observed proportions p_A and p_B and defining $q_A = 1 - p_A$ and $q_B = 1 - p_B$ an alternative χ_1^2 formula is:

$$\chi_1^2 = \frac{(p_A - p_B)^2 \cdot N^2}{(1/N_A + 1/N_B)\ (N_A p_A + N_B p_B) \cdot (N_A q_A + N_B q_B)}. \qquad (20.8)$$

Using eqn (20.8) then the data in Table 20.1 yields:

$$\chi_1^2 = \frac{(0.56 - 0.36)^2 \cdot (112)^2}{(1/59 + 1/53) \cdot (52) \cdot (60)} = 4.490, \qquad (20.9)$$

which would lead to the same conclusions derived above. This result is different than that given by eqn (20.5) because of rounding error.

For smaller sample sizes a factor known as a continuity correction is used in eqns (20.5) and (20.8) by rewriting the numerator in eqn (20.5) as $(|S_A \cdot F_B - S_B \cdot F_A| - \frac{1}{2}N)^2 \cdot N$ and in (20.8) as $(|p_A - p_B| - \frac{1}{2}(1/N_A + 1/N_B))^2 \cdot N^2$. Using this correction factor in (20.5) and re-computing χ_1^2 for our CHOP versus BCOP example, we have $\chi_1^2 = 3.756$ which makes the data significant in a two-sided situation at the 0.054 level. This is a good example of how nonsensical it may be to base all decisions to reject or not to reject on a 0.05 significance level. Would one change their decision if the chance of observing an event was 5.4 times in 100 rather than five times in 100? Although the continuity correction may not be needed at sample sizes of 50 or greater, this example serves well to caution us not to base all decisions on one significance level.

We see by (20.7) that the two-sided test is more stringent than the one-sided test. In most clinical trial situations the two-sided test is more appropriate. Clearly by our example the one-sided test ignores the possibility that CHOP is significantly worse than BCOP. If such were actually the case that inference would be possible only via the two-sided test and one would be obligated to report that result to their colleagues. The situation can be generalized to comparing a standard to a new therapy. An investigator may only be interested in the new therapy if it is superior to the standard. However, if the opposite is true he/she should provide for that possibility by reporting the two sided results. For further discussion of the one-sided versus the two-sided test see Fleiss (1973, Chapter 2).

Fisher's exact test

In situations where the sample size is inadequate for use of the χ^2 statistic, an alternate method is Fisher's exact procedure to test if the responses in each treatment group are equal. It involves calculating exact probabilities and counting combinations. For example, the probability of a table such as Table 20.7 is

$$\frac{N_A!N_B!(S_A+S_B)!(F_A+F_B)!}{S_A!S_B!F_A!F_B!N!} \tag{20.10}$$

where $N! = N \cdot (N-1) \cdot (N-2) \cdots 1$.

Given any observed table we can calculate the probabilities of all tables with the same marginal totals and the significance level can be calculated by summation. This is best seen by example. Suppose we have the following table.

Table 20.8.

	Response	No response	Total
Treatment A	2	16	18
Treatment B	4	13	17
Total	6	29	35

The marginal totals are 18, 17, 6, and 29 or in our notation N_A, N_B, $S_A + S_B$ and $F_A + F_B$. There are seven possible tables having these marginal totals since S_A or S_B can only take values between 0 and 6 inclusive. The seven possible tables are:

(observed table)

(1)	0	18	18	(2)	1	17	18	(3)	2	16	18
	6	11	17		5	12	17		4	13	17
	6	29	35		6	29	35		6	29	35

(4)	3	15	18	(5)	4	14	18	(6)	5	13	18
	3	14	17		2	15	17		1	16	17
	6	29	35		6	29	35		6	29	35

and

(7)	6	12	18
	0	17	17
	6	29	35

We then use (20.10) repeatedly to compute the probability of each of the seven tables or equivalently that S_A takes the values from 0 to 6.

Table 20.9.

Table	S_A	Probability
1	0	0.00762
2	1	0.06862
3*	2	0.22434
4	3	0.34185
5	4	0.25639
6	5	0.08974
7	6	0.01144
		1.00000

* The probability of the observed Table 20.8 is 0.22434.

The significance level for a one-sided test is calculated by adding the probabilities as extreme as or more extreme than 0.224434 in the same tail or

$$\text{Prob} = 0.22434 + 0.06862 + 0.00762 = 0.30058.$$

The probability or significance level for the two-sided test is computed by summing the probabilities as extreme as or more extreme than the observed 0.22434 in both tails or

$$\text{Prob} = 0.22434 + 0.06862 + 0.00762 + 0.08974 + 0.01144 = 0.40176.$$

In either case we would not reject the hypothesis that the treatments are equally effective.

The chi-square value for Table 20.8 with continuity correction is 0.24995 which has significance level 0.38027. This differs from the exact value by 0.02149. Thus, the exact test is probably more appropriate for this case. For larger sample sizes the χ_1^2 results are fairly consistent with the exact test. For example, in our BCOP/CHOP study the Fisher's exact test two-sided significance value is 0.038. Recall, using (20.4) the significance level was 0.033. As the sample size and possible number of 2×2 tables increase the calculations for the exact test become extensive and we require the use of an electronic computer. For further discussion of this exact procedure see Fisher (1934), Irwin (1935), Cox (1970), and Armitage (1971).

Combining information from several 2 × 2 tables

In a clinical trial to compare melphalan plus prednisone (Pam-Pred) with BCNU, cytoxan, and prednisone (BCP) for remission induction in multiple myeloma, the following 2×2 tables were generated according to age group as in Table 20.10.

Table 20.10.

	Response (%)		No response (%)		Total
(1) Age < 60					
BCP	41	(53.9%)	35	(46.1%)	76
Pam-Pred	43	(53.8%)	37	(46.2%)	80
Total	84		72		156
(2) 60 ≤ Age < 70					
BCP	38	(51%)	36	(49%)	74
Pam-Pred	30	(52%)	28	(48%)	58
Total	68		64		132
(3) Age ≥ 70					
BCP	11	(30%)	26	(70%)	37
Pam-Pred	21	(44%)	27	(56%)	48
Total	32		53		85

The natural questions to ask are: (a) is there an overall association between treatment and response? (b) whatever the degree of association, is it consistent from one age group to the next?

One method proposed by Cochran (1954) to address question (a) is to compute eqn (20.5) for each table and add the chi-square values so that we have a pooled chi-square statistic on three degrees of freedom.

Table	χ_1^2
(1)	0.00016
(2)	0.01302
(3)	1.74458

or

$$\chi^2_{\text{pooled}} = 0.00016 + 0.01302 + 1.74458$$
$$= 1.75776$$

which on three degrees of freedom has a significance level of 0.625. Also, none of the individual chi-squares is significant below the 0.1 level. Thus, we would conclude that there is perhaps no association of treatment and response within the three age groups.

Another way of pooling is to combine all the data into one table and compute a chi-square on one degree of freedom which would yield $\chi^2_{\text{comb}} = 0.2165$ which has significance level 0.646 (see Ostle and Mensing 1975, Chapter 6).

A quantity which is used to test the consistency of association among the three tables is the homogeneity chi-square which is

$$\chi^2_{\text{homog}} = \chi^2_{\text{pooled}} - \chi^2_{\text{comb}}. \tag{20.11}$$

To get the degrees of freedom (d.f.) for χ^2_{homog} you merely subtract one from the pooled degrees of freedom or in our case this is $3 - 1 = 2$, and

$$\chi^2_{\text{homog}} = 1.7577 - 0.2165 = 1.5412,$$

which on 2 d.f. has significance level 0.534. Thus, we conclude that although the older age group seems to fare more poorly with respect to response, the association between treatment and response is not significantly inconsistent among the three age groups.

For a further discussion of this methodology when applied to tables containing smaller sample sizes, see Mantel and Haenszel (1959) and Mantel (1963). In particular, Fleiss (1973, Chapter 10) points out some good examples of how this method of summing chi-squares may be applied inappropriately to sample sizes of a large magnitude or when sample sizes differ in magnitude.

The odds ratio

Another methodology for measuring associations in the fourfold table, especially for retrospective studies, is via the odds ratio. To best demonstrate the use of this tool we refer to Table 20.6 and define some notation. Let

$C =$ event of having lung cancer,
$\bar{C} =$ event of not having lung cancer,
$S =$ event of being a smoker,
$\bar{S} =$ event of being a non-smoker,

$P(C|S)$ = the probability of having lung cancer given that one is a smoker,

and

$P(C|\bar{S})$ = the probability of having lung cancer given that one is a non-smoker.

It is clear from Table 20.6 that the data readily yield the estimates of $P(S|C)$ and $P(\bar{S}|C)$ which are

$$p(S|C) = 56/66 = 0.85$$

and

$$p(\bar{S}|C) = 10/66 = 0.15,$$

where we use lower case p to denote the estimate of the probability or proportion P. We define

$$\Omega_c = P(S|C)/P(\bar{S}|C)$$

which is the odds that S will occur given C. We denote the estimate of Ω_c as

$$O_c = p(S|C)/p(\bar{S}|C) \qquad (20.12)$$
$$= 5.6.$$

Likewise $\Omega_{\bar{c}} = P(S|\bar{C})/P(\bar{S}|\bar{C})$ or the odds that S occurs given $\bar{C}$. The estimate of $\Omega_{\bar{c}}$ from Table 20.6 is

$$O_{\bar{c}} = p(S|\bar{C})/p(\bar{S}|\bar{C}) \qquad (20.13)$$
$$= 27/39/12/39$$
$$= 27/12$$
$$= 2.25.$$

So the odds ratio (sometimes referred to as relative risk) of being a smoker conditional on having lung cancer versus not having lung cancer is $\Omega_c/\Omega_{\bar{c}}$ which is estimated by

$$O_c/O_{\bar{c}} = \frac{p(S|C)\ p(\bar{S}|\bar{C})}{p(\bar{S}|C)\ p(S|\bar{C})} = 5.6/2.25 = 2.49.$$

However, recall that we are interested in $P(C|S)$ and $P(C|\bar{S})$ and the odds ratio or relative risk of having lung cancer conditional on being a smoker versus being a non-smoker or

$$\Omega_s/\Omega_{\bar{s}} = \frac{P(C|S)/P(\bar{C}|S)}{P(C|\bar{S})/P(\bar{C}|\bar{S})} \qquad (20.14)$$

$$= \frac{P(C|S)\ P(\bar{C}|\bar{S})}{P(C|\bar{S})\ P(\bar{C}|S)}.$$

It can be shown mathematically that

$$\Omega_s/\Omega_{\bar{s}} = \Omega_c/\Omega_{\bar{c}}. \qquad (20.15)$$

Thus we can use $O_c/O_{\bar{c}}$ to estimate (20.14) or equivalently stated 'the odds of smokers having lung cancer is 2.49 times that of non-smokers'.

Given the discussion at the end of Part II, we see that one has to be very careful in interpreting the results of fourfold tables, especially when compiled in a retrospective manner. See Berkson (1958) for added examples of how caution must be exercised when using the odds ratio. For further discussion of the odds ratio, see Goodman and Kruskal (1954, 1959, 1963).

Another way of examining the odds ratio and relative risk is through the use of the logistic model. However, it is beyond the scope of this chapter to attempt to cover the wide application and use of the logistic model in testing and comparison of rates and proportions. For further details on the subject, see Cox (1958; 1970), Grizzle (1961, 1963), Zelen (1971, 1972), and Lee (1974).

Comparison of several proportions (K × 2 tables)

The situation for estimating and comparing proportions in the fourfold table is extended in some respects to the case in which we have $k > 2$ treatments and a binary response. Let us reconsider the data in Table 20.3, our non-small-cell lung cancer data. We want to compare the three treatments with respect to their ability to achieve a response, CR or PR. We rewrite the Table 20.3 as Table 20.11 below.

Table 20.11.

	CR or PR (%)		No response (%)		Total
CAMF	13	(13.3%)	85	(86.7%)	98
CAP	9	(8%)	104	(92%)	113
CA	4	(3%)	124	(97%)	128
Total	26		313		339

Table 20.11 is a $k \times 2$ table for $k = 3$. The general form of the $k \times 2$ table is

Table 20.12.

Treatment	Success	No success	Total
1	O_{11}	O_{12}	N_1
2	O_{21}	O_{22}	N_2
.	.	.	.
.	.	.	.
.	.	.	.
k	O_{k1}	O_{k2}	N_k
Total	C_1	C_2	$N = \sum_{i=1}^{k} N_i$

where O_{ij} is the number or frequency in the ith row and j^{th} column. In Table 20.11 above for example, $O_{11}=13$, $O_{12}=85$, and $N_1=O_{11}+O_{12}=98$.

The general hypothesis H under test is that the proportion of success in each treatment group is the same versus the alternative $\bar{H}$ that they are different. To test this hypothesis we use the formula

$$\chi^2_{k-1} = \sum_{i=1}^{k} \sum_{j=1}^{2} (O_{ij}-E_{ij})^2/E_{ij}, \tag{20.16}$$

where E_{ij} is the expected cell count for the ij^{th} cell and is defined

$$E_{ij}=N_i C_j/N.$$

So in Table 20.11 for example,

$$E_{11} = \frac{(98)\,(26)}{339} = 7.52 \qquad E_{12} = \frac{(98)\,(313)}{339} = 90.48$$

$$E_{21} = \frac{(113)\,(26)}{339} = 8.67 \qquad E_{22} = \frac{(113)\,(313)}{339} = 104.33 \qquad (20.17)$$

$$E_{31} = \frac{(128)\,(26)}{339} = 9.82 \qquad E_{32} = \frac{(128)\,(313)}{339} = 118.18.$$

Then (20.16) is

$$\chi^2_{k-1} = \frac{(13-7.52)^2}{7.52} + \frac{(85-90.48)^2}{90.48} + \frac{(9-8.67)^2}{8.67} + \frac{(104-104.33)^2}{104.33}$$

$$+ \frac{(4-9.82)^2}{9.82} + \frac{(124-118.18)^2}{118.18}$$

$$= 3.99 + 0.3319 + 0.0126 + 0.0010 + 3.449 + 0.2866$$
$$= 8.07,$$

which when we refer to a chi-square table on $k-1=2$ d.f. is significant at the 0.019 level. Therefore, the treatments as presented in the table are not equally effective in achieving a response and we would reject H.

K × M tables

The formulation in eqn (20.16) can be extended to accommodate further classifications (more than two) of response or various levels of toxicity. For example, suppose we wish to compare the three lung treatments with respect to granulocyte toxicity. We define our levels of granulocyte toxicity as follows in Table 20.13.

Table 20.13.

Decrease (%) in absolute granulocyte count	
Level	Count
Mild	$<25\%$
Moderate	$25-<50\%$
Severe	$50-<75\%$
Life threatening	$\geq 75\%$

The data results are as in Table 20.14.

Table 20.14.

		Level of granulocyte toxicity				
Treatment	None	Mild	Moderate	Severe	Life threatening	Total
CAMP	42	11	15	18	18	104
CAP	56	11	15	21	11	114
CA	61	13	22	23	16	135
Total	159	35	52	62	45	353*

* In this particular trial there were 14 patients evaluable for toxicity but not for response.

We now have a $k \times m$ table ($k=3$, $m=5$). The hypothesis under test is that the proportion of patients achieving a specific level of toxicity is the same for each treatment group. The chi-square statistic for the $k \times m$ setting is now:

$$\chi^2_{(k-1)(m-1)} = \sum_{i=1}^{k} \sum_{j=1}^{m} (O_{ij}-E_{ij})^2/E_{ij} \tag{20.18}$$

with $(k-1)\cdot(m-1)$ degrees of freedom. For Table 20.14

$$\chi^2_8 = 4.251,$$

which is significant at the 0.83 level on 8 degrees of freedom. Thus we would not reject the hypothesis under test. In general this is not a good test for comparing the average degree of toxicity in the treatment groups. We discuss the technique for doing so in the next section.

A restriction placed on Tables of the form 20.12 and 20.14 for the use of the chi-square test is that $E_{ij} \geq 5$. Tables 20.11 and 20.14 satisfy this requirement. If the requirement is not satisfied, the usual technique is to pool or combine some cells if this can be done meaningfully.

COMPARISON OF DEGREE OF RESPONSE OR TOXICITY (TEST FOR TREND)

The types of hypotheses we have been considering have dealt with the equality of proportions of success across treatment groups. In some trials we have considered success as a PR or CR and compared only the percentage of successes in each treatment group. By doing this we have ignored the distinction between CR or PR and between stable and progression. Sylvester (1980) has stated that: 'Important differences may be missed if the treatment differences depend on the inherent ordering of the response categories which reflect the degree of tumour change'. Let us consider an SECSG trial in metastatic sarcoma comparing adriamycin, cytoxan and methotrexate (ACM) versus the same combination with Amphotericin B (AMB). The response results are set out in Table 20.15.

Table 20.15.

Treatment	CR	PR	Stable	Progression	Total
ACM	1	10	9	17	37
ACM + AMB	0	4	13	26	43
Total	1	14	22	43	80

If one compares the percentage of responders (CR or PR) in each treatment group, we have $11/37 = 30$ per cent on ACM and $4/43 = 9$ per cent on ACM + AMB. The chi-square result corrected for continuity is:

$$\chi_1^2 = 4.188.$$ The 'two-sided' significance level is 0.032.

So, we may conclude that the two treatments differ in their ability to achieve a CR or PR. However, what else may we conclude from these results? To address this question we consider the following development which is an application of a methodology discussed by Cochran (1954), Armitage (1955, 1971), and Sylvester (1980). Let us rewrite Table 20.15 as Table 20.16.

Table 20.16.

Treatment	CR		PR		Stable		Progression		Total
ACM	1	(100%)	10	(71%)	9	(41%)	17	(40%)	37
ACM + AMB	0	(0%)	4	(29%)	13	(59%)	26	(60%)	43
Total	1	(100%)	14	(100%)	22	(100%)	43	(100%)	80

The percentages now are the percentage of patients at each level of response receiving a particular treatment. For example, 71 per cent of the PRs were on ACM and 29 per cent received ACM + AMB. Now if the treatments are truly different when we take the ordering of the response categories into account, then for the superior treatment one would expect these percentages to increase linearly as one goes from progression to stable to PR to CR and for the opposite trend to hold for the inferior treatment. To test for this linear trend one has to assign scores to each of the response categories. If all categories are of equal importance the scores may be equi-spaced. For example, one can assign 3 to a CR, 2 to a PR, 1 to a stable, and 0 to progression. Other scores could be 4, 3, 2, 1 or 3, 1, -1, -3, etc. The selection is quite arbitrary. Once the scores are assigned, we can write a general version of Table 20.15.

Table 20.17.

Response category	CR	PR	Stable	Progression	Total
Score	s_1	s_2	s_3	s_4	
ACM	c_1	c_2	c_3	c_4	C
ACM + AMB	$n_1 - c_1$	$n_2 - c_2$	$n_3 - c_3$	$n_4 - c_4$	$N - C$
Total	n_1	n_2	n_3	n_4	N

Where c_i $(i=1, \ldots, 4)$ is the number of patients on ACM who are in that particular response category. For example, in Table 20.15 $c_2 = 10$ or 10 PRs on ACM. n_i is the total number of patients in a response category or $n_2 = 14$ in Table 20.15. So naturally $n_i - c_i$ are the number of patients on ACM + AMB in response category i or $n_2 - c_2 = 4$. C is the total number of patients on ACM, $C = 37$. N is the total patient count in the table, $N = 80$, and therefore $N - C$ is the total number of patients on ACM + AMB or $N - C = 80 - 37 = 43$. $s_i (i = 1, \ldots, 4)$ is the score assigned to the ith response category. For our case let $s_1 = 3$, $s_2 = 2$, $s_3 = 1$, $s_4 = 0$.

So to test for the linear trend one computes:

$$\chi_{1,t}^2 = \frac{N\left(N \sum_{i=1}^m c_i s_i - C \sum_{i=1}^m n_i s_i\right)^2}{C(N-C)\left[N \sum_{i=1}^m n_i s_i^2 - \left(\sum_{i=1}^m n_i s_i\right)^2\right]} \tag{20.19}$$

which is distributed approximately as chi-square with 1 degree of freedom under the null hypothesis of no trend. Equation 20.19 is a general formula for testing of a linear trend in m categories for any two treatments. The t in $\chi_{1,t}^2$ denotes the chi-square computed to test for a trend. In our case $m = 4$ and

$$\chi_{1,t}^2 = \frac{80(80(3 + 20 + 9 + 0) - 37(4 + 28 + 22 + 0))^2}{(37)(43) \, [80(9 + 56 + 22 + 0) - (4 + 28 + 22 + 0)^2]} \tag{20.20}$$

$$= \frac{80(2560 - 1.998)^2}{1591 \, [6960 - 2916]}$$

$$= 3.927,$$

which is significant at the 0.048 level so we would reject the hypothesis of no linear trend. Even if we were to combine the CR and PR categories to have adequate expected cell frequencies, the result would be approximately the same. To test for a departure from a linear trend we apply eqn (20.18) to Table 20.15 for $k=2$ and $m=3$ ($m=3$ because we combine CRs and PRs to have adequate expected cell frequencies as discussed above) and we have $\chi^2_{m-1}=\chi^2_2=5.451$. Thus a test for departure from a linear trend is

$$\chi^2_{m-2}=\chi^2_{m-1}-\chi^2_{1,t} \tag{20.21}$$
$$=5.451-3.927$$
$$=1.524$$

which for $m=3$ is not significant and we would not reject the null hypothesis of no departure from linear trend. If there were enough CRs in Table 20.15 to allow for adequate expected cell counts then we would compute eqn (20.18) for $m=4$.

This methodology is very useful when comparing treatments for patterns of response especially for the case in which treatments may not differ significantly when comparing proportions of CRs or PRs only but do differ significantly in linear trend seen when we apply eqn (20.19). See Sylvester (1980) where such is, in fact, the case. Also a significant test for trend in response comparisons between two treatments can be interpreted as indicating that the average response on one treatment is higher than the average response on the other.

This technique is also applicable to situations, say, where treatments may not differ in overall response but do exhibit significantly different trends in toxicity. One such example is a metastatic cancer protocol with blinded treatments A and B. When comparing CR + PR rates, the significance level was 0.70 with no linear trend in response. The granulocyte toxicity table was as follows in Table 20.18.

Table 20.18.

Toxicity level	None or mild		Moderate		Severe		Life threat		Total
Score	4		3		2		1		
Treatment A	10	(58%)	7	(54%)	15	(39%)	12	(28%)	44
Treatment B	7	(42%)	6	(46%)	23	(61%)	31	(72%)	67*
Total	17	(100%)	13	(100%)	28	(100%)	43	(100%)	111

* When the study was initiated there was an imbalanced randomization in favour of treatment B.

The test for a linear trend in toxicity yielded

$$\chi^2_{1,t}=6.072 \tag{20.22}$$

which is significant at the 0.015 level. The overall test for the equality of the four proportions (using eqn 20.18, $k = 2$, $n = 4$) resulted in

$$\chi^2_{4-1} = \chi^2_3 = 6.1949 \tag{20.23}$$

with significance level 0.103 which would be considered non-significant by most standards. The test result for departure from the linear trend is

$$\chi^2_2 = \chi^2_3 - \chi^2_{1,t} = 0.123 \tag{20.24}$$

with significance level equal to 0.94 or there is no departure from a linear trend in rate of toxicity. Therefore, we conclude that although A and B do not differ with respect to proportions of patients responding, it appears that toxicities increase linearly in B and decrease likewise in A. Similarly treatment B appears to have a significantly higher average rate of toxicity.

For the case in which there are more than two treatments one can extend the above procedure by comparing the average scores per treatment using a non-parametric test. The Kruskal–Wallis H test would be an example of this procedure. For a discussion of this technique see Kruskal and Wallis (1952), Siegel (1956), Hollander and Wolfe (1973), and Lee (1980, Chapter 5).

SOME THOUGHTS ON MULTIPLE COMPARISONS

The multiple comparison problem that we discuss here deals primarily with the attempt to gain a vast amount of information from a single study. One purpose may be to identify important factors for stratification for future studies or to identify subgroups of patients for whom particular clinical studies may be designed. The multiple comparison discussion usually centres on a retrospective look at data to attempt to identify factors associated with a disease. Our purpose here is to show how it may apply when we want to determine a factor–response relationship. As in all retrospective analyses the results are not conclusive, but are only leads for future directions. Such analyses may yield valid inference when confirmed by data from similar studies.

When a large phase III trial is completed, it is often very tempting for investigators to retrospectively seek out subgroups of patients whom they can identify as good or poor risk patients, or simply those most likely to respond or not to respond. One wishes, say, to look at various factors associated with response holding other factors, or series of factors, fixed. It is obvious that there are potentially many comparisons that one could attempt. Mantel and Haenszel (1959) point out that using a reasonable significance level to do all those tests will, with a high degree of probability, result in some comparisons being significant, even if there is no real association. This can be seen in an attempt to associate some factors in a univariate fashion to the achievement of a complete remission in an adult acute myelogenous leukaemia study in which over 250 patients were entered. There were 22 pre-treatment characteristics considered in addition to induction treatment. These characteristics are set out in Table 20.19.

Table 20.19.

Categorical	Quantitative	
1. Sex	9. Marrow (% blasts)	18. BUN
2. Race	10. Haemoglobin	19. Age
Presence or absence of:	11. Reticulocyte count	20. Uric acid
3. Fever	12. Platelets	21. Surface area
4. Infection	13. White blood cell	22. Serum Alkaline
5. Weight loss (> 10%)	14. Circulating blasts (%)	phosphatase
6. Haemorrhage	15. SGOT	
7. Splenomegaly	16. LDH	
8. Hepatomegaly	17. Bilirubin	

The two major factors testing significant at 0.05 or less and with real association to response were age and BUN; the results are:

	CR		No CR		Total
Age < 50	52	(55%)	43	(45%)	95
Age > 50	38	(23%)	130	(77%)	168
Total	90		173		263

$\chi_1^2 = 27.80$, significance level $p = 0.0001$

	CR		No CR		Total
Normal BUN	67	(39%)	103	(61%)	170
Elevated BUN	23	(25%)	70	(75%)	93
Total	90		173		263

$\chi_1^2 = 5.54$, significance level $p = 0.02$.

Also as anticipated, some minor factors with little associative value to response tested significantly (0.05 or less). One such factor was weight loss ($p = 0.014$). When examining the data set more closely one sees that the association of weight loss for response is really due to its own association with the major factors. Only 27 per cent of the younger age group (less than 50 years of age) had weight loss, while 46 per cent of the older age group had weight loss of 10 per cent or more ($p = 0.01$). Likewise 35 per cent of the patients with no

BUN elevation had weight loss, while over 50 per cent of patients with BUN elevation had weight loss ($p = 0.03$). This is an example in which we are able to detect underlying reasons why some associations in a multiple comparison setting do occur. There are times when factors will test significantly and the reason is not readily discernible.

There are several solutions to the multiple comparison questions which have been proposed:

(a) one solution is to test all comparisons at extreme levels of significance, say less than 0.05, which would reduce the number of associations being made incorrectly. Mantel and Haenszel (1959), however, have pointed out that this would possibly hamper efforts to detect real associations. In our example above if we had set the significance level at 0.01 and rejected the null hypothesis for only levels less than or equal to 0.01 then we would have missed the BUN effect.

(b) Secondly, provided you know what were major and minor factors, one could test the major factors at higher significance levels than one would test the minor factors.

(c) The third solution, which has wide appeal in large co-operative group studies, is to apply multivariate techniques to the data set. The most popular model now used to associate prognostic factors with response is the linear logistic model of Cox (1970). Application of this model to our adult AML data confirmed the importance of our major factors including age and BUN while weight loss was not a significant factor in the model. This procedure of identifying major prognostic factors while adjusting for factors of less importance is discussed elsewhere in this book and we do not pursue it further here. For further discussion of the logistic model see Lee (1974, 1980).

ACKNOWLEDGEMENTS

The author would like to thank Mr Robert Birch, Dr Seng-Jaw Soong and Dr John R. Durant for helpful discussions, Ms Billie Graham for her patience in the typing of this manuscript, and Ms Sandra Mosley and Ms Susan Belvin for their assistance in gathering reference materials for this article. Also, thanks to the editors for their efforts in compiling this book. The author's research was supported in part by NIH–NCI research grant CA-24456.

REFERENCES

Anscombe, F. J. (1963). Sequential medical trials. *J. Am. Statist. Ass.* **58**, 364–83.
Armitage, P. (1955). Tests for linear trends in proportions and frequencies. *Biometrics* **11**, 375–85.
—— (1971). *Statistical methods in medical research.* Blackwell Scientific Publications, Oxford.
Berkson, J. (1958). Smoking and lung cancer: some observations on two recent reports. *J. Am. statist. Ass.* **53**, 28–38.

Calvert, R. L. (1955). The determination of confidence intervals for probabilities of proper, dud and premature operation. *Sandia Corp. Tech. Memo SCTM* 213–55–31. Alburquerque, New Mexico.

Clopper, C. J. and Pearson, E. S. (1934). The use of confidence or fiducial limits in the case of the binomial. *Biometrika* **26**, 404–13.

Cochran, W. G. (1954). Some methods of strengthening the common χ^2 tests. *Biometrics* **10**, 417–51.

Colton, R. (1963). A model for selecting one of two medical treatments. *J. Am. statist. Ass.* **58**, 388–400.

Cornfield, J. (1966). A Bayesian test of some classical hypotheses—with applications to sequential medical trials. *J. Am. statist. Ass.* **61**, 577–94.

——— (1969). The Bayesian outlook and its applications. *Biometrics* **25**, 617–57.

——— Halperin, M., and Greenhouse, S. W. (1969). An adaptive procedure for sequential clinical trials. *J. Am. statist. Ass.* **64**, 759–70.

Cox, D. R. (1958). The regression analysis of binary sequences. *Jl R. statist. Soc. Series B* **20**, 215–42.

——— (1970). *Analysis of binary data*. Methuen, London.

Fisher, R. A. (1934). *Statistical methods for research workers*, 5th edn. Oliver and Boyd, Edinburgh.

Fleiss, J. L. (1973). *Statistical methods for rates and proportions*. John Wiley and Sons, New York.

Goodman, L. A. and Kruskal, W. H. (1954). Measures of association for cross classifications. *J. Am. statist. Ass.* **49**, 732–64.

——— (1959). Measures of association for cross classifications. II. Further discussion and references. *J. Am. statist. Ass.* **54**, 123–63.

——— (1963). Measures of association for cross classifications. III. Approximate sampling theory. *J. Am. statist. Ass.* **58**, 310–64.

Grizzle, J. E. (1961). A new method of testing hypotheses and estimating parameters for the logistic model. *Biometrics* **17**, 372–85.

——— (1963). Tests of linear hypotheses when the data are proportions. *Am. J. pub. Health* **53**, 970–6.

Gunel, E. and Dickey, J. (1974). Bayes factors for independence in contingency tables. *Biometrika* **61**, 545–57.

Hald, A. (1952). *Statistical tables and formulas*. Wiley, New York.

Hayward, J. L., Carbone, P. P., Heuson, J. C., Kimaoka, S., Segaloff, A., and Rubens, R. D. (1977). Assessment of response to therapy in advanced breast cancer. *Cancer* **39**, 1289–94.

Hollander, M. and Wolfe, D. D. (1973). *Nonparametric statistical methods*. Wiley, New York.

Irwin, J. O. (1935). Tests of significance for differences between percentages based on small numbers. *Metron* **12**, 83–94.

Kruskal, W. H., and Wallis, W. A. (1952). Use of ranks in one-criterion variance analysis. *J. Am. statist. Ass.* **47**, 583–621.

Lee, E. T. (1974). A computer program for linear logistic regression analysis. *Comput. Programs in Biomed.* **4**, 80–92.

——— (1980). *Statistical methods for survival data analysis*. Wadsworth Inc., Belmont, California.

Lindley, D. V. (1964). The Bayesian analysis of contingency tables. *Ann. math. Statist.* **35**, 1622–43.

Mantel, N. (1963). Chi-square tests with one degree of freedom: extensions of the Mantel–Haenszel procedure. *J. Am. statist. Ass.* **58**, 690–700.

—— and Haenszel, W. (1959). Statistical aspects of the analysis of data from retrospective studies of disease. *J. natn. Cancer Inst.* **22**, 719–48.

Muench, J. O. (1960). A confidence limit computer. *Sandia Corp. Monogr. SCR–159*, Alburquerque, New Mexico.

Ostle, B. and Mensing, R. W. (1975). *Statistics in research*, 3rd edn. The Iowa State University Press, Ames, Iowa.

Siegel, S. (1956). *Nonparametric statistics for the behavioral sciences*. McGraw-Hill, New York.

Sylvester, R. (1980). On the analysis of response rates in studies of advanced disease. *Breast cancer—experimental and clinical aspects*, pp. 5–7. Published as Supplement No. 1, 1980 to the *European Journal of Cancer*.

Walker, S. H. and Duncan, D. B. (1967). Estimation of the probability of an event as a function of several independent variables. *Biometrika* **54**, 167–79.

Zelen, M. (1969). Play the winner rule and the controlled trial. *J. Am. statist. Ass.* **64**, 131–46.

—— (1971). The analysis of several 2×2 contingency tables. *Biometrika* **58**, 129–37.

—— (1972). Exact significance tests for contingency tables embedded in a 2^n classification. In *Proceedings of Sixth Berkeley Symposium on Probability and Statistics* Vol. 1, pp. 737–58.

21 The calculation and interpretation of survival curves

Julian Peto

INTRODUCTION

The prognosis of patients with a chronic disease can be summarized by a single figure, such as the survival or recurrence rate five years after diagnosis, but only the whole survival curve shows the complete time course of the disease. The importance of looking at the overall pattern of recurrence or survival is illustrated in Fig. 21.1, which shows the disease-free survival rate in boys with acute lymphoblastic leukaemia who had already received continuous

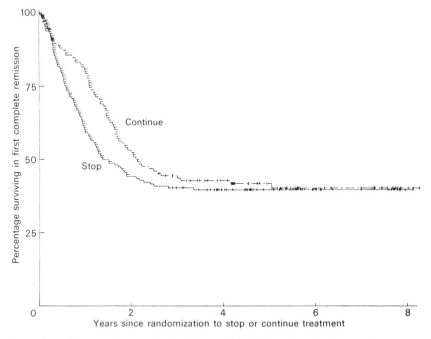

Fig. 21.1. Disease-free survival of boys with ALL randomly allocated to stop or continue treatment. The graph begins at the time of randomization, which was between 18 months and 2 years after starting treatment (279 patients).

chemotherapy for about 2 years, and then either stopped or continued treatment (MRC 1982). The relapse rate increased when treatment stopped, but patients whose chemotherapy continued suffered a similar relapse rate when their treatment stopped about a year later, and the long-term disease-free survival was not affected. Thus, although relapse was significantly delayed, the survival curves suggest that there was little or no eventual advantage in longer treatment.

Survival curves usually show the probability at different times of surviving, or of not having suffered recurrence, but the same methods can be used to analyse the time to any event. A 'survival curve' can thus be calculated for the time of first deviation from a protocol, or even, for certain chronic conditions, the time to disappearance of the disease. All such curves are simply referred to as survival curves in this chapter, both to emphasize that the same statistical methodology is used, and to avoid cumbersome expressions such as 'the probability at successive times that an event has not occurred'.

The following sections describe the calculation of the survival curve and its standard error. Simple mortality data are used to illustrate these methods to avoid the statistical and methodological difficulties (which are discussed later) that can arise when survival curves for a particular cause of death or type of recurrence are calculated, or when patients are withdrawn or re-classified.

CALCULATION OF THE ACTUARIAL SURVIVAL CURVE

For most clinical studies there is only one sensible way to estimate the survival curve. This is variously called the 'actuarial' curve, the 'product-limit' curve, the 'Kaplan–Meier' curve, or simply the survival curve (Kaplan and Meier 1958). If data are grouped into weeks or months rather than exact days, a modified, but essentially identical method, the 'life-table' estimate, is used (Sylvester, Machin, and Staquet 1978).

The method of calculating the actuarial survival curve follows immediately from the observation that to survive a year a patient must survive the first day, and the second, and the third, and so on to the 365th day. The separate probabilities of surviving each day are multiplied together, giving

Probability of surviving 365 days = (probability for day 1) × (probability for day 2) × . . . × (probability for day 364) × (probability for day 365).

This is analogous to the calculation of the probability of throwing four sixes in four throws of a die, which is $1/6 \times 1/6 \times 1/6 \times 1/6$, or $1/1296$.

All the patients in a study are observed on the first day of the trial, so $E(1)$, the estimated probability of surviving day 1, is simply

$$E(1) = \frac{\text{no. of patients} - \text{number of deaths on day 1}}{\text{no. of patients}}$$

The number actually observed on subsequent days will be less, however. For day 100, for example, patients who died before day 100, those who were lost to follow-up before day 100, and those who entered the study less than 100 days ago, contribute no information on the probability of surviving the 100th day, and $E(100)$, the estimated probability of surviving the 100th day for patients who have already survived 99 days, is

$$E(100) = \frac{\text{no. 'at risk' on day } 100 - \text{no. of deaths on day } 100}{\text{no. of patients 'at risk' on day } 100.} \quad (21.1)$$

The number of patients 'at risk' on day 100, $R(100)$, is the number who were still alive and under observation at the beginning of the 100th day. Patients lost sight of on day 100 are thus 'at risk' on day 100, but not on day 101 or later.

Denoting the number of deaths on day 1, 2, ... by $D(1)$, $D(2)$ ..., the actuarial survival curve at the end of the 100th day, $P(100)$, is thus

$$P(100) = E(1) \times E(2) \times \ldots \times E(99) \times E(100) \quad (21.2)$$

$$= \frac{(R(1) - D(1))}{R(1)} \times \frac{(R(2) - D(2))}{R(2)} \times \ldots$$

$$\times \frac{(R(99) - D(99))}{R(99)} \times \frac{(R(100) - D(100))}{R(100)}$$

This simple formula provides the best estimate of the probability of survival. On average it will give the right answer and is subject to less random variation than any alternative formula. (In statistical jargon, it is the minimum variance unbiased estimator, and is the curve which maximises the likelihood of the observed data).

An example

The data in the left-hand side of Table 21.1 give the dates of diagnosis and death, and the corresponding survival times of 25 patients with inoperable lung cancer. All have been followed up to death, and their survival curve is simply 96 per cent after the first death, 92 per cent after the second, 88 per cent after the third, and so on, falling to zero after the last death (continuous steps; Fig. 21.2). This is clearly a sensible representation of the data, but it is not immediately obvious that it corresponds to the formula for the survival curve given in eqn (21.2). R, the number of patients 'at risk', is 25 when the first death occurs, 24 when the second occurs, and so on, and D, the number of deaths, is either one or none on each day. Successive terms in eqn (21.2) thus cancel, giving:

Time	Equation 21.2		Survival curve
Day 0			(100%)
Day 22 (1st death)	24/25	=	24/25 (96%)

Time	Equation 21.2		Survival curve	
Day 27 (2nd death)	$24/25 \times 23/24$	=	23/25	(92%)
Day 50 (3rd death)	$24/25 \times 23/24$			
	$\times 22/23$	=	22/25	(88%)

The curve does not alter on days when no death occurs, as D is zero, and $(R-D)/R$ for such days (eqn 21.2) is simply R/R, or 1.

To calculate the survival curve at the end of a particular day as the product of the observed probabilities of surviving successive days up to and including that day, it is convenient to re-arrange the patients in the way shown in Table 21.1 in ascending order of survival or loss to follow-up. It would be unusual in practice to have followed every patient to death, and the right-hand side of Table 21.1 shows the analysis of those data that would have been available on 31 March 1980, 15 months after the first patient was diagnosed in January 1979 and three months after the last entered the study in December 1979. Twelve patients were then still alive, and it is interesting to compare the corresponding survival curve (broken steps; Fig. 21.2) with the curve obtained when all the patients had died (continuous steps; Fig. 21.2). The curves are identical for the first 3 months, as all patients had been followed up for at least 3 months by 31 March 1980, but further on the broken curve is based on fewer deaths, changes in larger steps, and is determined less precisely. It is sometimes higher and sometimes lower than the original more accurate curve, but is not *systematically* too high or too low—it is made less precise, but is not *biased*, by being based on shorter follow-up and fewer deaths.

The meaning of the statement that the actuarial curve is unbiased can

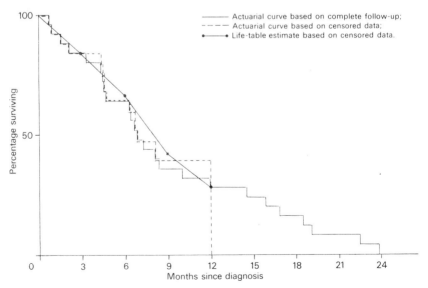

Fig. 21.2. Actuarial and life table survival curves for 25 patients with lung cancer.

Table 21.1. *Survival data on 25 patients with inoperable lung cancer*

Basic data					Survival curve based on complete follow-up			Survival curve based on follow-up to 31/3/1980			
Patient no.	Date of diagnosis	Date of death	Days to death	Days to 31/3/1980	Patient no.	Days to death	Survival curve	Patient no.	Days to follow-up or death	No. still 'at risk' (R)	Survival curve
1	11/1/79	30/5/79	139		12	22	0.96	12	22	25	$24/25 \times 1.000 = 0.9600$
2	23/1/79	21/1/80	363		5	27	0.92	5	27	24	$23/24 \times 0.9600 = 0.9200$
3	15/2/79	27/8/79	193		10	50	0.88	10	50	23	$22/23 \times 0.9200 = 0.8800$
4	7/3/79	10/11/79	248		21	68	0.84	21	68	22	$21/22 \times 0.8800 = 0.8400$
5	12/3/79	8/4/79	27		25	101	0.80	25	99 (alive)	21	0.8400
6	25/3/79	21/10/79	210		7	134	0.76	24	108 (alive)	20	0.8400
7	4/4/79	16/8/79	134		15	136	0.72	23	121 (alive)	19	0.8400
8	30/4/79	19/11/79	203		1	139	0.68	22	131 (alive)	18	0.8400
9	16/5/79	9/5/81	724	320	20	144	0.64	7	134	17	$16/17 \times 0.8400 = 0.7906$
10	26/5/79	15/7/79	50		19	191	0.60	15	136	16	$15/16 \times 0.7906 = 0.7412$
11	30/5/79	22/10/80	511	306	3	193	0.56	1	139	15	$14/15 \times 0.7412 = 0.6918$
12	3/6/79	25/6/79	22		8	203	0.52	20	144	14	$13/14 \times 0.6918 = 0.6424$
13	15/6/79	27/12/80	561	290	6	210	0.48	19	186 (alive)	13	0.6424
14	29/6/79	29/1/81	580	276	17	224	0.44	3	193	12	$11/12 \times 0.6424 = 0.5888$
15	1/7/79	14/11/79	136		4	248	0.40	18	198 (alive)	11	0.5888
16	13/8/79	16/6/80	308	231	23	256	0.36	8	203	10	$9/10 \times 0.5888 = 0.5299$
17	27/8/79	7/4/80	224	217	16	308	0.32	6	210	9	$8/9 \times 0.5299 = 0.4711$
18	15/9/79	9/1/81	482	198	2	363	0.28	17	217 (alive)	8	0.4711
19	27/9/79	5/4/80	191	186	24	441	0.24	16	231 (alive)	7	0.4711
20	11/10/79	3/3/80	144		18	482	0.20	4	248	6	$5/6 \times 0.4711 = 0.3925$
21	17/11/79	24/1/80	68		11	511	0.16	14	276 (alive)	5	0.3925
22	21/11/79	4/10/81	683	131	13	561	0.12	13	290 (alive)	4	0.3925
23	1/12/79	13/8/80	256	121	14	580	0.08	11	306 (alive)	3	0.3925
24	14/12/79	27/2/81	441	108	22	683	0.04	9	320 (alive)	2	0.3925
25	23/12/79	2/4/80	101	99	9	724	0.00	2	363	1	$0/1 \times 0.3925 = 0.0000$

perhaps be illustrated by a more extreme example. The best estimate of the 3-month survival rate based on these data is obviously 84 per cent—all patients were followed up for 3 months or longer, and four (16 per cent) died within 3 months. Suppose that we were to to calculate 25 separate actuarial survival curves, one for each patient. Four of these curves would fall from 100 to 0 per cent at some point before 3 months, and the other 21 would still be at 100 per cent at 3 months. One such graph, showing a 3-month survival of either 0 or 100 per cent, would be almost worthless, but by averaging them we would still estimate the 3-month survival rate correctly; $(4 \times 0\% + 21 \times 100\%)/25$ gives a 3-month survival estimate of 84 per cent. The actuarial survival curve, even if it is based on only one patient, is thus still unbiased.

THE LIFE-TABLE ESTIMATE: SIMULTANEOUS DEATHS AND LOSSES AND GROUPED DATA

In many studies patients are followed up periodically, and the exact day when a patient was lost to follow-up cannot be accurately determined. If patients are seen every 3 months, for example, several deaths and losses to follow-up may occur between successive follow-ups, and the number 'at risk' when the deaths occurred will not be known exactly. It will be, on average, less than the number last seen alive at the previous follow-up 3 months before, and be greater than this number minus the number lost since the last follow-up. A reasonable approximation is to average these numbers (see Appendix); thus, the number R 'at risk' in an interval is taken to be the number 'at risk' at the start of the interval minus half the number lost during the interval. The probability E of surviving the interval is calculated as before as $E = (R - D)/R$, where D is the number of deaths in the interval, and the estimated survival curve at the end of each interval is the product of these probabilities of surviving each preceding interval as in eqn 21.2. The calculation is shown in Table 21.2 for the lung cancer survival times with incomplete follow-up from Table 21.1. The life-table is calculated after grouping deaths and losses to follow-up in three-month periods, and the resulting survival curve, represented by points at 3, 6, 9, and 12 months, is shown in Fig. 21.2. Comparison against the actuarial curves, with and without losses to follow-up based on the same data, shows that the life-table estimates are similar to the actuarial curves up to 9 months. At 12 months, however, the life-table survival estimate is 28 per cent, but the actuarial estimate, calculated from the censored data, is zero, because the patient followed up the longest happened to die. This should not be regarded as evidence that either method of calculation is unsatisfactory; the correct conclusion, and one which cannot be emphasized too strongly, is that the tails of survival curves are so unstable that they are hardly worth plotting. A sensible rule of thumb which largely avoids this difficulty is to stop the curve at the point where only five patients are still being followed up.

The life-table estimates of the survival curve at the ends of successive

Table 21.2. *Life-table analysis of data from Table 21.1, in 3-month intervals*

Patient no.	Days to follow-up or death	No. 'at risk' at start of interval	Dead	Lost	Average 'at risk'	Survival curve at end of interval
12	22	25	4	0	25	$1.0000 \times 21/25$
5	27					$= 0.8400$ at 3 months
10	50					
21	68					
25	99 (alive)					
24	108 (alive)					
23	121 (alive)					
22	131 (alive)	21	4	4	19	$0.8400 \times 15/19$
7	134					$= 0.6632$ at 6 months
15	136					
1	139					
20	144					
19	186 (alive)					
3	193					
18	198 (alive)					
8	203	13	4	4	11	$0.6632 \times 7/11$
6	210					$= 0.4220$ at 9 months
17	217 (alive)					
16	231 (alive)					
4	248					
14	276 (alive)					
13	290 (alive)					
11	306 (alive)	5	1	4	3	$0.4220 \times 2/3$
9	320 (alive)					$= 0.2813$ at 12 months
2	363					

intervals can be joined by straight lines to make the curve easier to look at, as in Fig. 21.2, but it is not good practice to draw a smooth line through the steps of an actuarial curve. The steps show that it is an actuarial rather than a life-table curve, and the size of each step reflects how many patients were followed up to that point or beyond. Incidentally, to draw a line either through the tops or through the bottoms of the steps is wrong; if you insist on smoothing the curve, the mid-points of the steps should be joined.

THE STANDARD ERROR OF THE SURVIVAL CURVE

The statement that there is a 'statistically significant' difference between the survival curves for two treatments means that the curves appear to differ in some way, not that a higher proportion of the patients on one treatment were necessarily cured, or even that their life expectancy was longer. Different statistical significance tests are designed to answer different questions, such as 'do the curves differ substantially at a specified point in time' (for example at 5 years), 'do the overall death rates differ', or 'does treatment delay, if not prevent, relapse or death'. For the curves in Fig. 21.1, for example, tests comparing overall or 5 year disease-free survival rates would show little or no difference between shorter or longer chemotherapy, but a test designed to detect a delay in relapse would give a highly significant result (MRC 1982).

In this chapter we are concerned with estimating and interpreting the survival curve rather than with efficient significance testing, which is discussed in detail in Chapter 22. We shall give a few formulae for estimating the precision of the survival curve, ranging from a crude rule-of-thumb which gives some feeling for the reliability of the curve to a reasonably precise estimate that can be used to draw 95 per cent confidence intervals, but none of these methods is sufficiently accurate to be used for formal significance testing.

The most useful formula for a clinician looking at a survival curve is that the range of error of the curve (± 2 standard errors) at a given time is roughly $\pm 1/\sqrt{(N')}$, where N' is the number of patients who have either already died or are followed up to that time. (If no losses to follow-up have occurred N' thus equals N, the total number of patients in the trial.) This formula overestimates the error if the curve is close to 100 or 0 per cent, but between about 20 and 80 per cent it gives a sensible estimate. Thus, for example, if a survival curve based on 100 patients with a long follow-up shows a 40 per cent 5-year survival, the true 5-year survival is likely to be within ± 0.10 (that is $\pm 1/\sqrt{100}$) of 40 per cent, between 30 and 50 per cent. The same curve based on 1000 patients would be accurate to ± 3 per cent, while if only 20 patients were observed the range of error would be ± 22 per cent. This last figure should perhaps be given special prominence, as trials with 20 or so patients in each treatment group are unfortunately quite common. A 40 per cent 5-year survival rate based on 20 patients means that the true 5-year survival lies somewhere between about 18 and 62 per cent, a range of error so wide that no useful comparison with standard treatment could possibly be made unless the new treatment constituted a miraculous breakthrough in the treatment of a usually fatal disease. Therefore small trials may do more harm than good, as they are very unlikely to detect even quite large improvements, and the few that are published because they happen to achieve statistical significance (often through a combination of chance and incorrect design or analysis) give grossly exaggerated estimates of the benefits of the therapeutic innovation.

The remainder of this section, which describes more accurate methods for estimating the standard error of the curve, can be missed by non-statisticians.

No losses to follow-up

When no losses to follow-up occur, the probability of still being alive at any point is estimated directly as

$$\hat{P} = \text{no. of patients still alive}/N,$$

where N is the total number of patients in the trial. (The estimated probability of survival is now denoted by $\hat{P}$ to distinguish it from P, the true value.) The standard error (S) of $\hat{P}$ is the square root of $P(1-P)/N$, and a good estimate of S is thus

$$\hat{S} = \sqrt{(\hat{P}(1-\hat{P})/N)}. \tag{21.3}$$

For the lung cancer survival data based on complete follow-up (continuous steps in Fig. 21.2), for example, the survival curve at 6 months is 0.64, and there were initially 25 patients in the trial. The estimated standard error of the curve at 6 months is thus

$$\hat{S} = \sqrt{(0.64(1-0.64)/25)} = 9.6\%,$$

and the 95 per cent confidence limits (survival curve ± 2 standard errors) for the 6-month survival rate are 44.8 and 83.2 per cent.

Losses to follow-up

A slight overestimate of the standard error of the actuarial survival curve for a study in which losses occur is given by a modified form of eqn (21.3),

$$\hat{S} = \sqrt{(\hat{P}(1-\hat{P})/N')}, \tag{21.4}$$

where $\hat{P}$ is the actuarial curve at the given time (at 6 months for example), and N' is the number of patients in the trial minus the number lost to follow-up before this time. For the censored lung cancer data (broken line in Fig. 21.2), four of the 25 patients were lost to follow-up before 6 months (Table 21.1) and $\hat{P}$, the actuarial curve at 6 months, is 64.24 per cent. N' is therefore 21, and eqn (21.4) gives

$$\hat{S} = \sqrt{(\hat{P}(1-\hat{P})/N')} = \sqrt{(0.6424(1-0.6424)/21)} = 10.5\%.$$

The confidence limits for the 6-month survival rate are thus 43.2 and 85.2 per cent.

Losses to follow-up—Greenwood's formula for the standard error

By using eqn (21.4), we are assuming, in effect, that patients already lost to follow-up contributed no information, and the resulting confidence limits are, therefore, slightly too wide. A better approximation is provided by Greenwood's (1926) formula,

$$\hat{S} = \sqrt{(\hat{P}^2 \Sigma_i (D_i/N_i(N_i - D_i)))} \tag{21.5}$$

where D_i is the number of deaths on the ith day, N_i is the number of patients still 'at risk' on the ith day, and Σ_i denotes summation up to and including the day at which the curve P is estimated. For the same actuarial curve at 6 months, for example (see right-hand side, Table 21.1), eqn (21.5) gives

$$\hat{S}^2 = 0.6424^2 \times (1/25 \times 24 + 1/24 \times 23 + 1/23 \times 22 + 1/22 \times 21$$
$$+ 1/17 \times 16 + 1/16 \times 15 + 1/15 \times 14 + 1/14 \times 13),$$

and

$$\hat{S} = 0.103, \text{ or } 10.3\%.$$

Greenwood's formula provides a good estimate of the precision of the curve when a reasonable number of patients are still being followed up, but not in the tail of the curve, where misleading plateaux often occur. The interpretation of such plateaux is discussed in the following section.

Asymmetrical confidence intervals

The approximate 95 per cent confidence intervals given above are simply ± 2 standard errors from the estimated value of the survival curve, a crude procedure based on the assumption of approximate normality, and hence symmetry. Whichever variance estimate is used to calculate the standard error, an ingenious and simple modification suggested by Rothman (1978) provides better estimates of the upper and lower confidence limits. For Greenwood's estimate, for example, the binomial sample size N, for which (21.3) would give the same estimate for $\hat{S}$ as eqn (21.5), is calculated, and defined as the 'effective sample size'. The usual exact or approximate methods for calculating binomial confidence limits can then be applied, giving confidence limits which are asymmetrical, as they should be, and which appear to perform well even for small sample sizes and survival curves close to 0 or 100 per cent.

More accurate estimates of the standard error of the survival curve, the asymptotic normality of the curve (Breslow and Crowley 1974), and significance tests for comparing survival curves at a fixed point (Thomas and Grunkemeier 1975), are beyond the scope of this chapter. Some of these issues are discussed in other chapters of this book; the most useful reference as a starting point for further reading is Thomas and Grunkemeier (1975), who describe simulation studies of significance tests for comparing survival curves at a fixed point.

MISINTERPRETATION OF A PLATEAU IN THE TAIL OF A SURVIVAL CURVE

For many cancers, most patients suffer recurrence within a few years or not at all. This knowledge contributes considerably to the interpretation of the survival curve, and for such diseases a long plateau in the tail of the survival curve provides a reasonable estimate of the proportion of patients who have been cured. This inference is justified, however, by prior knowledge rather than statistical considerations. The tail of a survival curve is extremely unstable, as can be seen from the broken line in Fig. 21.2, which remains at 39 per cent from 8 months to a year and then falls to zero when the last patient relapsed. If this patient had happened to survive to the follow-up date, this survival curve might have been interpreted as showing that about 39 per cent of patients had been cured, a reasonable interpretation if these were patients with non-metastatic oral cancer, but not for inoperable lung cancer. Many statistical and interpretational difficulties with survival curves relate to the tail of the curve, and most can be avoided by the simple expedient described above of stopping the curve when less than five patients are still 'at risk'. For example in this case the broken line in Fig. 21.2 would then be truncated at 9 months, giving a useful estimate of prognosis up to 9 months, and removing both the meaningless plateau from 9 to 12 months and the meaningless drop from 39 to 0 per cent at 12 months based on a single patient. In the same way, life-table analysis of these data in 3-month periods can give either an estimate of 28 per cent for the 12-month survival (Table 21.2) or an estimate of 0 per cent if a different method of analysis is used (see Appendix). Neither estimate is wrong, but both are worthless; there are simply too few patients followed up beyond 9 months to provide any useful estimate of the later relapse rate. This last part of the curve is not ignored when carrying out a significance test, however; the last few relapses will carry more or less the same weight as the first in assessing the overall relapse rate.

OTHER METHODS FOR CALCULATING THE SURVIVAL CURVE

The survival curve can be estimated by fitting a mathematical model to the data, but this approach is beyond the scope of this chapter. Fitted curves should not be presented instead of the summary of the actual data provided by the actuarial curve, but they may provide a useful basis for extrapolation, or for testing a biological hypothesis which predicts a specific pattern of relapse (Sylvester *et al.* 1978).

The 'reduced-sample' estimate of the survival curve, for which patients who have not been followed up to the time at which the curve is calculated are excluded, should not be used (Sylvester *et al.* 1978). It is less precise than the actuarial estimate and has the rather silly property of sometimes increasing with time, so that the estimate of survival at 2 years can be greater than the estimate at 1 year.

DEFINING 'TIME OF ENTRY' CORRECTLY

The calculation of the survival curve depends on: (1) correct recording of time of entry to the study; (2) correct recording of time of loss to follow-up or death; and (3) the assumption that a patient's chance of being lost or withdrawn is unrelated to his risk of dying. These three apparently trivial conditions are frequently not met, leading to serious bias in the survival curve and sometimes to bias in the comparison of treatments.

The period from a patient's entry to his loss or death is called his period 'at risk'; it is simply the period during which his death would have been noted and included in the analysis if it had occurred. Date of entry to a study is, therefore, defined accordingly. If the patient had died the day before his entry date he would not have been in the study at all, but if he had died on, or after it, his death would have been counted.

The commonest error in defining date of entry arises when patients are re-classified after starting treatment. Suppose, for example, that you wish to plot the survival curve of patients with slow methotrexate absorption, and this assay is carried out 3 months after starting treatment. Patients who die within 3 months will not be included, and if date of entry is taken to be the beginning of treatment the survival curve will have a spurious plateau at 100 per cent up to 3 months. The date of entry must be the date when the assay was performed.

A similar problem arises in the analysis of the number of courses of chemotherapy that have been given in full, or the number that have been reduced or omitted due to toxicity. If date of entry is taken to be the date of first treatment, such analyses may suggest that patients who have taken many courses live longer than those who have not, and that patients whose dose was reduced many times live longer than those with fewer dose reductions. The reason for this absurd contradiction is that you have to live quite a long time to be able to have a larger number of dose reductions or full courses of treatment. This source of bias is avoided by classifying patients by the amount of chemotherapy given during, say, the first 6 months of treatment and taking the date of entry to be 6 months after starting treatment. Thus patients who die before 6 months are excluded and treatment deviations after 6 months are ignored.

RECURRENCE, PERIOD 'AT RISK', AND TIME OF LOSS TO FOLLOW-UP

Discussion has so far been largely restricted to the analysis of mortality data, where each patient is classified unambiguously as dead, or followed up and still alive (censored). The analysis of disease-free survival is calculated, in principle, in exactly the same way, as each patient is classified as either alive and disease-free or not, but in practice recurrence may be detected more readily in patients who are investigated intensively. It should always be borne in mind that any patient whose cancer recurs was never in fact 'disease-free'; his residual disease was not detected clinically between the time of 'complete remission' and 'recurrence', but it might well have been detected earlier by more intensive investigation.

The two commonest schemes for systematic follow-up are (1) to see all patients at fixed intervals after diagnosis (for example at 3 months, 6 months, 1 year and then annually, and (2) to follow up all patients to a certain date (31 March 1980 in the example in Table 21.1). The first scheme, under which patients are followed up periodically, is often incorrectly analysed (Peto 1980). Suppose, for simplicity, that patients are investigated annually for disease recurrence, and recurrence is never diagnosed except at annual follow-up. The probability of suffering recurrence by the end of the first year should be estimated by the life-table method described above, dividing the number of recurrences detected at the end of the first year by the number of patients who have been followed up to the end of the year. It is, however, common practice to record the date of the examination at which recurrence was detected as the date of recurrence for patients who have relapsed, and the date of the last routine examination as the date 'lost sight of' for those still free of disease. If these data are simply fed into a computer program which calculates the product-limit survival curve, the resulting estimate of the risk of recurrence can be seriously exaggerated. Suppose, for example, that 100 patients are examined at roughly 1 year and four are found to have suffered a recurrence, giving the data shown in Table 21.3. It is obvious that the correct estimate of the recurrence-free survival curve at 1 year is 96 per cent, but the product-limit

Table 21.3. *Results of annual examination of 100 patients for recurrence, and resulting incorrect actuarial estimate of disease-free survival; the correct estimate is 96 per cent*

Days from entry to 'annual' examination	No. 'at risk'	No. examined	No. of recurrences detected	Incorrect actuarial curve
363	100	25	1	$1.000 \times 99/100 = 0.9900$
364	75	25	1	$0.9900 \times 74/75 = 0.9768$
365	50	25	1	$0.9768 \times 49/50 = 0.9573$
366	25	25	1	$0.9573 \times 24/25 = 0.9190$

estimate is $99/100$ on day 363, $99/100 \times 74/75$ on day 364, $99/100 \times 74/75 \times 49/50$ on day 365, and $99/100 \times 74/75 \times 49/50 \times 24/25$ on day 366, which equals 92 per cent. The reason for this curious bias is that the date of recurrence is not in fact the day of the examination, but some unknown day during the previous year. Ninety-seven patients were therefore 'at risk' when the fourth recurrence occurred (that is 100 minus three who had recurred already), not 25, and the recurrence-free survival rate at day 366 is actually $(99/100) \times (98/99) \times (97/98) \times (96/97) = 96$ per cent. These data should be analysed either by re-coding all annual examination dates to exactly 365 days, so that a standard survival curve program will calculate the recurrence-free survival rate on day 365 as 96/100, or by re-coding the date of any recurrence to slightly less than a year so that the correct denominator is used. This problem arises only in the calculation of recurrence rates; if a patient dies between annual follow-ups his date of death will, of course, be recorded exactly.

The fact that recurrences and deaths are often reported between annual follow-ups is also a source of potential bias, as patients with no overt symptoms will be recorded as 'followed up' only to their previous annual examination. Follow-up is thus extended selectively for those who relapse or die, again exaggerating the calculated risk of death or relapse. This can be avoided by calculating each patient's 'date lost sight of' as his date of last routine follow-up, and ignoring subsequent events.

Patients who cannot be traced are usually regarded as 'lost sight of' on the day when they were last known to be alive and well. This is an unsatisfactory but unavoidable compromise. They may be lost because they have died, or because they felt so well that they did not bother to attend the clinic, and biases resulting from incomplete follow-up can be thus in either direction. This does not mean that they will cancel each other, however, and strenuous efforts should be made to trace every patient. This is particularly important when comparing treatment protocols which differ in the frequency with which patients are seen.

In certain circumstances it may be informative to restrict analysis by withdrawing or excluding certain patients, although the analysis should always be repeated with these patients included to ensure that the gross biases this can lead to (which are discussed in the next section) are not dominating the analysis. There is an important difference between withdrawal and exclusion. A patient should be excluded from analysis only if he is a priori ineligible. Thus, for example, a patient whose pre-treatment clinical records indicate that his disease may not have been diagnosed correctly can be excluded. Withdrawal is based on subsequent events, such as gross deviation from treatment due to clinical whim or error, or failure to provide adequate documentation. Therefore, patients who are withdrawn must be analysed as being 'lost to follow-up' from the date of withdrawal, not excluded. If they had relapsed or died before the problem arose they would not have been withdrawn, and they must therefore contribute to the number 'at risk' up to that point to avoid overestimating the risk of relapse or death. Neither exclusion nor withdrawal is ever wholly satisfactory, however, except for exclusions which are identified by blind review of information available at entry. A patient tentatively classified as having acute lymphoblastic leukaemia, who later relapses with acute myeloid leukaemia, is likely to be excluded, but even this introduces a small bias as any such patient who does not relapse will be left in the trial, and the relapse-free survival rate will be slightly exaggerated.

WITHDRAWALS AND EXCLUSIONS IN RANDOMIZED TRIALS

In randomized trials, *post hoc* exclusions or withdrawals should not be permitted. It is remarkable how often statistically significant differences between treatments are balanced by an opposite difference among excluded patients, suggesting at the very least a possible treatment danger which will be concealed if full results on all randomized patients are not published. The importance in a controlled trial of never withdrawing or, worse still, transferring patients between treatment groups cannot be emphasised too strongly. If there is a tendency not to give an intensive treatment to moribund patients for example, their exclusion from the treated group will bias the results, and if they are then added to the untreated group the error will be doubled. This is a major source of serious disagreement between clinicians and statisticians. Many clinicians simply cannot accept that analysis according to what patients were supposed to receive can give a more accurate estimate of the effect of treatment than analysis according to how they were actually treated, particularly when analysis according to 'actual' treatment shows a statistically significant (and hence publishable) effect, while analysis by allocated treatment does not. No referee or editor should accept an article describing a randomized trial of cancer therapy which does not include an analysis of all eligible randomized patients according to allocated treatment. Those who do not accept this cardinal principle should examine the results of the Coronary Drug Project Research Group (1980), which showed that patients who failed to take their placebo, like those who failed to take their clofibrate, suffered significantly higher mortality than 'properly treated' patients who did take their placebo.

MULTIPLE END-POINTS

If the only end-point in an analysis is death, the survival curve simply gives the probability of survival, but if more than one type of end-point is considered the interpretation of the curve is less direct. In calculating a survival curve for cancer mortality for example, cancer deaths are regarded as 'events', but deaths due to other causes are 'losses to follow-up'. This raises two difficulties. The classification of deaths, as due to cancer or not, may not be entirely objective, so the analysis is intrinsically less reliable than the overall survival curve, and the curve does not simply portray the probability of not dying of cancer, but the probability of not dying of cancer 'in the absence of other causes of death'. It is not uncommon, particularly in the treatment of solid tumours, for more intensive chemotherapy to reduce the death rate 'due to cancer' (or to increase the 'objective remission rate') without any improvement in overall survival. This is often interpreted as evidence of a real benefit of therapy offset by increased toxicity, but the sceptic is entitled to suggest that neither cause of death nor remission can really be classified objectively, and the prognosis of the average patient is certainly not improved in such studies. Actuarial curves showing cancer mortality or recurrence are often useful, but overall survival should always be plotted as well to ensure that the 'other causes of death' are not also treatment related.

Studies in which different types or causes of recurrence are interrelated are still more difficult to analyse and interpret. In acute lymphoblastic leukaemia for example, both CNS and marrow relapse rates are important measures of treatment failure, although marrow relapse is the more serious. The effects of treatment can thus be portrayed in different ways, as in Figs 21.3, 21.4, and 21.5 which give three alternative analyses of the effect of CNS prophylaxis. Figure 21.3 shows the risk of marrow relapse not preceded by CNS relapse; Fig. 21.4 shows the risk of marrow relapse at any time, including marrow relapses occurring after CNS relapse, and Fig. 21.5 shows the risk of relapse of either type. CNS relapses are thus treated as 'losses to follow-up' in Fig. 21.3, completely ignored in Fig. 21.4, and regarded as 'events' in Fig. 21.5, and CNS prophylaxis appears to be harmful in Fig. 21.3, ineffectual in Fig. 21.4, and beneficial in Fig. 21.5. The reason for these apparently inconsistent results seems to be that patients at high risk of CNS relapse are also at high risk of marrow relapse. CNS prophylaxis delays or prevents CNS relapse, and those high-risk patients who would otherwise have been 'lost to follow-up' because of early CNS relapse remain 'at risk', increasing the probability shown in Fig. 21.3 that first remission will be terminated by marrow relapse (Peto 1981). The

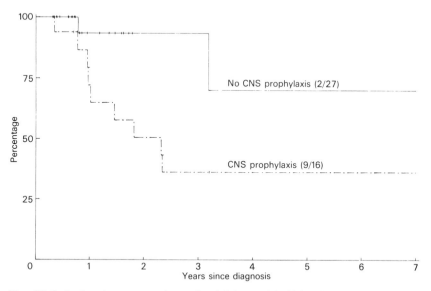

Fig. 21.3. Isolated marrow relapse in children with ALL with initial WBC over 20 000. Patients are censored at CNS relapse, death in remission, or at last follow-up.

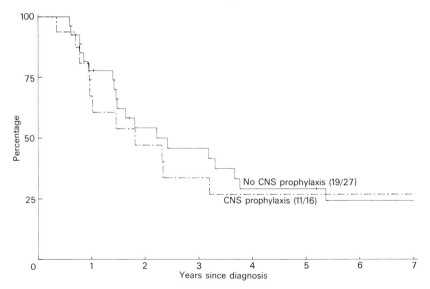

Fig. 21.4. Marrow relapse in children with ALL with initial WBC over 20 000. CNS relapse is ignored and patients are censored only at death or at last follow-up.

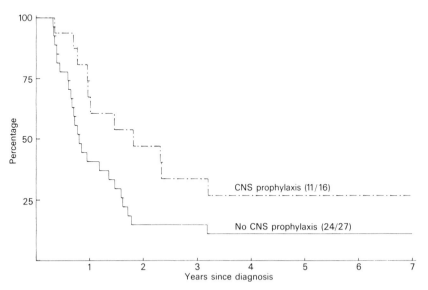

Fig. 21.5. CNS or marrow relapse in children with ALL with initial WBC over 20 000. CNS relapse is treated as an 'event'.

overall relapse rate is reduced because not all patients whose CNS relapse is prevented will suffer marrow relapse (Fig. 21.5); CNS prophylaxis appears to have little direct effect on the risk of marrow relapse (Fig. 21.4).

The difficulties that arise in survival analysis, when events are not independent, cannot be adequately discussed in a few paragraphs. None of the three analyses shown in Figs 21.3, 21.4, and 21.5 is wrong, but all three are required to give any clear idea of the overall pattern of response to treatment.

DISPLAYING MULTIPLE EVENTS ON ONE GRAPH

Survival curves similar to those shown in Fig. 21.3 do not give the probability that a particular event, such as bone marrow relapse, will terminate the first remission. Rather, such curves give the probability of marrow relapse in the absence of other events. It may sometimes be more useful to calculate simple probabilities for different events which correspond to a more natural definition of probability. Thus, for example, a clinician may wish to know what percentage of his patients' first remissions will be terminated by marrow relapse, and what percentage by CNS relapse; these two percentages should add up to the overall probability of relapse. This sort of analysis is shown in Fig. 21.6. The bottom curve, which shows the proportion of women still using intrauterine contraceptive devices, is a conventional actuarial survival curve, calculated by regarding cessation of use for any reason as an 'event' (Bull 1983). Each step in this overall curve is then classified according to the reason for that patient's termination of use, and the successive curves above the

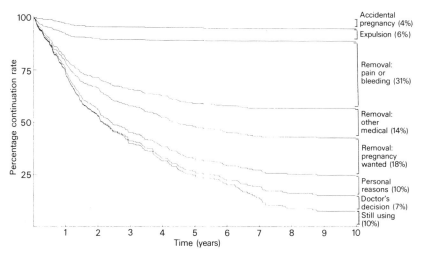

Fig. 21.6. Probabilities of ceasing IUD use for various reasons. Only the bottom (overall) curve is a true actuarial curve. The probabilities for each reason for termination are given by the distances between successive lines (9-year values in parentheses).

overall curve are calculated by simply adding all steps in the overall curve corresponding to the first reason (accidental pregnancy), all steps corresponding to the first or second reasons (accidental pregnancy or expulsion), and so on. These are not survival curves in the usual sense. The distance between successive pairs of lines gives the probability for each reason. The fourth line, denoting termination for any medical reason, has fallen to 45 per cent by 9 years, showing that 55 per cent of women will have lost their device for some medical reason within 9 years.

CONCLUSION

Clinical studies, and particularly randomized trials, constitute the chief source of reliable information on prognosis and treatment. There is now almost universal agreement, at least among statisticians, on the way in which clinical trials should be designed, conducted, and analysed, yet biased exclusion or withdrawal, selective reporting, and inadequate analysis and presentation are still quite common. The design and conduct of trials, which are discussed in other chapters, determine the quality of the data, but even the largest and best conducted studies are not always published in the most informative way. Sophisticated analyses may provide the best answers to particular questions, but it is often impossible to re-analyse and combine or compare published studies. A survival curve provides reasonably complete information on a particular aspect of treatment or prognosis, but if full use is to be made of available data, the results on each patient, including remission, survival, and treatment and prognostic factors, should be published as an appendix to the main report on a trial.

APPENDIX 1

An alternative to the conventional life-table estimate

The probability of surviving an interval can be calculated on the assumption that the death and loss rates r_d and r_l are constant during each interval. The combined death or loss rate r equals $r_d + r_l$, and the observed probability $(N - l - d)/N$ of not being lost or dying can be equated to $\exp(-r)$, giving $\hat{r} = -\log((N - l - d)/N)$, where N is the number alive at the beginning of the interval, and l and d are the respective numbers of losses and deaths in the interval. The death rate r_d is estimated by $\hat{r}_d = \hat{r} \cdot d/(d + l)$, and the estimated probability of not dying in the interval, $\exp(-\hat{r}_d)$, is thus $\exp[(d/(d + l)) \cdot \log((N - l - d)/N)]$.

The difference between the methods is shown in the following Table 21.4, where P_{ave} denotes the conventional estimate described in the text based on the number initially at risk minus half the number lost. The conventional estimate tends to overestimate the survival curve, although the error is small unless a high proportion of patients are lost or die in a single interval. Note that the alternative method always gives a survival probability of zero for an interval in which any deaths occur and all patients are lost or die. If no losses occur, both methods reduce to the usual actuarial estimate.

Table 21.4.

				Estimates of probability of surviving the interval	
N	l	d	Average number 'at risk'	P_{ave}	$\exp(-\hat{r}_d)$
10	4	5	8	0.375	0.278
10	5	1	7.5	0.867	0.858
10	1	5	9.5	0.474	0.466
10	1	9	9.5	0.053	0.000
10	9	1	5.5	0.818	0.000

REFERENCES

Breslow, N. and Crowley, J. (1974). A large sample study of the life-table and product limit estimates under random censorship. *Am. Statist.* **2**, 437–53.

Bull, M. J. V. (1983). A life table analysis technique for the evaluation of intrauterine contraceptive devices. *Jl. R. Coll. gen. Pract.* **33**, 403–7.

Coronary Drug Project Research Group (1980). Influence of adherence to treatment and response of cholesterol on mortality in the coronary drug project. *N. Engl. J. Med.* **303**, 1038–41.

Greenwood, M. (1926). *The natural duration of cancer.* Reports on Public Health and Medical Subjects number 33. HMSO, London.

Kaplan, E. L. and Meier, P. (1958). Nonparametric estimation from incomplete observations. *J. Am. statist. Ass.* **53**, 457–81.

Medical Research Council (1973). Treatment of acute lymphoblastic leukaemia: effect of prophylactic therapy against central nervous system leukaemia. *Br. med. J.* **2**, 381–4.

—— (1982). Duration of chemotherapy in childhood acute lymphoblastic leukaemia. *Med. Ped. Oncol.* **10**, 511–20.

Peto, J. (1981). C.N.S. relapse in childhood leukaemia. (Letter) *Lancet*, **ii**, 753–4.

Peto, R. (1980). Monitoring cancer patients need not be precise. In *Cancer: assessment and monitoring.* (ed. T. Symington and A. E. Williams). pp. 377–81. Churchill Livingstone, Edinburgh.

Rothman, K. J. (1978). Estimation of confidence limits for the cumulative probability of survival in life table analysis. *J. chron. Dis.* **31**, 557–60.

Sylvester, R. J., Machin, D., and Staquet, M. J. (1978). A comparison of the alternative methods of calculating survival curves arising from clinical trials. *Biomedicine* (Special Issue) **28**, 49–53.

Thomas, D. R. and Grunkemeier, G. L. (1975). Confidence interval estimation of survival probabilities for censored data. *J. Am. Statist. Ass.* **70**, 865–71.

22 Comparison of survival curves

Norman Breslow

INTRODUCTION

The value of anti-cancer therapy is usually measured by the elapsed time between the onset of treatment and the occurrence of any of several end-points: local recurrence or distant metastasis; progression of disease to new sites; death due to the tumour, its treatment, or unrelated causes. Since treatments may have different effects upon each end-point, a comprehensive analysis will often involve several separate comparisons. Two treatment groups may differ markedly with respect to relapse rates for example, but if relapses which occur with the apparently inferior treatment are easily retrieved, there may be little difference in survival itself.

Once the end-point has been selected, the treatment comparison is of two or more survival curves, where survival is interpreted in a generic sense to mean observation until the designated event. The first step in the analysis is the estimation and graphical display of the curves for each treatment group using the methods described in the preceding chapter. Then, in order to distinguish real treatment effects from sampling fluctuations, it is usually necessary to carry out more formal statistical tests of the observed differences. This chapter discusses a number of tests which are widely used by biostatisticians in the cancer field.

CHOOSING A VALID STATISTICAL TEST

Two basic criteria govern the choice of a statistical test. The first concern is for a valid test in the sense of one which rejects the null hypothesis in the nominally specified percentage of samples when, in fact, the hypothesis holds. Unfortunately, many of the common tests are invalid when applied to survival data. Secondly, the test should be sensitive to the types of alternatives to the null hypothesis which are of medical importance and likely to be observed.

The problem of censorship

The major complicating feature of survival data is the presence of censored observations. For patients who are still alive at the time of analysis, or who were lost to follow-up during the trial, all one knows about their lifetime is that it exceeds the recorded value. This effectively rules out such powerful statistical procedures as t-tests, analyses of variance, and least-squares regression, all of which involve averages of the observations. The sample mean tends to underestimate by an indeterminate amount the mean survival time which would be observed if all patients were completely followed up until death. If the treatment groups differ in their average duration of follow-up, as would occur with a historical control, a comparison based on averages could be seriously misleading. Even in the randomized trial, in which censorship patterns are fairly equal, comparison of mean survival times may obscure important treatment differences.

Comparisons of the crude proportions of survivors in each treatment group are invalid for precisely the same reasons. If one takes as an estimate of 5-year survival, the number of patients surviving 5 years divided by the total number treated, the result will be too low unless everyone has the opportunity for a full 5 years of follow-up. Likewise the number of deaths before 5 years, divided by that number plus the number of survivors beyond 5 years, yields an overestimate of mortality. Only by using life-tables or actuarial methods can correct estimates be obtained.

Comparison of survival curves at a single point in time

The simplest valid test for the equality of survival curves is to compare them at a fixed point in time, say 2 or 5 years after treatment. The Kaplan–Meier estimates and Greenwood standard errors described in the previous chapter are suitable for this purpose. Obvious weaknesses of the approach are its sensitivity to the (arbitrary) choice of the time point and its inefficiency for detecting differences likely to occur in practice.

Figure 22.1 shows schematically three ways in which survival curves for two treatments A and B could differ. In (a) the instantaneous mortality or hazard rates for B exceed those for A at all times; this is also illustrated in Fig. 22.2a. Comparison of such curves at a single point in time wastes valuable information about the survival differences which occur earlier or later. If the two survival curves are exponential, meaning they have constant mortality rates, and if patient entry is uniform over time, results of Armitage (1959) indicate that the efficiency of this method is at most 82 per cent in comparison with a parametric analysis, and may be substantially less if the time point is not optimally chosen.

In Figure 22.1b both treatments have identical long-term survival rates, but such deaths as do occur are delayed by treatment A. Survival curves with flat tails occur with several childhood solid tumours and some forms of leukaemia. Then it is reasonable to use the proportion of long-term survivors or 'cures' as the major end-point for evaluation. If previous work has established that few tumour deaths occur after 3 years for example, comparison of the curves at this point makes good sense. Of course one should be careful not to interpret a flat tail on the estimated survival curves as evidence for such a shape unless large

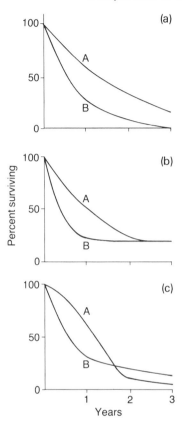

Fig. 22.1. Schematic drawing showing three ways in which the survival curves for two treatments A and B may differ. (a) A uniformly superior to B; (b) percentage of long-term survivors equal but deaths occur earlier on B; (c) initial superiority of A reversed in the long run.

numbers of patients have been followed beyond the point of apparent flattening. Other statistical tests may be used to detect early differences in the curves as shown in the figure, but these will usually be of subsidiary interest.

Figure 22.1c depicts a more complicated situation where A is evidently to be preferred in the early post-treatment period, while B is superior later on. Here it is unlikely that any single statistical test will render a satisfactory verdict regarding the treatment differences. One remedy is to divide the follow-up period into two or three intervals and to make separate statements about the A and B mortality rates in each one. Close attention to the causes of death or failure in the different time periods is called for, since these may explain the apparently aberrant behavior. For example, B might have both toxic and therapeutic effects, producing high early mortality due to the treatment but also a decrease in tumour deaths among those who survived it.

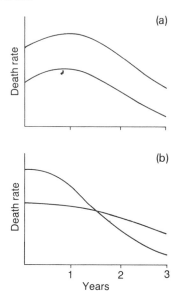

Fig. 22.2. Schematic drawing showing two ways in which the mortality rate (hazard) functions for two treatments may differ. (a) Proportional hazards (PH) situation in which one rate is a constant multiple of the other (constant difference on log scale); (b) 'crossing hazards' situation in which the difference in mortality rates changes sign.

Maximum difference between survival curves

A somewhat more satisfactory approach is to consider the maximum difference between the curves over time. This yields a generalization of the famous Smirnov test (Koziol and Byar 1975). Unfortunately, its distribution depends in a rather complicated way on the censorship patterns. A modified version of the test has been proposed by Fleming, O'Fallon, O'Brien, and Harrington (1980), who support the use of an asymptotic distribution with Monte Carlo experiments. However, since it involves rather complex calculations, and since it has had only limited testing as yet, their test is not developed in detail here.

Comparison of medians

The median is often used as an alternative to the mean for measuring the location of a distribution and would seem particularly suitable for survival data. It is easily obtained as that time, or interval of times, for which the actuarially estimated survival proportion equals one-half. Moreover, once follow-up is complete to this point for all patients, the value of the median does not change with further observation.

The main drawback of the median is its variability, which is substantial unless the survival curve is based on a large number of deaths and falls quickly through the fiftieth percentile (Reid 1981). For cancers with a high fraction of long term survivors, it may not even be estimable. Hence, while a median-based test for equality of survival distributions is available, it cannot be recommended for routine general use (Brookmeyer and Crowley 1982).

Parametric methods

The earliest methods assumed a parametric form for the survival distribution such as the exponential (Bartholomew 1957), log-normal (Sampford and Taylor 1959), or Weibull (Pike 1966). Kalbfleisch and Prentice (1980) present a comprehensive review of these models in the context of regression analysis and indicate how they may be imbedded in a generalized log-gamma model which allows testing of distributional shape in addition to a comparison of treatment groups.

Unfortunately, when applied to censored survival data, the parametric methods involve the complicated iterative calculations of general maximum likelihood estimation. An exception is the test for equality of two exponential distributions. Denote by S_1 and S_2 the total observed survival time (sum of the censored and uncensored observations) in groups 1 and 2, and by D_1 and D_2 the number of deaths (uncensored observations) in each. The test statistic $(D_2 S_1)/(S_2 D_1)$, which also measures the ratio λ_2/λ_1 of death rates in the two samples, is usually referred to F tables with $2D_2$ and $2D_1$ degress of freedom. However, with the type of censored data which arise in clinical trials, this F distribution is only approximate (Regal 1980).

The main value of the parametric models seems to lie in the possibility they offer for extrapolation beyond the range of the observed data. They also may be of special interest when modelling the probability of cure (Fig. 22.1b). Farewell's (1977) model for example, assumes exponential survivals and allows the treatment to influence both the proportion cured and the duration of survival for those who are not. A similar hybrid model based on the log-normal distribution was proposed earlier by Boag (1949). However, in view of the computational complexities, the fact that the reference distributions are only known asymptotically, and the usual doubts which attend any specific distributional assumptions, biostaticians have looked beyond the parametric models in their search for robust tests which are valid in a wide variety of circumstances.

Non-parametric tests

An event of major importance for clinical trials statisticians was the independent discovery by Gilbert (1962) and Gehan (1965) of a censored data analogue of the Wilcoxon rank sum test. Shortly thereafter Mantel (1966) demonstrated that the Mantel–Haenszel procedure (Mantel and Haenszel 1959) could be adapted to survival data. Essentially the same statistic was later advocated by Peto and Peto (1972) and Cox (1972), who also noted that it generalized the exponential scores or Savage rank test. Efron (1967) pointed out that the Gehan–Gilbert procedure made inefficient use of the censored observations and suggested an alternative statistic which is calculated from the Kaplan–Meier estimates of the survival curves for each treatment group. However technical difficulties preclude its use in practice. Peto and Peto (1972) and Prentice (1978) derived another analogue to the Wilcoxon statistic which is practicable and which captures Efron's central idea (Latta 1977).

Censored data rank statistics provide valid comparisons of all types of survival curves and are sensitive to clinically meaningful differences. The remainder of this chapter is devoted to a detailed description of their construction and use.

TWO SAMPLE RANK TESTS FOR CENSORED DATA

Linear rank statistics for the comparison of two distributions in the absence of censorship are constructed by assigning scores to the ranked observations in the combined sample and summing these over the second sample (Hajek 1969). The scores may be chosen so as to maximize the statistical power against alternatives of a change in location or scale in a known error distribution. For example, using the ranks themselves as scores leads to the common Wilcoxon or rank sum test which is optimal for detecting shifts in the location of a logistic distribution.

Two general approaches to the construction of optimal rank tests for censored samples have been outlined by Peto and Peto (1972) and by Prentice (1978). Both consider the joint ranking of the uncensored observations and assign separate scores to the censored and the uncensored observations at each rank. Before a precise definition can be given, however, we need to introduce some notation.

Notation and definition

Denote by $t_1 < t_2 < \ldots < t_I$ the ordered, distinct uncensored survival times for the combined sample. Suppose that d_i deaths occur at t_i and that there are e_i exits, or censored observations, in the interval $[t_i, t_{i+1})$. The number of patients 'at risk' of death at t_i, that is still alive and under observation just prior to that time, is defined by $n_i = \sum_{j=i}^{I}(d_j + e_j)$. Censored observations which occur before t_1 and hence contribute no information to the comparison are discarded, and we take as a definition of the total sample size $N = n_1$.

A second subscript $k = 1$ or 2 is used with the quantities d_i, e_i, and n_i to denote the numbers of deaths, exits, and 'at risk' in each of the $K = 2$ samples at

t_i. Likewise $N = N_1 + N_2$ gives the breakdown of the total sample size. The general linear rank statistic for censored data is then defined

$$W = \sum_{i=1}^{I} (d_{i2}a_i + e_{i2}A_i), \tag{22.1}$$

as a sum over the second sample of scores a_i assigned to the uncensored observations at t_i and scores A_i assigned to the censored observations just beyond that point.

A condition satisfied by all the scoring systems considered here is

$$n_i A_{i-1} = d_i a_i + (n_i - d_i)A_i, \tag{22.2}$$

which may be interpreted as a preservation of the total score at each t_i (Prentice and Marek 1979). In this case, with $w_i = a_i - A_i = n_i(A_{i-1} - A_i)/d_i$ denoting 'weights' associated with each time of death, the statistic also may be expressed

$$W = \sum_{i=1}^{I} w_i(d_{i2} - n_{i2}d_i/n_i) \tag{22.3}$$

as a weighted sum of the observed number of deaths in sample two at t_i minus an 'expected' number (Tarone and Ware 1977; Thomas, Breslow, and Gart 1977). This alternative formula for W facilitates variance estimation and the derivation of asymptotic normality under arbitrary patterns of censorship (Gill 1980; Andersen, Borgan, Gill, and Keiding 1982). A key assumption in this development is that the scores a_i and A_i depend on the pattern of deaths and exits only up to and including time t_i.

In order to carry out the statistical test based on W, one must determine its probability distribution under the null hypothesis that survival times are equally distributed in the two samples. A permutation model is available, but it is applicable only when the censoring patterns in the two samples are also equal (see below). Therefore, most statisticians use the asymptotic distribution of W, which is normal with mean 0 and variance V. An approximate two-tailed test is obtained by referring $\chi_1^2 = W^2/V$ to tables of the chi-square distribution with one degree of freedom. Two methods of calculating V are considered next.

Estimation of the variance

One way to obtain a reference distribution for W under the null hypothesis, which parallels the classical theory of rank tests, is to consider each of the $\binom{N}{N_2}$ possible assignments of both censored and uncensored observations to sample two as equally likely. Provided that the total score $\sum_{i=1}^{I} d_i a_i + e_i A_i$ equals zero, which may be arranged simply by adding a constant to each a_i and A_i, the exact variance of this permutation distribution (Hajek 1969) is

$$V_P = \frac{N_1 N_2}{N(N-1)} \sum_{i=1}^{I} d_i a_i^2 + e_i A_i^2. \tag{22.4}$$

It is applicable whenever the censorship patterns for the two samples are equal, as would usually be the case when comparing randomized treatment groups in a Phase III trial.

In other contexts, for example in retrospective analyses of prognostic factors or when making historical comparisons of different treatments, censorship may be much heavier in one sample than another. Then it is more appropriate to use (22.3) to derive the 'conditional' variance of the asymptotic normal distribution. The intuitive idea is to construct a 2×2 table of deaths and survivors at each time point (Table 22.1 with $K=2$). Conditional on the marginal totals, d_{i2} has under the null hypothesis a hypergeometric distribution with expectation $n_{i2}d_i/n_i$. Since these tables have properties analogous to those of statistical independence (Gill 1980), the corresponding variance of W is a weighted sum of hypergeometric variances

$$V_C = \sum_{i=1}^{I} w_i^2 \frac{n_{i1}n_{i2}d_i(n_i - d_i)}{n_i^2(n_i - 1)}. \tag{22.5}$$

$|W|$ and V_C are correlated in small samples (Morton 1978) and it could be advantageous therefore to replace V_C by a suitable expectation. For example, under equal censorship the conditional expectation of $n_{i1}n_{i2}$ given n_i is $n_i(n_i - 1) N_1 N_2 / \{N(N-1)\}$. This leads to the formula

$$V_C^* = \frac{N_1 N_2}{N(N-1)} \sum_{i=1}^{I} \frac{w_i^2 d_i(n_i - d_i)}{n_i}, \tag{22.6}$$

which, as it turns out, is just another way of writing V_P. We recommend the conditional variance V_C for routine use since fewer assumptions are involved in its derivation.

The Mantel–Haenszel or logrank test

When the mortality rates in the two treatment groups have a constant ratio over time, which is the famous 'proportional hazards' (PH) assumption, uniform weights yield the most powerful test. This means substituting $w_i = 1$ in (22.3) or $a_i = 1 - \sum_{j=1}^{i} d_j/n_j$ and $A_i = -\sum_{j=1}^{i} d_j/n_j$ in (22.1). An attractive feature of the statistic is that it may be written $W_L = \sum_{i=1}^{I}(d_{i2} - n_{i2}d_i/n_i) = O_2 - E_2$ as the difference between the observed $O_2 = \sum_{i=1}^{I} d_{i2}$ and a conditionally expected $E_2 = \sum_{i=1}^{I} n_{i2}d_i/n_i$ number of deaths in sample two. Moreover, defining O_1 and $E_1 = O_1 + O_2 - E_2$ to be the analogous quantities for sample one, one obtains a rough and ready estimator $\hat{\psi} = (O_2 E_1)/(O_1 E_2)$ for the mortality rate ratio in sample two versus sample one (Bernstein, Anderson, and Pike 1981). The variance of W_L is obtained from (22.5) or (22.6) with all $w_i = 1$.

This test is known variously in the literature as the Mantel–Haenszel, logrank or Cox test following its proponents as cited previously. Due to the simplicity of its construction and interpretation, and the fact that PH alternatives are of particular importance in medical research, it has become the standard test for comparison of survival curves.

The generalized Wilcoxon tests

The first widely-used censored data test was the Gehan (1965) and Gilbert (1962) generalized Wilcoxon statistic $W_G = \sum_{i=1}^{I} n_i(d_{i2} - n_{i2}d_i/n_i)$ obtained by setting $w_i = n_i$ in (22.3) or equivalently $a_i = n_i - \sum_{j=1}^{i} d_j$ and $A_i = -\sum_{j=1}^{i} d_j$ in (22.1). Here the score assigned to an observation at t_i is the number of survival times which are known definitely to be greater minus the number known definitely to be smaller. The two variances

$$V_C = \sum_{i=1}^{I} \{n_{i1}n_{i2}d_i(n_i - d_i)/(n_i - 1)\}$$

and

$$V_P = N_1 N_2 \sum_{i=1}^{I} n_i d_i(n_i - d_i)/\{N(N-1)\},$$

obtained by substitution of $w_i = n_i$ in (22.5) and (22.6), are roughly equal in large samples of continuous data to those shown in formulae (15) and (16) of Breslow (1970). The expressions for V_P and V_C given here are more accurate for small samples.

Several authors have pointed out a defect in W_G which, although not a serious problem for randomized clinical trials, may limit its applicability in certain other contexts. Since the weights $w_i = n_i$ involve the numbers 'at risk' at each time point, they may depend more on the censorship patterns imposed by the particular experimental design than on any inherent property of the survival curves being compared. For this reason the Peto and Peto (1972) and Prentice (1975) statistic $W_P = \sum_{i=1}^{I} \tilde{F}_i(d_{i2} - n_{i2}d_i/n_i)$ has been gaining favour recently as a Wilcoxon analogue. It is defined by substituting $w_i = \tilde{F}_i$ in (22.3), or alternatively $a_i = 2\tilde{F}_i - 1$ and $A_i = \tilde{F}_i - 1$ in (22.1) where

$$\tilde{F}_i = \prod_{j=1}^{i} \frac{n_j}{(n_j + d_j)} \qquad (22.7)$$

is an estimate of the survival curve for the combined sample at t_i analogous to the Kaplan–Meier estimate considered in Chapter 21 of this book. V_C and V_P are found by substitution of $w_i = \tilde{F}_i$ in (22.5) or (22.6).

Tarone (1981) has derived the asymptotic joint distribution of the maximum of the two chi-square statistics based on W_L and W_G with conditional variance. This is useful as a means of resolving the multiple comparisons issue which arises when both tests are applied to the same data. A similar adjustment is possible when W_P is used in place of W_G (Tarone, personal communication).

Monte-Carlo investigations

A number of Monte-Carlo studies have investigated the actual size and power of W_L, W_G and W_P in various contexts using either permutation or conditional variances (Lee, Desu, and Gehan 1975; Lininger, Gail, Green, and Byar 1979; Latta 1981). These confirm the superior performance of the logrank test against PH alternatives, the advantages of the Wilcoxon analogues in certain other situations, and the aberrant behaviour possible from W_G with extreme forms of censorship. However, in more typical circumstances there may be little difference between the three tests. None of them are designed to detect acceleration or crossing hazards alternatives for example. W_G and W_P give more weight to differences in the survival curves which appear early in the course of follow-up, while W_L is more powerful for detecting a later separation of the curves.

Tied observations

The definitions of test statistics and variances given here account adequately for the presence of tied observations provided that the numbers of deaths d_i are generally small relative to the numbers at risk n_i. Typically this will be the case with survival data of the type encountered in clinical trials. Grouping of the data into large intervals prior to analysis is not recommended since it can introduce bias when the censorship patterns differ (Mantel 1967; Breslow 1970).

An alternative approach to ties similar to that used with rank tests for uncensored data is also available. This is to consider the scores which would have been assigned at each t_i if the uncensored observations were separated by an infinitesimal amount. One then defines a_i to be the average of the d_i scores so generated, and A_i as the single score assigned to the e_i censored observations, all of which are assumed to exceed t_i.

A test for acceleration

Cox (1972) noted that a test for the type of acceleration or crossing hazards alternative illustrated in Figs 22.1c and 22.2b could be obtained by incorporation of a treatment × time covariable in the PH model. His suggestion is put into practice easily by applying Breslow's (1976) method for regression analysis of the log odds ratio to the series of 2×2 tables constructed at each t_i (Table 22.1). A key role is played by the expectations $\mu_i(\psi) = E(d_{i2}|d_i, n_{i1}, n_{i2}; \psi)$ and variances $\sigma_i^2(\psi) = Var(d_{i2}|d_i, n_{i1}, n_{i2}; \psi)$ of the exact distributions

Table 22.1. $2 \times K$ *table of deaths and survivors at time* t_i

	Sample				Totals
	1	2	...	K	
Deaths	d_{i1}	d_{i2}	...	d_{iK}	d_i
Survivors	$n_{i1} - d_{i1}$	$n_{i2} - d_{i2}$	...	$n_{iK} - d_{iK}$	$n_i - d_i$
'At risk'	n_{i1}	n_{i2}	...	n_{iK}	n_i

of d_{i2} in each table conditional on fixed values for the marginal totals. These are non-central hypergeometric distributions which depend only on the odds ratio or relative risk parameter ψ, assumed to remain constant from table to table under the PH model.

To carry out the test, one first determines the maximum likelihood estimate $\hat{\psi}$ as the solution to $\sum_{i=1}^{I} d_{i2} = \sum_{i=1}^{I} \mu_i(\psi)$. The score statistic (Rao 1965; 6c.3) for a trend in the mortality rate ratio at t_i with the index i is

$$\frac{\left[\sum_{i=1}^{I} i\{d_{i2} - \mu_i(\hat{\psi})\} \right]^2}{\sum_{i=1}^{I} i^2 \sigma_i^2(\hat{\psi}) - \left\{ \sum_{i=1}^{I} i\sigma_i^2(\hat{\psi}) \right\}^2 / \sum_{i=1}^{I} \sigma_i^2(\hat{\psi})}, \tag{22.8}$$

which also has an approximate χ_1^2 distribution under the null hypothesis. Any other covariable z_i which depends on information available at t_i could of course be substituted for i in this expression, for example t_i itself. However $z_i = i$ is used in the examples which follow in keeping with our emphasis on rank methods.

An alternative form of this statistic uses the approximation to the exact conditional likelihood suggested by Peto and Peto (1972) and Breslow (1975). Here the quantities $d_i n_{i2} \psi / (n_{i1} + n_{i2}\psi)$ and $d_i n_{i1} n_{i2} \psi / (n_{i1} + n_{i2}\psi)^2$ replace $\mu_i(\psi)$ and $\sigma_i^2(\psi)$, respectively, both for determination of $\hat{\psi}$ and in the statistic (22.8). This approximation should be adequate in the typical situation where the d_i are small relative to the n_i, and is exact if $d_i = 1$.

Two examples

Fleming, O'Fallan, O'Brien, and Harrington (1980) present data on time from treatment to progression of disease for 35 patients with Stage II or IIA ovarian cancer treated at the Mayo Clinic. For 15 patients with low grade tumours these times were 28, 89, 175, 195, 309, 377$^+$, 393$^+$, 421$^+$, 447$^+$, 462, 709$^+$, 744$^+$, 770$^+$, 1106$^+$, and 1206$^+$ days, where $+$ denotes a censored observation.

Twenty patients with high grade tumours had times to progression of 34, 88, 137, 199, 280, 291, 299$^+$, 300$^+$, 309, 351, 358, 369, 369, 370, 375, 382, 392, 429$^+$, 451, and 1119$^+$ days. The graphical display in Figure 22.3a shows that grade influences the rate of progression only towards the end of the time scale. Therefore, we expect the logrank test to perform better than the Wilcoxon analogues, and that there will be some evidence of acceleration.

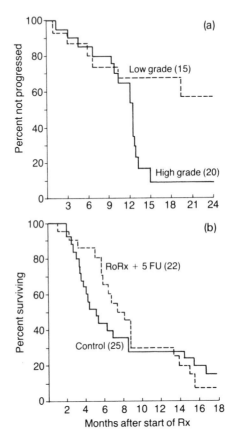

Fig. 22.3. (a) Curves of time to progression of disease for patients with low-grade and high-grade ovarian carcinoma. (b) Survival curves for bile duct cancer patients receiving radiation and 5-FU versus those in a control sample. (Reproduced with permission, from Fleming *et al.* 1980.)

Intermediate quantities needed for calculation of the various test statistics are shown in Table 22.2. Observed and expected numbers of 'deaths' in the two groups are $O_1 = 6$, $O_2 = 16$, $E_1 = 11.33$ and $E_2 = 10.67$, yielding a rough estimate of $(16 \times 11.33)/(6 \times 10.67) = 2.83$ for the hazard rate ratio. This may be contrasted with the estimate $\hat{\psi} = 3.09$ obtained by maximization of the exact

Table 22.2. *Comparison of time-to-progression curves for patients with low and high grade ovarian cancers**

i	t_i	n_i	d_i	$\tilde{F}_i$	n_{i1}	d_{i1}	n_{i2}	d_{i2}	$\sigma_i^2(\hat{\psi})$	$\mu_i(\hat{\psi})$
			Combined sample		High grade		Low grade		Acceleration test†	
1	28	35	1	0.972	20	0	15	1	0.157	0.20
2	34	34	1	0.944	20	1	14	0	0.151	0.18
3	88	33	1	0.917	19	1	14	0	0.155	0.19
4	89	32	1	0.889	18	0	14	1	0.161	0.20
5	137	31	1	0.861	18	1	13	0	0.154	0.19
6	175	30	1	0.833	17	0	13	1	0.159	0.20
7	195	29	1	0.806	17	0	12	1	0.151	0.19
8	199	28	1	0.778	17	1	11	0	0.143	0.17
9	280	27	1	0.750	16	1	11	0	0.149	0.18
10	291	26	1	0.722	15	1	11	0	0.155	0.19
11	309	23	2	0.664	12	1	11	1	0.350	0.47
12	351	21	1	0.634	11	1	10	0	0.176	0.23
13	358	20	1	0.604	10	1	10	0	0.185	0.24
14	369	19	2	0.547	9	2	10	0	0.382	0.55
15	370	17	1	0.516	7	1	10	0	0.216	0.32
16	375	16	1	0.486	6	1	10	0	0.228	0.35
17	382	14	1	0.453	5	1	9	0	0.233	0.37
18	392	13	1	0.421	4	1	9	0	0.244	0.42
19	451	8	1	0.374	2	1	6	0	0.250	0.49
20	462	7	1	0.327	1	0	6	1	0.224	0.66

* See Fig. 22.3a. Data from Fleming *et al.* (1980).
† $\hat{\psi} = 3.09$ (see text).

conditional likelihood. The permutation and conditional variances for $W_L = O_2 - E_2 = 5.33$ are $V_P = 5.21$ and $V_C = 5.11$, yielding χ_1^2 test statistics of 5.46 ($p = 0.019$) and 5.57 ($p = 0.018$). The test for acceleration (22.8) is likewise significant with $\chi_1^2 = 5.73$ ($p = 0.017$). As anticipated, however, neither W_G nor W_P are as sensitive to this type of late difference in the curves. W_G with permutation variance yields $p = 0.203$ and with conditional variance $p = 0.134$. The corresponding p values for W_P are 0.160 and 0.099.

Another example by the same authors consists of survival times for patients with bile duct cancer. The days to death for 22 patients treated with radiation and chemotherapy (5-FU) are 30, 67, 79$^+$, 82$^+$, 95, 148, 170, 171, 176, 193, 200, 221, 243, 261, 262, 263, 399, 414, 446, 446$^+$, 464, and 777, while for 25 patients in a control group they are 57, 58, 74, 79, 89, 98, 101, 104, 110, 118, 125, 132, 154, 159, 188, 203, 257, 257, 431, 461, 497, 723, 747, 1313, and 2636. The plotted curves (Fig. 22.3b) display the crossing-over behaviour typified by Fig. 22.1c in which an early treatment advantage is eliminated or even reversed in the long run. Although none of the usual rank tests are specifically designed to detect such effects, the Wilcoxon procedures weigh more heavily the early separation.

Significance levels for the three tests based on W_L, W_G and W_P with conditional variance are $p = 0.836, 0.254$, and 0.260. However, the acceleration test does achieve significance with $\chi_1^2 = 4.93$ $(p = 0.026)$. Hence, one would conclude that the crossing-over of hazard rates is real and that the survival distributions in the two groups are indeed different.

For completeness, we mention that the Smirnov-type test procedures proposed by Fleming *et al.* (1980) yield a two-sided significance level of $p = 0.002$ for the ovarian cases and a one-sided level of $p = 0.046$ for the bile duct cases. However the asymptotic approximation especially for the first example may be in doubt since the maximum separation between the curves was observed in the tail area where censorship was heavy. All p values reported for the rank tests developed here are based on χ^2 and hence two-sided.

EXTENSIONS TO K SAMPLES

Many clinical trials involve randomization of eligible patients to more than two treatment groups. In some contexts each of these may represent a distinct approach to patient management, in which case a global test of the null hypothesis that the K survival curves are equal is appropriate. In other problems the different groups may have a natural order corresponding to increasing doses of radiation or chemotherapy. Then one needs a trend test which is particularly sensitive to a decrease in mortality rates with increasing dose.

Notation and definition

Extension of the previous results for use with K samples is straightforward. Firstly the data are arranged in a series of $2 \times K$ tables with tabular entries denoted as in Table 22.1. For a given system of weights $\{w_i\}$ the total score for the kth sample is defined

$$W_k = \sum_{i=1}^{I} w_i(d_{ik} - n_{ik}d_i/n_i) \tag{22.9}$$

as a weighted sum of observed minus conditionally expected deaths analogous to (22.3). The null covariance matrix for the data in the ith $2 \times K$ table, given the marginal totals, has (k,l) component

$$\|\mathbf{V}_i\|_{k,l} = Cov(d_{ik}, d_{il}) = \begin{cases} \dfrac{n_{ik}(n_i - n_{ik})d_i(n_i - d_i)}{n_i^2(n_i - 1)}, & k = l \\[4mm] \dfrac{-n_{ik}n_{il}d_i(n_i - d_i)}{n_i^2(n_i - 1)}, & k \neq l \end{cases} \tag{22.10}$$

and the conditional covariance matrix for the vector $\mathbf{W} = (W_1, \ldots, W_K)^T$ of scores is thus $\mathbf{V}_C = \sum_{i=1}^{I} w_i^2 \mathbf{V}_i$ (Thomas *et al.* 1977). Replacing $n_{ik} n_{il}$ in (22.10) by its conditional expectation given n_i under equal censorship, the alternative covariance matrix is obtained as

$$\|\mathbf{V}_P\|_{k,l} = \frac{\sum_{i=1}^{I} w_i^2 d_i (n_i - d_i)/n_i}{N(N-1)} \times \begin{cases} N_k(N - N_k), & k = l \\ -N_k N_l, & k \neq l \end{cases} \tag{22.11}$$

where $N = N_1 + \ldots + N_K$ denote the totals 'at risk' just prior to t_1. This may also be derived from the permutation arguments of Hajek (1969) by assuming the corresponding scores a_i and A_i are randomly distributed among the K samples.

Statistics for testing the global null hypothesis are defined by $\mathbf{W}^T \mathbf{V}_C^- \mathbf{W}$ for the case of unequal censorship and by

$$\mathbf{W}^T \mathbf{V}_P^- \mathbf{W} = \frac{(N-1) \sum_{k=1}^{K} W_k^2/N_k}{\sum_{i=1}^{I} w_i^2 d_i(n_i - d_i)/n_i} \tag{22.12}$$

for equally censored samples (Breslow 1970). Here $\mathbf{V}^-$ denotes a generalized inverse (Rao 1965, 1b.5) of the covariance matrix $\mathbf{V}$. In practice the test based on the conditional variance is obtained by deleting the last (Kth) element of $\mathbf{W}$ and the last row and column of $\mathbf{V}_C$ and using ordinary matrix inversion applied to the $(K-1) \times (K-1)$ dimensional problem. The resulting statistic has an asymptotic chi-square distribution with $K-1$ degrees of freedom under the null hypothesis that the mortality rates in the K treatment groups are equal. This is true for the more easily calculated statistic (22.12) only under the additional hypothesis that the censoring patterns in the K samples are also equal.

When there are no ties or censorship, the statistic (22.12) reduces to a classical test for analysis of variance based on ranks. For example, with $w_i = n_i$, $d_i = 1$ and $e_i = 0$, it is identical to the test proposed by Kruskal and Wallis (1952).

Conservative approximations

Since the test statistic for unequal censorship requires matrix inversion, a simpler version may be useful in some applications. Following the arguments of Peto and Pike (1973) and Crowley and Breslow (1975), $\mathbf{V}_C$ is replaced in this version by the approximate covariance matrix

$$\|\mathbf{V}_A\|_{k,l} = \left(\sum_{i=1}^{I} \alpha_i \right) \times \begin{cases} P_k(1 - P_k), & k = l \\ -P_k P_l, & k \neq l \end{cases}$$

where $P_k = \sum_{i=1}^{I} \alpha_i(n_{ik}/n_i) / \sum_{i=1}^{I} \alpha_i$ and $\alpha_i = w_i^2 d_i(n_i - d_i)/(n_i - 1)$. The statistic

$$\mathbf{W}^T \mathbf{V}_A^- \mathbf{W} = \sum_{k=1}^{K} \frac{W_k^2}{\sum_{i=1}^{I} \dfrac{w_i^2 n_{ik} d_i(n_i - d_i)}{n_i(n_i - 1)}} \tag{22.13}$$

is conservative in the sense that it never exceeds $\mathbf{W}^T \mathbf{V}_C^- \mathbf{W}$, but is reasonably close to it unless there are marked differences in the censorship patterns among the treatment groups. When $w_i \equiv d_i \equiv 1$ (22.13) yields the simple formula $\sum_{k=1}^{K} (O_k - E_k)^2 / E_k$ for the logrank statistic, where $O_k = \sum_{i=1}^{I} d_{ik}$ and $E_k = \sum_{i=1}^{I} n_{ik} d_i / n_i$ (Peto, 1977). The $\sum_{k=1}^{K} (O_k - E_k)^2 / E_k$ statistic is even more conservative than (22.13) in the presence of ties ($d_i > 1$ for some i).

Testing for trend

If the K samples have a natural order related to mortality, a more powerful test can be achieved by partitioning from the global chi-square a single degree of freedom statistic which represents the linear regression of the W_k scores on a quantitative variable x_k. A common choice in practice is simply to set $x_k = k$ to indicate the order of the samples. However if the treatment groups correspond to doses of an investigational drug for example, the actual dose levels or some suitable transformation of them may be used instead.

The basic form of the trend test is

$$\frac{\left(\sum_{k=1}^{I} x_k W_k \right)^2}{\mathbf{x}^T \mathbf{V} \mathbf{x}}, \tag{22.14}$$

where $\mathbf{x} = (x_1, \ldots x_K)^T$ is the vector of quantitative values and $\mathbf{V}$ is the covariance matrix of $\mathbf{W}$. Either $\mathbf{V}_C$ or $\mathbf{V}_P$ may be substituted in this expression depending on the assumptions made about the censorship patterns. When $\mathbf{V}_P$ is used the statistic becomes

$$\frac{(N-1)\left(\sum_{k=1}^{K} x_k W_k \right)^2}{\left\{ \sum_{i=1}^{I} w_i^2 d_i(n_i - d_i)/n_i \right\} \left\{ \sum_{k=1}^{K} x_k^2 N_k - \left(\sum_{k=1}^{K} x_k N_k \right)^2 / \sum_{k=1}^{K} N_k \right\}}. \tag{22.15}$$

An analogous form exists when the approximate matrix $\mathbf{V}_A$ is substituted for $\mathbf{V}_C$. For example, for the special case of the logrank test in the absence of ties ($w_i = 1$, $d_i = 1$), a conservative version of the trend statistic is

$$\frac{\left\{ \sum_{k=1}^{K} x_k(O_k - E_k) \right\}^2}{\left\{ \sum_{k=1}^{K} x_k^2 E_k - \left(\sum_{k=1}^{K} x_k E_k \right)^2 / \sum_{k=1}^{K} E_k \right\}}. \tag{22.16}$$

Use of the trend statistic (22.14) with the logrank scores ($w_i = 1$) has been defended theoretically by Tarone (1975) in terms of the PH model. However some modification of the procedure may be desirable when it is used with the Gehan–Gilbert scores ($w_i = n_i$) since these are heavily influenced by the size of the sample in each group. Miller (1981) suggests in this case that $x_k^* = x_k/\{N_k(N - N_k)\}$ be substituted for x_k in (22.14). Of course this modification will have little effect for randomized trials with approximately equal sample sizes.

The difference between the global χ^2 and the single degree of freedom trend statistic may be used in a rough and ready fashion to decide whether most of the variation between treatment groups is explainable by the linear regression. There is an obvious analogy here with the usual analysis of variance applied to regression (Armitage 1971, 9.1). However, in the present context the difference between the two chi-squares has no formal justification as a test for deviations from linearity. A more rigorous approach necessitates use of the regression models considered later in the book.

Pairwise comparisons

As a complement to the test of the global null hypothesis, one often wishes to identify which specific pairs of the K survival curves are significantly different from each other. Pairwise comparisons based on the joint ranking of data from K uncensored samples can yield anomalous results (Miller 1966, 4.6) however, and this drawback extends to the censored data statistics presented here. Thus it is preferable to consider the series of two-sample tests comparing each pair of curves without regard to the others. Koziol and Reid (1977) suggest two conservative procedures which account for the multiplicity of comparisons being made. Bonferroni's method simply multiplies the observed p values by the number of comparisons, in this case $K(K - 1)/2$. Another slightly less conservative procedure is to treat the comparisons as independent, which increases the significance level from p to $1 - (1 - p)^{K(K-1)/2}$. For example, if the attained significance level comparing the first two of $K = 5$ samples was $p = 0.012$, the Bonferroni procedure would adjust this upwards to $10 \times 0.012 = 0.120$ and the alternative procedure to $1 - 0.988^{10} = 0.114$. However, for larger values of K, such adjustments are usually so conservative as to be of dubious value.

The same series of two-sample statistics may be used to construct a test for trend in accordance with the ideas of Jonckheere (1954). If W_{kl} denotes the sum of the scores (22.3) comparing sample k with sample l, and if the samples are arranged in order of increasing dose, an alternative trend statistic is defined by $\sum_{k=1}^{K} \sum_{l=k+1}^{K} W_{kl}/(N_k N_l)$. The variance is somewhat complex since dependencies among the W_{kl} statistics must be accounted for; explicit variances for the Gehan–Gilbert scores are given by Patel and Hoel (1973). Crowley

(1979) considers an analogous test of the form $\sum_{k=1}^{K} W^k$, where the W^k are scores comparing the kth sample with pooled samples $k+1$ through K. Since these are uncorrelated, an appropriate chi-square statistic is $(\sum_{k=1}^{K} W^k)^2 / \sum_{k=1}^{K} V^k$, where $V^k = Var(W^k)$.

An example

Heyn, Holland, Newton, Tefft, Breslow, and Hartman (1974) conducted a randomized trial to evaluate the role of combination chemotherapy (AMD + VCR) in the prevention of metatasis or recurrence following surgery for childhood rhabdomyosarcoma. The months to relapse for 15 children in the control group were 2, 3, 9, 10, 10, 12^+, 15, 15^+, 16, 18^+, 24^+, 30, 36^+, 40^+, and 45^+ while for 17 treated children they were 9, 12^+, 16, 19, 19^+, 20^+, 20^+, 24^+, 24^+, 30^+, 31^+, 34^+, 42^+, 44^+, 53^+, 59^+, and 62^+. Both these randomized groups had completely resected disease. Eleven patients with microscopic residual disease formed a third group whose remission duration times were 25^+, 28^+, 29^+, 37, 38^+, 42^+, 45^+, 47^+, 48^+, 50^+, and 52^+.

Table 22.3 summarizes the results of applying the various $K = 3$ sample test statistics to these data. The observed numbers of deaths of 8, 3, and 1 contrast with conditionally expected numbers of 3.11, 4.99, and 3.90. Thus, the simple $\sum_{k=1}^{K} (O_k - E_k)^2 / E_k$ version of the logrank test yields 10.64, which is slightly more conservative than the value of 10.77 achieved with V_A due to the presence of ties. While the results based on the permutation variances are less significant, there is good agreement among all three scoring methods for these data. Note that the W_G scores have been divided by $(N+1) = 44$ in order to make them comparable in value to W_L and W_P. This normalization is particularly important when conducting a stratified analysis (see below).

Since there is no natural order among the three treatment groups in this example, it makes no sense to carry out the usual test for trend. However, one contrast of interest is between the control and the two treatment groups. The 'trend' test with $x_1 = 0$ and $x_2 = x_3 = 1$ is identical with the two-sample test comparing sample one with the combined samples two and three. This is easily obtained from the data in Table 22.3 by adding together the scores from the second and third treatment groups for comparison with the first. The values of the two sample W_L, W_G and W_P tests with conditional variance are thus $4.89^2/2.22 = 10.78$, $4.07^2/1.53 = 10.84$, and $4.25^2/1.64 = 11.02$, each of them nearly as large as that of the corresponding two degree-of-freedom test. Thus, the contrast between the control and the combination of the treated groups accounts for nearly all of the variation observed between the three samples.

STRATIFIED ANALYSES

Cancer clinical trials frequently employ a restricted form of randomization which ensures that approximately equal numbers of patients are assigned to

Table 22.3. *Results of applying the K-sample tests to data on children with rhabdomyosarcoma*

	Method of analysis								
	Logrank (W_L)			Gehan–Gilbert (W_G)*			Peto–Prentice (W_P)		
Sample†	1	2	3	1	2	3	1	2	3
Scores (W)	4.89	−1.99	−2.90	4.07	−1.55	−2.52	4.25	−1.73	−2.52
Covariance Matrix (V_C)	2.22	−1.27	−0.94	1.53	−0.90	−0.62	1.64	−0.96	−0.68
		2.86	−1.59		1.85	−0.94		2.05	−1.09
			2.53			1.57			1.78
Test statistics									
$W^T V_C^- W$	11.10	($p=0.004$)		11.41	($p=0.003$)		11.40	($p=0.003$)	
$W^T V_A^- W$	10.77	($p=0.005$)		11.20	($p=0.004$)		(not calculated)		
$W^T V_P^- W$	9.49	($p=0.009$)		8.57	($p=0.014$)		8.54	($p=0.015$)	

* W_G scores divided by $(N+1)=44$, V_C by $(N+1)^2=1936$ as an appropriate normalization.
† First sample, control; second, treatment; third, microscopic residual.

each treatment arm within subgroups of the population, defined usually by one or more prognostic variables. This design feature suggests that the data be analysed as a stratified rather than as a simple random sample in order to make precise inferences about treatment effects. Even if restricted randomization has not been used in the design, *post hoc* stratification on the major prognostic factors at the time of analysis helps to ensure that any imbalance between treatment groups which may have arisen by chance is appropriately controlled, and that measured differences reflect the effects of treatment alone. Such control is even more important when making non-randomized comparisons, where imbalance between treatment groups on prognostic factors is to be expected. However, there are limitations on the degree to which several potentially confounding variables may be accounted for simultaneously with this approach. More complete control in a multi-variable framework is available using the statistical models discussed elsewhere.

One advantage of stratification as a method of adjustment is that it forces the data analyst to consider the separate treatment effects within each stratum. Observed differences often provide important clues that a particular treatment may be benefiting one segment of the patient population but not another. However a word of caution should be inserted about overinterpretation of these data, since chance fluctuations can also be expected to result in apparent differences among stratum-specific treatment effects. Formal statistical methods are available for testing and quantifying such treatment × covariable interactions, but these also require the fitting of models.

Adjusted rank tests

Stratification of the sample is a very simple way to adjust the censored data rank tests for the confounding effects of other variables. A separate calculation of the score vector W and covariance matrix V_C or V_P is made within each stratum, usually in conjunction with a visual examination of the survival curves for each treatment. The scores and covariance matrices are then aggregated by summing up the contributions from each stratum so as to obtain an adjusted set of scores and covariance matrix. These are inserted in the usual formulae (for example 22.12 or 22.14) to provide adjusted test statistics for comparing two or more samples, or for testing against alternatives of trend.

In the case of the logrank and Peto–Prentice scores, the adjusted test statistics may be derived from likelihood considerations. Each stratum makes a separate contribution to the log-likelihood function, and the aggregation of the scores and covariance matrices as described amounts to a summation of the appropriate log-likelihood derivatives. However, van Elteren's (1960) results for uncensored samples suggest that W_G be divided by one plus the stratum-specific sample size $(N + 1)$ before summation, so that it has the same order of magnitude as W_L and W_P (Mantel and Ciminera 1979). The stratum-specific covariance matrix for W_G is normalized by division by $(N+1)^2$. With this modification, adjusted analyses based on W_G and W_P are identical for untied, uncensored data, as was already true for unadjusted analyses.

An example

Table 22.4 presents interim data from an early study of maintenance chemotherapy for childhood acute lymphocytic leukaemia (Miller, Sonley, Karon, Breslow, and Hammond 1974). Three treatment regimens having a total of 152 patients employed AMD with or without other drugs as an additive to the standard maintenance chemotherapy, whereas two regimens having 116 patients did not. The end-point used for evaluation was relapse following induction into a state of complete remission. Even though the treatments had been assigned at random, a smaller fraction of AMD-treated patients were *a priori* at high risk of relapse due to an elevated diagnostic white blood count (WBC). Thus an adjusted analysis was needed to determine how much of the apparent effect of AMD could be ascribed to differences in WBC.

Table 22.4. *Stratified analysis of remission duration for 268 children with acute lymphocytic leukaemia*

	Unadjusted analysis	Adjusted analysis			
		Stratum (WBC)			
		0–	5000–	20 000–	Total
Sample sizes					
N_1	152	51	58	43	152
N_2	116	36	37	43	116
Logrank scores					
O_1	100	25	38	37	100
O_2	81	18	28	35	81
E_1	113.00	27.08	44.84	39.04	110.96
E_2	68.00	15.92	21.16	32.96	70.04
V_C	41.66	9.81	13.89	17.65	41.35
p	0.044	0.506	0.066	0.236	0.089
Gehan–Gilbert scores*					
W_G	9.86	2.11	4.72	2.05	8.88
V_C	19.26	5.04	6.47	6.88	18.39
p	0.025	0.346	0.064	0.435	0.038
Peto–Prentice scores					
W_P	10.10	1.98	4.87	1.99	8.84
V_C	19.99	5.67	6.61	6.94	19.22
p	0.024	0.405	0.058	0.449	0.044

* W_G scores in each stratum divided by $(N+1)$ and V_C by $(N+1)^2$ as appropriate normalization.

Table 22.4 contrasts the rank statistic scores and variances obtained without stratification (left-hand column) to those obtained after stratification into three WBC categories of approximately equal size (right-hand column). It is clear that the effect of stratification is to reduce the size of the apparent treatment effect, for example $O_2 - E_2 = 81 - 68.00 = 13.00$ before versus $81 - 70.04 = 10.96$ after. The significance levels of all three tests are approximately doubled after stratification, and that for the logrank statistic moves from $p < 0.05$ to $p > 0.05$ in the process.

Examination of the stratum-specific results shows that the benefit of treatment with AMD is apparently confined to the middle group of patients with WBC in the range from 5000 to 20 000. However, the data are quite insufficient to conclude that such a differential effect is real. For example, a test based on the PH model for homogeneity of the relative relapse rates in the three strata yields $\chi_2^2 = 1.62$ ($p = 0.45$). In view of the marginal significance of the overall effect of AMD, and the fact that it shows no clear trend with improving prognosis, it is prudent in this and similar examples to regard the stratum to stratum difference in relative relapse rates as being the result of random statistical fluctuations rather than of a real treatment × covariable interaction.

An approximate version of the adjusted logrank statistic may be obtained from the adjusted **O** and **E** vectors using the standard formula $\sum_{k=1}^K (O_k - E_k)^2 / E_k$. The resulting value in this example, $(100 - 110.96)^2 / 110.96 + (81 - 70.04)^2 / 70.04 = 2.80$, is only slightly less than that based on V_C, namely $(81 - 70.04)^2 / 41.35 = 2.90$. Similar approximate versions of the adjusted Wilcoxon tests may be derived using a formula analogous to (22.13), but where the denominator sums are over strata in addition to times t_i within strata. However these are more complicated and hence less useful in practice.

In this example the generalized Wilcoxon tests gave a more significant result than the logrank. One possible explanation is that the additive treatment had a more pronounced effect on relapse rates during the early phases of maintenance therapy than later on. Results of a further analysis with stratification on study time in addition to WBC, shown in Table 22.5, confirm this interpretation. Entries in the first column (early period) were obtained by treating all remission times of 270 days or more as censored. The second column figures were based on the reduced samples of 109 treated and 64 control patients still in remission and under observation at 270 days, and considered only relapses which occurred at that time or later. All three tests indicate a positive effect of treatment during the early period, but virtually no difference between relapse rates in the later one. Even here, however, it would be desirable to evaluate somewhat more formally the apparent treatment × time interaction.

One interesting aspect of Table 22.5 is the total column, which agrees with that of Table 22.4 only for the logrank test. The usual normalization of the W_G

Table 22.5. *Analysis of remission duration for 268 children with acute leukaemia: stratification on follow-up time in addition to WBC*

	Early period (under 270 days)	Late period (270 days and over)	Total
Sample sizes			
N_1	152	109	152
N_2	116	64	116
Logrank scores*			
O_1	42	58	100
O_2	51	30	81
E_1	54.19	56.77	110.96
E_2	38.81	31.23	70.04
V_C	22.12	19.23	41.35
p	0.010	0.779	0.089
Gehan–Gilbert scores (normalized)*			
W_G	9.76	−1.85	7.91†
V_C	14.64	8.83	23.47
p	0.011	0.535	0.103
Peto–Prentice scores*			
W_p	9.67	−1.78	7.89†
V_C	14.56	10.35	24.91
p	0.011	0.575	0.114

* Adjusted for WBC in three strata.

† Inappropriate for use as a summary statistic (see text).

and W_P statistics is inappropriate when strata correspond to different time intervals rather than separate samples. The correct summary statistics for the combined time period, shown in Table 22.4, give less weight to the later relapses. This discrepancy does not arise with the uniform weighting which generates the logrank scores.

SUMMARY

Rank tests for censored data offer a robust approach to the comparison of survival curves. They are most easily calculated as a weighted sum of the observed minus a conditionally expected number of deaths in each sample, a representation which also facilitates estimation of the variance. The Mantel–Haenszel or logrank statistic, which uses uniform weights, is most appropriate for proportional hazard (PH) alternatives. The generalized Wilcoxon statistics perform better when the survival curves show a greater separation in the early post-treatment period than they do later on, and since the original version of Gehan and Gilbert is sensitive to extreme forms of censorship, that suggested later by Peto and Prentice is now to be preferred. A different statistic is proposed to test for acceleration, wherein the difference in the mortality rates for two samples changes sign as time progresses.

The censored data rank tests are easily extended for use with K samples, whether testing the general hypothesis of homogeneity or more specifically against alternatives of trend. Two different variance formulae are available, with the choice between them depending upon whether or not the censoring patterns for the various samples are assumed to be equal; however, it is usually prudent to assume that they are not. Adjustment for covariable effects is easily carried out by stratification of the sample into homogeneous subgroups and aggregation of the rank test scores and variances calculated separately within each one.

ACKNOWLEDGEMENTS

Research supported by grants 1–K07CA–00723 and 2–R10CA–11722 from the US Public Health Service.

REFERENCES

Andersen, P. K., Borgan, O., Gill, R., and Keiding, N. (1982). Linear non parametric tests for comparison of counting processes, with applications to censored survival data. *Int. Statist. Rev.* **50**, 219–58.

Armitage, P. (1959). The comparison of survival curves. *Proc. R. statist. Soc.* **A122**, 279–300.

—— (1971). *Statistical methods in medical research.* Blackwell Scientific Publications, Oxford.

Bartholomew, D. J. (1957). A problem in life testing. *J. Am. statist. Ass.* **52**, 350–5.

Bernstein, L., Anderson, J., and Pike, M. C. (1981). Estimation of the proportional hazard in two-treatment-group clinical trials. *Biometrics* **37**, 513–19.

Boag, J. W. (1949). Maximum likelihood estimates of the proportion of patients cured by cancer therapy. *Jl R. statist. Soc.* **B11**, 15–23.

Breslow, N. (1970). A generalized Kruskal–Wallis test for comparing K samples subject to unequal patterns of censorship. *Biometrika* **57**, 579–94.

—— (1975). Analysis of survival data under the proportional hazards model. *Int. statist. Rev.* **43**, 45–58.

—— (1976). Regression analysis of the log odds ratio: a method for retrospective studies. *Biometrics* **32**, 409–16.

Brookmeyer, R. and Crowley, J. (1982). A k-sample median test for censored data. *J. Am. statist. Ass.* **77**, 433–40.

Cox, D. R. (1972). Regression models and life-tables (with discussion). *Jl R. statist. Soc.* **B34**, 187–220.

Crowley, J. (1979). Some extensions of the logrank test. In *Clinical trials in early breast cancer* (eds. H. R. Scheurlen, G. Weckesser, and J. Armbuster) Vol. 4, pp. 213–23. Springer-Verlag, Berlin.

—— and Breslow, N. (1975). Remarks on the conservatism of $\Sigma(O - E)^2/E$ in survival data. *Biometrics* **31**, 957–61.

Efron, B. (1967). The two sample problem with censored data. In *Proceedings of the fifth Berkeley symposium* (ed. J. Newman) Vol. 4, pp. 831–54. University of California Press, Berkeley.

Farewell, V. T. (1977). A model for a binary variable with time-censored observations. *Biometrika* **64,** 43–6.

Fleming, T. R., O'Fallon, J. R., O'Brien, P. C., and Harrington, D. P. (1980). Modified Kolmogorov–Smirnov test procedures with application to arbitrarily right-censored data. *Biometrics* **36,** 607–25.

Gehan, E. A. (1965). A generalized Wilcoxon test for comparing arbitrarily singly-censored samples. *Biometrika* **52,** 203–23.

Gilbert, J. P. (1962). *Random censorship.* Ph.D. Dissertation. University of Chicago, Chicago.

Gill, R. D. (1980). *Censoring and stochastic integrals.* Mathematical Centre Tracts 124. Mathematisch Centrum, Amsterdam.

Hajek, J. (1969). *A course in nonparametric statistics.* Holden Day, San Francisco.

Heyn, R. M., Holland, R., Newton, W. A., Jr, Tefft, M., Breslow, N., and Hartmann, J. R. (1974). The role of combined chemotherapy in the treatment of rhabdomyosarcoma in children. *Cancer* **34,** 2128–42.

Jonckheere, A. R. (1954). A distribution-free K-sample test against ordered alternatives. *Biometrika* **41,** 133–45.

Kalbfleisch, J. D. and Prentice, R. L. (1980). *The statistical analysis of failure time data.* Wiley, New York.

Koziol, J. A. and Byar, David P. (1975). Percentage points of the asymptotic distributions of one and two sample K-S statistics for truncated or censored data. *Technometrics* **17,** 507–10.

—— and Reid, N. (1977). On multiple comparisons among *K* samples subject to unequal patterns of censorship. *Communs Statist.—Theory Meth.* **A6** (12), 1149–64.

Kruskal, W. H. and Wallis, W. A. (1952). Use of ranks in one-criterion analysis of variance. *J. Am. statist. Ass.* **47,** 583–621.

Latta, R. B. (1977). Generalized Wilcoxon statistics for the two-sample problem with censored data. *Biometrika* **64,** 633–5.

—— (1981). A Monte Carlo study of some two-sample rank tests with censored data. *J. Am. statist. Ass.* **76,** 713–19.

Lee, E. T., Desu, M. M., and Gehan, E. A. (1975). A Monte Carlo study of the power of some two-sample tests. *Biometrika* **62,** 425–32.

Lininger, L., Gail, M. H., Green, S. B., and Byar, D. P. (1979). Comparison of four tests for the equality of survival curves in the presence of stratification and censoring. *Biometrika* **66,** 419–28.

Mantel, N. (1966). Evaluation of survival data and two new rank order statistics arising in its consideration. *Cancer Chemother. Rep.* **50,** 163–70.

—— (1967). Ranking procedures for arbitrarily restricted observations. *Biometrics* **23,** 65–78.

—— and Ciminera, J. L. (1979). Use of logrank scores in the analysis of litter-matched data on time to tumor appearance. *Cancer Res.* **39,** 4308–15.

—— and Haenszel, W. (1959). Statistical aspects of the analysis of data from retrospective studies of disease. *J. natn. Cancer Inst.* **22,** 719–48.

Miller, D. R., Sonley, M., Karon, M., Breslow, N., and Hammond, D. (1974). Additive therapy in the maintenance of remission in acute lymphoblastic leukemia of childhood: the effect of the intial leukocyte count. *Cancer* **34,** 508–17.

Miller, Jr, R. G. (1966). *Simultaneous statistical inference.* McGraw-Hill, New York.

—— (1981). *Survival analysis.* John Wiley and Sons, New York.

Morton, R. (1978). Regression analysis of life tables and related non-parametric tests. *Biometrika* **65,** 329–33.

Patel, K. M. and Hoel, D. G. (1973). A generalized Jonckheere *k*-sample test against ordered alternatives when observations are subject to arbitrary right censorship. *Communs Statist.* **2,** 373–80.

Peto, R. (1977). Contribution to the discussion on the paper of D. R. Cox (1972). *Jl R. Statist Soc.* **B34,** 205–7.

—— and Peto, J. (1972). Asymptotically efficient rank invariant test procedures. *Jl. R. statist. Soc.* **A135,** 185–206.

—— and Pike, M. C. (1973). Conservatism of the approximation $\Sigma(O-E)^2/E$ in the logrank test for survival data or tumor incidence data. *Biometrics* **29,** 579–84.

—— —— Armitage, P., Breslow, N. E., Cox, D. R., Howard, S. V., Mantel, N., McPherson, K., Peto, J., and Smith, P. G. (1977). Design and analysis of randomized clinical trials requiring prolonged observation of each patient. II. Analysis and examples. *Br. J. Cancer* **35,** 1–39.

Pike, M. C. (1966). A method of analysis of a certain class of experiments in carcinogenesis. *Biometrics* **22,** 142–61.

Prentice, R. L. (1978). Linear rank tests with right censored data. *Biometrika* **65,** 167–79.

—— and Marek, P. (1979). A qualitative discrepancy between censored data rank tests. *Biometrics* **35,** 861–7.

Rao, C. R. (1965). *Linear statistical inference and its applications.* Wiley, New York.

Regal, R. (1980). The *F* test with time-censored data. *Biometrika* **67,** 479–81.

Reid, N. (1981). Estimating the median survival time. *Biometrika* **68,** 601–8.

Sampford, M. R. and Taylor, J. (1959). Censored observations in randomized block experiments. *Jl R. statist. Soc.* **B21,** 214–37.

Tarone, R. E. (1975). Tests for trend in life table analysis. *Biometrika* **62,** 679–82.

—— (1981). On the distribution of the maximum of the logrank statistic and the modified Wilcoxon statistic. *Biometrics* **37,** 79–85.

—— and Ware, J. (1977). On distribution-free tests for equality of survival distributions. *Biometrika* **64,** 156–60.

Thomas, D. G., Breslow, N., and Gart, J. J. (1977). Trend and homogeneity analyses of proportion and life table data. *Comput. biomed. Res.* **10,** 373–81.

van Elteren, P. H. (1960). On the combination of independent two-sample tests of Wilcoxon. *Bull. Int. statist. Inst.* **37,** 351–61.

23 Interim analysis and stopping rules

Klim McPherson

INTRODUCTION

In most clinical trials of cancer therapy, the patients who will participate arrive for treatment over the course of a long period of time. A researcher wishing to compare two treatments for early breast cancer will not be able to allocate randomly the two treatments to the required number of women at a single point in time, because such patients are not available in sufficiently large numbers: he will have to wait for suitable patients to present themselves. This characteristic of the design of clinical trials naturally raises certain special issues which do not arise when the complete sample size is available for entry in the trial at one point in time. Firstly, it is often tempting to examine one's accumulated results at various stages during the trial to see whether or not enough patients have been included to demonstrate a reportable or interesting result. Secondly, in a situation of genuine agnosticism it seems desirable, in principle, to include only the minimum number of patients necessary to demonstrate a real difference in the effectiveness of treatments in order that subsequent patients can be given the superior treatment. The first of these considerations is based on pragmatic reasoning, since it is clear that no researcher would want to undertake a clinical trial lasting 3 years when one of a single year would provide nearly as convincing a result. The second is primarily an ethical matter: patient welfare demands clear answers to the clinical question as soon as possible. A concern with the patients' best interests is the major motivation for carrying out interim analyses in clinical trials. In fact, though, the development of the theory of sequential trials (Wald 1947) stemmed mainly from a need for speed in reaching a decision during the Second World War when it was important to be able to test the physical attributes of devices as quickly as possible by experimentation, without being misled by the habitual use of samples which were too small.

Although a fixed sample size for the trial may be specified prior to its start, whenever interim analyses are performed the ultimate sample size is no longer fixed in advance, but depends on the outcome of the individual analyses. In practice this means that at a number of stages during the accumulation of data the results are analysed with a view to taking either of two courses of action, namely: collect more data and continue the trial, or stop the trial and conclude either that the treatments are equally effective or that they are not.

In general, whenever an inference is made from a sample to a defined population, the strength of that inference increases as the sample size increases. This is measured by the width of the confidence limits on estimates of the differences in response to treatment. If these are narrow then one is correspondingly reasonably sure that a particular effect is in reality what the observations in the sample seem to indicate. Statistical inference generally takes the form of measuring, in probability terms, how likely certain outcomes of a trial are when the true effectiveness assumes particular values. A null hypothesis will specify zero effectiveness, or no difference between treatments, and interest will lie in the probability of particular results occurring on the basis of that assumption. This provides a starting point for considering the place of interim analysis in clinical trials.

OPTIONAL STOPPING

In order to achieve the ethical ideal of being in a position to give patients the superior treatment as soon as it has been identified, it might seem (at first sight) desirable to evaluate the results of a trial at intervals until a difference between the treatments emerges which is significant at a certain acceptable level (usually 5 per cent) using a fixed sample size test. It is clear that the more patients that are included, the narrower the confidence limits will be on estimates of treatment differences and, therefore, the more likely that a given difference will achieve statistical significance. If the evaluations are performed sufficiently frequently then the experimenter may appear to be reasonably certain that he will finish his trial at the earliest opportunity, from the point of view of being satisfied that a real effect (that is difference between treatments) exists. He can then allocate all subsequent patients to whichever treatment is superior. This procedure appears to be ideal from the clinical point of view since two distinct objectives may then be seen to have been fulfilled. Firstly, the original question of which treatment works best will be answered. Secondly, a rational decision will have been made as quickly as possible about how to treat subsequent patients who have the disease.

The above framework for analysing clinical trials evidently has a flaw somewhere, for if there were none it would constitute a panacea for resolving many of the ethical and practical problems of clinical experimentation. The main problem is that the level of statistical significance (the p value associated with the null hypothesis) is calculated with respect to a particular sampling framework. In general, it is assumed that the sample size is fixed in advance of an experiment and, in particular, that it will not be dependent on the results of the trial. Achieving, at some stage or other with interim analysis, a significant result using a fixed sample-size test does not allow the experimenter to quote a p value as if that sample size had been fixed at the outset. Imaginary repeats of that sampling framework will certainly yield different sample sizes and thus the conventional (that is fixed sample size) tests of significance will not apply. In fact, the situation is actually more serious than the mere application of inappropriate methods may imply. It can be proved (Kintchine 1924) that should an investigator carry out such a procedure he is absolutely certain to eventually achieve some small level of nominal significance (for example $p < 0.000001$), even when the population from which he is sampling conforms exactly to the specifications of the null hypothesis. (Nominal significance is used here to refer to the use of fixed sample-size p values when carrying out an interim analysis. This p value may be smaller than the true level of statistical significance.) This puts a rather strange light on the original idea that the experimenter will finish his trial as soon as he can be sure that a real effect exists. If he is certain to reach any level of nominal significance, even when there is no difference between the two treatments being compared, he obviously cannot be too sure that there is a *real* effect when a small p value is obtained. The extent to which he can be certain that the effect is real can be measured by the probability of achieving, within the prescribed duration of the clinical trial, a given level of nominal significance when the null hypothesis is true. If this is low, notwithstanding the sequential sampling framework, then he can be reasonably certain that there is a real treatment effect.

As an example of the extent of this problem in practice, let us consider briefly by how much interim analysis can exaggerate the true p value for repeated analysis of accumulating data. This general phenomenum is known as 'optional stopping' because it has been cited (Feller 1940) as an explanation for particularly favourable results in the reporting of experiments in extra-sensory perception. In Table 23.1 we show the probability in repeated sampling of achieving a trial result which has a *fixed sample-size p* value (called the nominal significance level) of 1, 5, or 10 per cent when there is no difference in the effect of the two treatments. That is, if we analyse a quite general class of clinical trials at equally spaced intervals during the accumulation of data with a view to stopping if the results appear significant at one of these nominal levels, then in the case of no treatment effect the chance of achieving such a

Table 23.1. *Overall probability of achieving a result with a given nominal significance after L repeated tests when there is no difference in the effects of two treatments (expressed as a percentage)*

Nominal significance level (%)	No. of repeated significance tests (L)								
	1	2	3	4	5	10	25	50	200
1	1	1.8	2.4	2.9	3.3	4.7	7.0	8.8	12.6
5	5	8.3	10.7	12.6	14.2	19.3	26.6	32.0	42.4
10	10	16.0	20.2	23.4	26.0	34.2	44.9	52.4	65.2

level sometime by L such analyses is given in the body of the table. Thus, for example, if an experimenter analyses his data on 10 (equally spaced) occasions during its collection and would stop the trial as soon as the results appeared to be significant at the 5 per cent level, then, even though the treatments are not different in a long sequence of clinical trials, such a strategy would lead to that level of nominal significance sometime in those 10 analyses in 19.3 per cent of trials. If more analyses are contemplated then the chance of achieving a given level of nominal significance is correspondingly enhanced.

The problems of optional stopping are well understood in terms of their frequency implications. That is to say that formal investigations of the probability of achieving results which are nominally significant in various clinical trial set-ups have been calculated and published. This has been done for various distributional forms of the measure of treatment response (Armitage, McPherson, and Rowe 1969) and, in particular, when the response variable is the time to death or recurrence of disease (Canner 1977). These calculations have been performed also for cases when the null hypothesis is not true, in order to investigate the power of clinical trials with interim analyses (McPherson and Armitage 1971). A feature of such investigations is that whatever the distributional form of the measure of treatment response the frequency properties of repeated significance tests at a constant nominal level are surprisingly similar when interim analyses are performed at equally-spaced intervals in the accumulation of data. This means in practice that Table 23.1 applies to many types of large clinical trials when interim analyses are contemplated and, therefore, that the true level of significance for L interim analyses is given by the body of Table 23.1. Moreover, if we require to compensate for the effects of optional stopping then a realistic strategy would be to decide in advance how many interim analyses to undertake and the level of nominal significance at which to stop. Thus, if we wanted to keep the overall false-positive rate low in spite of performing interim analyses we would need to adopt more stringent stopping criteria. Such criteria are shown in Table 23.2. From this Table we can see that for five looks ($L=5$), each of which could cause the cessation of the study, the trial could be fairly reported with an overall p value of 5 per cent only if the nominal significance level was as low as 1.59 per cent. In a strict sense such a strategy would lead to the rejection of a true null hypothesis at any one of these analyses in only 5 per cent of the trials.

These statistical considerations are, in essence, the reason that sequential methods in clinical trials require theoretical and practical frameworks which are so different from a fixed sample-size trial. It is also the reason for giving explicit consideration to the frequency implications of even a few interim analyses in clinical trials.

However, we ought not to lose sight of the reason for wanting to look at accumulating clinical trial data. When designing a study we are concerned with the dilemma of choosing a realistic treatment effect from which to calculate the sample size of a clinical trial with a given power. This is a real

Table 23.2. *Value of the nominal significance level necessary to achieve a given true level of significance after L repeated tests (expressed as a percentage)*

True level of significance	No. of repeated significance tests (L)													
(%)	1	2	3	4	·5	6	7	8	9	10	15	20	100
1	1	0.56	0.41	0.33	0.28	0.25	0.23	0.21	0.20	0.19	0.15	0.13	0.06
5	5	2.96	2.21	1.83	1.59	1.42	1.30	1.20	1.13	1.07	0.86	0.75	0.32
10	10	6.01	4.62	3.85	3.37	3.04	2.80	2.60	2.45	2.32	1.88	1.66	0.72

dilemma because, on the one hand, we would like to choose this effect sufficiently small, which requires a large number of patients. But, on the other hand, we would be unwilling to recruit new patients to a trial which already showed strong evidence in favour of one of the treatments. The point is, of course, that at the design stage of a large trial we do not know which treatment is better or, if there is a difference, the magnitude of any therapeutic effect. It is precisely for this reason that it is usually essential to plan for some interim analyses during the accumulation of the clinical trial data—just in case the effect is greater than anticipated.

Therefore, in terms of the normal significance testing framework it is essential to plan in advance of a clinical trial the number and frequency of interim analyses. For if this is not done, and there is any chance that an interim analysis will be undertaken, then strict interpretation of the results in a significance testing framework will be very problematic. It need not be emphasized that the circumstances under which an interim analysis will never be undertaken are essentially non-existent. Consider, for instance, the normal circumstances in which a trial is undertaken where there is considerable uncertainty about the relative merits of competing treatments. A certain difference is considered to be worthy of detection and therefore a high power is incorporated into the design. It is clearly always possible that such a difference is an underestimate of the true difference and, therefore, that at some time during the collection of data informal analyses may well indicate a strong therapeutic difference. Even if it is not an underestimate chance allocation of patients may give rise to important-looking effects and in these circumstances it will be difficult to resist the temptation to analyse the data.

It is, thus, a matter of simple logic that where interim analysis is possible then it is as well to plan for it in advance so that the results can be correctly reported. Indeed if it is generally the case that there is an overriding temptation to analyse results during clinical trials if they begin to look 'significant' then the fact that such analysis is not undertaken in a particular trial, because the data do not look 'significant' at any stage, does not necessarily allow the participants to report the trial as if they did no interim analyses, unless they were completely ignorant of all comparative data until the final analysis. This is because not undertaking a statistical analysis when the results are known not to yield a significant result is equivalent in probability to undertaking an analysis and not stopping because the results are non-significant.

It must be said that these kinds of considerations lead to some absurd examples however. The most quoted example of this absurdity (Hacking 1965) is the case of two collaborating experimenters one of whom had decided to examine his data 10 times and stop if the results were significant at 1.07 per cent (see Table 23.2). The other planned only to analyse the data at the end of the trial and report those results. Many different outcomes can be imagined for such a state of affairs, but the one that elicits the most interest is when no interim analyses achieve a nominal significance level of 1.07 per cent but the final analysis is just significant at 5 per cent. Clearly the first experimenter would report his results as significant at 19.3 per cent (Table 23.1) and the second at 5 per cent in spite of being in possession of the same data. It is obviously not possible to dismiss such a paradox by appealing to the rarity in practice of such an outcome, or by suggesting that the second experimenter would have been persuaded by a *p* value as low as 1.07 per cent if he had been faced with the ethical dilemma of stopping or continuing. He may have had perfectly sensible grounds for preferring to continue until the end, whatever the interim results may have turned out to be.

It is the case, therefore, that by using conventional significance testing the inference that one makes is somewhat dependent on the stopping rule chosen. This is an unattractive characteristic and derives directly from the implicit assumption that strength of evidence is measured only by frequency probabilities of particular outcomes when the null hypothesis is true. Alternative schemes of making inferences can overome this characteristic but only by placing less weight on the evidence provided by *p* values (McPherson 1971).

For example, examining data in terms of likelihood ratios, and making an inference based on critical values of likelihood ratios, yields tests which are independent of the stopping rule chosen (Cornfield 1966). Moreover, inter-pretating data in terms of posterior distributions formed with Bayes' theorem (Lindley 1965) from prior distributions and the likelihood function will be independent again of the stopping rule. In both cases however, no control of probabilities of error need be implied by these forms of inference and it will remain true that these probabilities will, in general, be dependent on the stopping rule chosen. Thus, while it is perfectly possible to adopt inferential schemes which are independent of the stopping rule used, some such rules may have probabilities of error which are absurdly high.

SEQUENTIAL EXPERIMENTATION

The main advantage which sequential experimentation offers to clinical trials in cancer is to ensure that the sample size is small, particularly when there is a large difference between treatments. This aim, of course, does not imply that sequential trials should always be used in medical experimentation. There is, for instance, a tendency to believe that because sequential trials can have the effect of allowing smaller samples in practice, then research can be conducted more expeditiously by their common use. This may not, however, be a sufficient justification. If one is investigating the relative efficacy of two treatments for the common cold for example, then the only advantage of a small sample is that the trial is finished quickly; the disadvantage is that the precision of any estimate of treatment differences is correspondingly low and therefore of less use. The justification for such a potential loss in precision should be commensurate with the extent of the ethical pressure to treat patients with the better of the two treatments. It is this latter consideration which is the real justification for sequential experiments, although other, more pragmatic, reasons may well play a part.

There are also some specific contra-indications to the use of interim analyses.

(1) If the response to treatment is observable only after a long period of time (long, that is to say, in relation to the expected duration of the trial) then sequential methods provide little advantage. This is because whenever a stopping boundary is reached there will be almost certainly a large number of patients still awaiting assessment of clinical response after treatment. The fact that a boundary has been crossed, thereby indicating that a significant difference between treatments has apparently been established, may well turn out to be irrelevant as soon as the outstanding clinical data become available.

(2) It may be important, for administrative reasons, to know in advance exactly how long the trial will take, a matter which is of particular importance in multi-centre trials.

(3) There may be several clinical response indicators of comparable importance. The sequential analysis of one of these may indicate that the trial should be stopped while analysis of one or more other indicators may not lead to this conclusion. The resolution of this problem will depend essentially on the ethical implications.

SEQUENTIAL TRIALS

Thus, since some kind of interim analysis is frequently indicated we will proceed to discuss two broad kinds of clinical trial design options. The first is a fully sequential design of the kind described by Armitage (1975). In these trials each observation of outcome from a clinical trial is tested along with all previous observations for a significant departure from the null hypothesis. In other words, the accumulating data is constantly being monitored against a stopping boundary for which the overall probabilities of error are fixed. These designs are fully described in Armitage's book and the interested reader is referred there for a detailed discussion. Moreover, these topics have been covered by Iglewicz in Chapter 19 of this book.

To be able to test the accumulating data continuously when comparing two treatments, patients are usually allocated in pairs so that each pair provides a measure of relative response. This is not always necessary, but sequential schemes are suited especially to clinical trials where paired observations are expected. In particular this will be true when a patient acts as his or her own control by, for instance, random allocation of the sequence treatment/placebo or placebo/treatment and comparing the response. Thus, fully sequential designs can be used without having to constrain the design to achieve paired observations where this would be difficult or inconvenient. However, for a variety of reasons, sequential trials have not been used often in practice. This has usually been attributed to complications of design and analysis (Pocock

1977). In fact the reasons are probably more deeply rooted in the wider practicalities of clinical experimentation. Sequential methods offer important advantages in large clinical trials where savings, in expense and in numbers of patients receiving an inferior treatment, can be substantial in absolute terms. However, large clinical trials are planned and undertaken only when the possibilities of large therapeutic effects are known to be remote. Thus, if a large effect is plausible then a small trial will be planned for obvious ethical and practical reasons. Indeed other important design constraints may well play a dominant part in the decision about sample-size requirements. Few clinicians would risk embarking on a trial to detect an important therapeutic effect which would take 2 years to complete when almost equally secure results could be obtained in 6 months. The point is that sequential methods offer substantial advantages mainly in large trials and then only when the estimated treatment effect turns out to have been pessimistic. In practice, estimates of treatment effect, if anything, tend to be optimistic. Hence, the circumstances in which the advantages of a sequential design can legitimately be expected to be substantial are, in practice, likely to be rare. At the same time the costs and inconvenience of unfamiliar methods, paired allocation, and assiduous analysis are often likely to appear substantial.

GROUP SEQUENTIAL SCHEMES

The choice of design does not, however, lie only between either sequential methods or a fixed sample-size trial. More recently a second type of design, known as group sequential designs, have been developed. These were first suggested in 1966 (Cutler 1966) as a reasonable compromise between the two extremes, offering some of the advantages of sequential methods with fewer of their perceived disadvantages. At the same time they can be used in experimental situations where the advantages can plausibly be realized. The notion is that the accumulated data from a clinical trial can be analysed several times during its course and if unexpected results emerge at any of these analyses then appropriate action can be taken.

These designs have been described by McPherson (1977) and Pocock (1977, 1982). Basically, the notion is that before a trial is started and after the maximum sample size has been fixed to correspond to acceptable probabilities of error against a meaningful alternative hypothesis, a fixed number of interim analyses are planned. Usually these interim analyses take place at equally spaced intervals during the collection of data. The reason for this is that not much is gained by varying the spacing, but there is a dramatic increase in the complexity of calculating the operating characteristics.

It is then generally the case that once the number of interim analyses has been decided upon the accumulated data can be examined using fixed sample-size tests, but using the more stringent nominal significance levels from Table 23.2 to allow for the repeated testing. Obviously, in order to maintain a particular probability of a type I error the nominal significance at which a trial should be stopped becomes lower as the number of interim analyses get bigger. As for the type II error (accepting the null hypothesis of no treatment effect when there is really a treatment effect of a stated amount), more interim analyses at lower levels of nominal significance tends to increase its probability. In other words, if the maximum sample size of a clinical trial is fixed and the number of interim analyses (hereafter called 'looks') is varied, then the consequence of more looks (and the necessity for more stringent nominal significance levels) is to reduce the power of the trial at all values of the treatment difference under test.

This is illustrated in Table 23.3 where results are presented for a Gaussian response variable whose variance is known. This table shows the operating characteristics of eight possible clinical trials for which the maximum sample size in each treatment group is 40, and for which the probability of a type I error is 5 per cent in each. The main part of the table tabulates the probability of achieving at least one result of an interim analysis which is significant at the stated nominal significance level. Thus δ is the mean treatment effect for a Gaussian response whose variance is scaled to unity (see below). A value of δ equal to zero corresponds to the case of no treatment effect and increasing treatment differences correspond to values of δ rising to 1.0, which represents a substantial effect relative to the intrinsic variability of the treatment response.

The nature of the assumptions here appear not to be important because qualitatively similar results are obtained for binomial and exponential

Table 23.3. *Operating characteristics of eight plans with constant type I error probability*

Maximum number of patients (N)	40	40	40	40	40	40	40	40
Group size (G)	1	2	4	5	8	10	20	40
No. of looks (L)	40	20	10	8	5	4	2	1
Nominal significance level (%)	0.56	0.74	1.05	1.21	1.55	1.78	3.00	5.00

Operating characteristics (overall probability (%) of achieving nominal significance levels)

Size of treatment difference $\lvert\delta\rvert$								
0.0	$\alpha =$	5	5	5	5	5	5	5	5
0.1		6	7	7	7	7	8	8	9
0.2		15	16	17	18	19	19	22	24
0.3		31	33	35	36	38	39	43	48
0.4		54	56	58	60	61	62	67	72
0.5	$(1-\beta)$	75	77	79	80	81	82	86	89
0.6		90	91	92	93	93	94	95	97
0.8		99	100	100	100	100	100	100	100
1.0		100	100	100	100	100	100	100	100

response variables. If, as is often the case in cancer trials, the response variate is the time between diagnosis and some event, such as death or recurrence, then such assumptions will not be strictly applicable. This is because in the first place some observations will be censored in the sense that patients will be known to be recurrence-free sometime after diagnosis. Secondly, of course, since any response measurement will take time to observe, the number of patients available for meaningful analysis will not correspond to the number of patients admitted. However, Canner (1977) has shown that the frequency properties of repeated significance tests on survival data are very similar to those illustrated in Table 23.1. Making appropriate changes in terminology the results reported here could, therefore, be used as qualitative guidance for the choice of the number of interim analyses, in the design of trials with a prolonged period of observation on each patient (Peto, Pike, Armitage, Breslow, Cox, Howard, Mantel, McPherson, Peto, and Smith 1976).

Of course survival data are usually analysed by non-parametric methods. Armitage (1975, Chapter 7) describes sequential analysis of follow-up studies including a sequential version of the logrank test. Moreover, Jones and Whitehead (1979) have investigated in detail sequential analogues of fixed sample-size analysis using the logrank test or Wilcoxon test (Gehan 1965) for censored survival data. These methods are illustrated in an application of a sequential trial comparing treatment for lung cancer (Jones, Newman, and Whitehead 1982), to which the interested reader is referred. If a clinical trial is comparing survival data then interim analyses could be undertaken by looking at the data at equally spaced intervals measured in terms of the number of events, as opposed to patients.

EXPECTED SAMPLE SIZE

The expected sample size is considerably reduced by many interim analyses, particularly for large values of the treatment difference. These values, together with the variance of the sample size, are shown in Table 23.4. It can be seen from this example that, compared with a fixed sample-size test, a halving of the expected sample size when $\delta = 0.6$ is obtained for 40 looks but (from Table 23.3 when $\delta = 0.6$) at the cost of a reduction of power from 97 to 90 per cent. In order to maintain the power characteristics for many looks at the accumulating data we would have to increase the maximum sample size to above 40. The questions we would like to address now are, firstly, by how much do we need to increase the maximum sample size in order to maintain power and, secondly, what would be the consequence for the expected sample size. Having solved the questions we would like to investigate the choice of number of looks when the probabilities of error of the two kinds (design characteristics) are held constant.

McPherson (1982*b*) has shown that the increase in maximum sample size necessary to maintain power, when many looks are contemplated, can be quite

Table 23.4. *Average sample size and variance of the sample size for the plans of Table 23.3*

Maximum number of patients (N)	40	40	40	40	40	40	40	40
Group size (G)	1	2	4	5	8	10	20	40
No. of looks (L)	40	20	10	8	5	4	2	1
Nominal significance level (%)	0.56	0.74	1.05	1.21	1.55	1.78	3.00	5.00

Average sample number (ASN)

	0.0	38.6	38.7	38.9	38.9	39.0	39.1	39.4	40
	0.1	38.2	38.3	38.4	38.4	38.6	38.7	39.1	40
	0.2	36.7	36.8	36.8	36.9	37.1	37.2	38.0	40
	0.3	33.9	33.9	33.9	34.0	34.3	34.6	35.9	40
	0.4	29.6	29.7	29.7	29.9	30.3	30.7	33.0	40
$|\delta|$	0.5	24.6	24.6	24.8	24.9	25.7	26.2	29.5	40
	0.6	19.6	19.7	20.0	20.0	21.2	21.9	26.1	40
	0.8	12.3	12.5	13.1	13.5	14.7	15.6	21.6	40
	1.0	8.2	8.6	9.4	9.7	11.2	12.3	20.2	40
	1.2	6.0	6.4	7.3	7.8	9.4	10.8	20.0	40

Variance of sample size

	0.0	42.5	37.1	31.7	30.1	24.3	21.4	11.6	0
	0.1	51.9	46.6	41.3	38.7	33.3	30.0	17.9	0
	0.2	80.2	75.4	69.8	65.5	59.9	55.3	36.7	0
	0.3	122.2	117.4	110.9	108.6	98.1	92.0	64.9	0
	0.4	158.7	152.9	144.6	139.2	129.8	123.1	91.2	0
$|\delta|$	0.5	165.4	158.5	149.0	145.3	135.5	129.7	99.7	0
	0.6	139.0	132.2	123.8	120.0	114.0	110.2	84.8	0
	0.8	65.0	61.6	57.9	55.3	54.6	52.8	31.9	0
	1.0	27.9	26.6	25.5	24.7	23.6	21.3	4.2	0
	1.2	14.0	13.2	12.8	12.2	10.2	7.5	0.3	0

substantial. However, for reasonably large treatment differences the savings in expected sample size, attributable to many looks, more than compensates for a larger maximum sample size. An example is shown in Table 23.5 which gives the expected sample size for eight different numbers of looks when testing a quantitative response variate. All these plans have an α level of 5 per cent and a 90 per cent power of detecting a difference of one-fifth of a standard deviation. It can be seen that for small differences (denoted by δ) the smallest expected sample size is achieved in a fixed sample-size test, because in such a trial a significant result is unlikely whatever the number of looks. However, as the difference approaches the value at which the power is 90 per cent ($\delta = 0.20$) then around eight looks yield the minimum expected sample size. Let us now investigate further the general problem of choosing the number of interim analyses in advance of a clinical trial for any repeated use of fixed sample-size criteria with appropriately adjusted use of nominal significance levels.

Table 23.5. *Average sample size for eight plans with varying numbers of looks, but the same probability of detecting a given treatment effect at the same level of overall significance*

Number of looks (L)	40	20	10	8	5	4	2	1
Maximum number of patients (N)	361	349	333	323	317	309	285	262
Nominal significance level (%)	0.56	0.74	1.05	1.21	1.55	1.78	3.00	5.00
$|\delta|$								
0.00	350	338	323	315	309	302	281	262
0.05	340	329	314	306	302	295	275	262
0.10	303	293	280	275	272	268	257	262
0.15	244	238	230	228	227	225	228	262
0.20	177	174	169	166	174	176	193	262
0.25	124	124	125	125	132	136	166	262
0.30	89	90	93	93	104	110	150	262
0.35	67	69	74	76	87	94	144	262
0.40	54	56	61	64	76	85	143	262

The minimum of each row is underlined.

CHOOSING THE NUMBER OF INTERIM ANALYSES

In essence the choice of the number of looks in a given clinical trial depends on how likely certain values of the treatment difference actually are. This in turn depends on the information available about the treatments to be compared. Evidence about plausible treatment effects comes generally from several possible sources: animal experiments, clinical experience, basic biology, and perhaps other clinical trials. Each of these is more or less reliable in extrapolating to the population of patients with cancer, and indeed the utility of each will vary markedly between diseases and treatment. Generally, however, previous randomized comparisons will provide a more secure basis for a sensible choice of the alternative hypothesis than will limited clinical experience of selected patients.

McPherson (1982*b*) considered the choice of the optimum number of looks from two points of view. The first was to minimize the expected sample size, integrated over some prior distribution representing the precision of prior knowledge concerning the treatment difference. The second was to minimize some linear function of the treatment differences, multiplied by the expected sample size integrated over the prior distribution. Very roughly the first represents a practical desire to minimize the number of patients in a clinical trial of given strength, and the second an ethical desire to treat as a few patients as possible with an inferior treatment—the more so when the treatments are very different.

A summary of the results for three plausible prior distributions (representing vague, moderate, and precise distributions) centred around no treatment effect and a precise distribution (centred between the null point and the alternative) are shown in Table 23.6. Generally ethical requirements need more looks than practical ones but, in fact, the losses associated with fewer looks according to the ethical criterion are very small.

A final strategy which has been advocated for the interim analysis of clinical trials is to adopt a very stringent criterion (that is low nominal p values) during the interim analyses. Then, if the data do not reach these low levels, the final analysis is performed using conventional fixed sample-size criteria. If the interim analysis criterion is sufficiently stringent then the interpretation at the end will not be affected much by optional stopping. Moreover, such a strategy fits in rather well with the requirements of large prospective trials where the interim analyses are simple and are primarily for ethical reassurance, whereas the final analysis is complex and usually a test of several hypotheses allowing for possible confounding and so on. Clearly such a strategy will not generally allow early stopping for moderate departures from no treatment effect, but gross underestimates of the expected treatment effect will be more likely to do so.

Table 23.7 (taken from McPherson 1982a) shows that if one decides to

Table 23.6. *Optimal number of looks for four degrees of prior knowledge*

	Number of looks	
Prior knowledge	Pragmatic	Ethical
Vague	8	40
Moderate	5	20
Precise	2	8
Precise and positive	2	10

Table 23.7. *Repeated significance test or group sequential schemes. A stopping rule for which the real significance level is 1 per cent followed at the end of the trial by analysis using fixed sample-size criteria. The realized level is the total probability of achieving a significant result either during interim analysis or at the end.*

Fixed sample-size level of significance at the end of trial (%)	Realized level (%)
5	5.4
4	4.4
2	2.5
1	1.6

adopt a stopping rule with an overall significance level of 1 per cent (Table 23.2, row one), then the effect on the actual significance level at the end of the trial is generally small. This is true however many interim analyses are planned so long as the critical p value allows for them.

CONCLUSIONS

Interim analysis in clinical trials is almost always desirable from some points of view and quite often necessary. We have seen that the statistical implications are often quite severe. If there is even a possibility that the interim results of clinical trials will be examined during the accrual of patients then, very roughly, the nominal levels of significance should be multiplied by a factor of between three and six when the trial is finally reported using fixed sample-size tests. Therefore, it is usually essential to explicitly allow for such a possibility in the design stage of a trial.

Maximum efficiency is not necessarily achieved by using fully sequential designs. In fact where prior knowledge of the treatment difference to be tested is fairly precise then the fewest expected number of patients is achieved with only two to three interim analyses at equally-spaced intervals. The use of repeated significance tests keeps the analysis of clinical trials in a comprehensible and widely accepted framework, which is less intimidating to the non-statistical specialists than complicated strategies with optimal characteristics.

REFERENCES

Armitage, P. (1975). *Sequential medical trials*, 2nd ed. Blackwell Scientific Publications, Oxford.
—— McPherson, K., and Rowe, B. C. (1969). Repeated significance tests on accumulating data. *Jl R. statist. Soc. Series A* **132**, 235–44.
Canner, P. L. (1977). Monitoring treatment differences in long-term clinical trials. *Biometrics* **33**, 603–15.
Cornfield, J. (1966). Sequential trials, sequential analysis and the likelihood principle. *Am. statist. Ass.* **20**, 18–23.
Cutler, S. J. *et al.* (1966). The rule of hypothesis testing in clinical trials. *Biometrics* seminar. *J. chron. Dis.* **19**, 857–82.
Feller, W. K. (1940). Statistical aspects of extra-sensory perception. *J. Parapsychol.* **4**, 271–98.
Gehen, E. A. (1965). A generalised Wilcoxon test for comparing arbitrarily singly-censored samples. *Biometrika* **52**, 202–23.
Hacking, I. (1965). *Logic of statistical inference*. Cambridge University Press, Cambridge.
Iglewicz, B. (1983). Alternative designs for phase III clinical trials. In *Cancer clinical trials: methods and practice* (eds. M. Buyse, R. Sylvester, and M. Staquet) pp. 311–34. Oxford University Press, London.
Jones, D., Newman, C. E., and Whitehead, J. (1982). The design of a sequential clinical trial for the comparison of two lung cancer treatments. *Statist. Med.* **1**, 73–82.
—— and Whitehead, J. (1979). Sequential forms of the log rank and modified Wilcoxon tests for censored data. *Biometrika* **66**, 105–13.

Kintchine, A. (1924). Uber einen satz der wahrscheinlichbeitstrechnueg. *Fundamenta Mathematical* **6**, 9–20.

Lindley, D. V. (1965). Introducing to probability and statistics from a Bayesian viewpoint. 2. Inference. Cambridge University Press, Cambridge.

McPherson, K. (1971). Some problems in sequential experimentation. Unpublished Ph.D. Thesis, University of London, London.

—— (1977). Sequential analysis in clinical trials. In *Clinical Trials* (ed. S. Johnson and F. N. Johnson) pp. 108–28. Blackwell Scientific Publications, Oxford.

—— (1982*a*). Discussion to Pocock, S. J. (1981). Interim analysis and stopping rules for clinical trials. In *Perspectives in medical statistics* (ed. J. F. Bithell and R. Coppi) pp. 191–214. Academic Press, London.

—— (1982*b*). On choosing the number of interim analyses in clinical trials. *Statist. Med.* **1**, 25–36.

—— and Armitage, P. (1971). Repeated significance tests on accumulating data when the null hypothesis is not true. *Jl R. statist. Soc.* **A134**, 15–25.

Peto, R., Pike, M. C., Armitage, P., Breslow, N. E., Cox, D. R., Howard, S. V., Mantel, N., McPherson, K., Peto, J., and Smith, P. G. (1976). Design and analysis of randomised clinical trials requiring prolonged observation on each patient. I. Introduction and Design. *Br. J. Cancer* **34**, 585–612.

Pocock, S. J. (1977). Group sequential methods in the design and analysis of clinical trials. *Biometrika* **64**, 191–9.

—— (1982). Interim analysis and stopping rules for clinical trials. In *Perspectives in medical statistics* (eds. J. F. Bithell and R. Coppi), pp. 191–214. Academic Press, London.

Wald, A. (1947). *Sequential analysis*. Wiley, New York.

24 Identification of prognostic factors

David P. Byar

INTRODUCTION

Since the beginning of time, man has wanted to prognosticate, or know before. This desire explains the popularity of oracles and astrologers in ancient times. Foreknowledge about the outcome of a battle or the yield of a harvest would be of obvious importance to a general or a ruler. We moderns might have been tempted to write 'foreknowledge about the *probable* outcome of a battle or the *probable* yield of a harvest', but this could have been wrong because it has been argued that there was no concept of chance until relatively recent times in the history of man (James 1977). This notion may explain the authority granted to seers in the past who were assumed to be interpreting the will of the gods, even if they were deciding an issue by casting lots or reading the future in the pattern of entrails of a sacrificed animal. Since the birth of the idea of chance, however, predictions of the future seem mainly to have fallen into the hands of statisticians, at least so far as the scientific world is concerned.

In studies of cancer and other diseases, identification of prognostic factors is perhaps the present-day equivalent of predicting the future. Our goals are somewhat different from those of the ancients. We know that we cannot predict exactly for individual patients but can only make statements of probability, and even these are certain to be more accurate for groups of patients than for individuals. Nevertheless, the study of prognostic factors plays an important role in analysis of clinical studies.

REASONS FOR STUDYING PROGNOSTIC FACTORS

Interest in the study of prognostic factors arises for several different but to some extent overlapping reasons. I shall discuss seven reasons separately.

Learning about the natural history of disease

It is often said that a knowledge of prognostic factors helps us understand the natural history of a disease. The term 'natural history' is often not very precisely defined and may appear to some to be a misnomer since it seems to carry the implication of how the disease would behave if it were untreated.

There are, of course, some diseases which do not require treatment because it is known that they are self-limited processes. This is particularly likely to be true if the disease does not produce any annoying symptoms. After making a diagnosis of such conditions, it is our knowledge of prognostic factors which allows us to assure the patient that the disease will disappear on its own and advise him about its probable duration and course. There are other diseases for which no curative treatments are available, but for which therapy is directed toward relief of symptoms. Here we may again speak meaningfully of the natural history of a disease. In diseases like cancer, however, we are seldom able to study the natural history because usually some form of therapy is applied in the hope that it will interfere with the natural history by curing the disease, avoiding or delaying symptoms (as opposed to relieving them), or at least increasing the survival of the patient. In this setting the study of natural history means an understanding of how the disease is likely to behave, including the effects of treatment on the course of the disease. We may say, for example, that the natural history of a tumour with a certain cell type is different from that of a tumour of the same organ having another cell type. The natural history then refers to the probable course of a disease in subgroups of patients defined by the prognostic factors. The identification of these prognostic factors may provide information useful to biologists trying to understand disease mechanisms and to physicians trying to devise new treatments.

Adjusting for imbalances in comparing treatments

One of the most important reasons for studying prognostic variables is that by definition they affect the outcome variable. If two treatment groups are being compared which are not nearly identical with respect to important prognostic variables, then apparent differences in the results of treatment may result from our failure to compare 'like with like', that is, they may be due to imbalances in the prognostic factors. In deciding whether or not a prognostic variable is balanced across treatment groups, it is common practice to form tables of treatment group versus categories of the variable and test these for independence. Although this procedure may be useful in detecting gross imbalances, it is an improper use of statistical significance testing (Dales and Ury 1978) because large imbalances in unimportant variables will not matter, but even small imbalances in important ones may seriously bias treatment comparisons.

In the last decade, sophisticated and flexible mathematical models have been developed which allow us to adjust to some extent for imbalances in prognostic factors. Many of these methods are reviewed by Simon in Chapter 25 of this book. Adjustment is most frequently needed when we are comparing groups whose treatments were not assigned by randomization, but even in randomized trials, if important imbalances are noted or if we are analysing subsets of patients resulting, for example, from the exclusion of protocol violations, adjustment procedures are often important.

Designing future studies

A knowledge of prognostic factors may assist in the design of future studies in several ways. For some planned treatment comparisons, it may be desirable to limit the patients studied to certain prognostic groups. There is an informal rule which states that treatments cannot be reasonably compared in patients who are either too sick or too well: if they are too sick, no treatment will help; if they are too well, the effects of treatment will not be apparent. Therefore, we may wish to confine our treatment comparisons to groups of patients in which there is a reasonable expectation that the treatments may affect outcome. A knowledge of prognostic factors also helps in determining necessary sample sizes, whether the response to be measured is a binomial variable (such as response versus no response), a measurement, or a time-to-response. If the outcome of interest is a binomial variable then the necessary sample size for comparing two different proportions depends on what those proportions are likely to be. If the outcome is a measurement (such as change in blood pressure or cholesterol level), then the required sample size depends on the mean difference expected between the treatment groups and the variation within each group. If the outcome of interest is a time-to-response (such as duration of remission or length of survival), then the required sample size depends heavily on the number of events (relapses or deaths) expected to be observed over the planned duration of the study. Predicting the necessary duration of a study and determining the required sample size to obtain reasonable statistical power are closely related concepts, and a knowledge of prognosis is useful in considering both design issues.

Another important use of prognostic variables in designing randomized studies is to determine which variables may be needed for stratified allocation or retrospectively stratified analysis. Stratified allocation usually means that one employs a form of restricted randomization designed to ensure that balance between treatment groups is achieved with respect to important prognostic variables. Such balance in the distribution of prognostic factors across treatment groups is considered essential because if it is not achieved, then some treatment group may appear superior to another, not because it is in fact superior, but simply because it contains a higher proportion of patients who had a more favourable prognosis before treatment.

Many schemes of stratified allocation have been proposed, ranging from simple randomization within blocks of patients determined by a few important prognostic variables, to fairly elaborate schemes of adaptive randomization (Simon 1977) designed to minimize the prognostic distance between treatment groups according to some reasonable measure of distance. The most extreme example of stratified allocation, termed 'minimization', replaces randomization entirely (Taves 1974).

It has been emphasized (Peto, Pike, Armitage, Breslow, Cox, Howard, Mantel, McPherson, Peto, and Smith 1976) that stratified allocation is scientifically unnecessary in reasonably large randomized clinical trials as long as retrospectively stratified analysis is planned. The same authors point out that stratified allocation is simply equivalent (from the point of view of statistical power) to having on average one more patient per stratum in the retrospectively stratified analysis, which adjusts for any serious imbalances in prognostic variables that do occur by chance in a particular trial. However, the only serious argument against stratified allocation is inconvenience, surely not a very persuasive argument, and therefore I believe that randomization in most clinical trials ought to be stratified on a few prognostic variables known to be of importance, particularly if the trial is relatively small.

However, stratifying on too many variables relative to the size of the study has been shown (Simon and Pocock 1975) to be equivalent to not stratifying at all. There are strong statistical reasons for preferring large trials whenever possible (Peto 1980), but frequently it is desirable to undertake randomized studies in settings where for practical reasons large trials are out of the question. Examples of such situations include study of rare forms of cancer, studies testing new drugs which may be very expensive and/or limited in supply (such as interferon), and studies carried out in isolated centres. In such situations, stratification is particularly important, because the occurrence of chance imbalances in prognostic factors sufficiently large to bias seriously the comparisons of treatments are much more likely in small studies than in large ones. One must remember, however, that whether or not allocation was stratified, the analysis should be. If allocation was not stratified, then a retrospectively stratified analysis will correct for any chance imbalances in the prognostic variables, while if allocation was stratified, then failure to take the stratification into account in the analysis will sacrifice statistical power (Green and Byar 1978).

A detailed and quantitative knowledge of prognostic factors is of even greater importance in situations where randomized trials are not possible because of ethical considerations, or because of philosophical preferences for non-randomized studies (Gehan and Freireich 1974). Here it is essential to apply the principle of comparing 'like with like'. The problem then is to select controls who are matched to the non-randomized patients receiving some new treatment as closely as possible with respect to all known important prognostic variables. Athough such an approach to comparing treatments is fraught with problems and uncertainties (Byar, Simon, Friedewald, Schlesselman, DeMets, Ellenberg, Gail, and Ware 1976; Byar 1979, Byar 1980, Byar 1981; Green 1981), a detailed knowledge of prognostic factors and a method of analysis which adequately accounts for them when comparing treatments provide the only available protection against serious bias.

Looking for treatment–covariate interactions

It is sometimes the case that treatments affect different kinds of patients differently (Byar and Green 1980). For example, if we were comparing treatments A and B, it might happen that treatment A is much more effective than treatment B in males but no difference is observed in females, or it may even be that treatment B is superior for females. In statistical language, such a situation is called an interaction between treatment and a covariate (in this example, gender). It is important to examine all treatment studied carefully for such situations, but because of the large number of ways we can subdivide the patients, one is likely to find apparent treatment–covariate interactions frequently by chance and special caution is therefore necessary in interpreting them (Peto, Pike, Armitage, Breslow, Cox, Howard, Mantel, McPherson, Peto, and Smith 1977; Peto 1982). Usually the variables employed to define such subclasses are prognostic when examined alone, but this need not be the case. It is certainly possible that a variable which does not appear prognostic when treatment is ignored may still be used to subdivide the total group of patients into classes showing important interactions with treatment.

Predicting the outcome for individual patients

Although I have mentioned above that our predictions for groups of patients are always more precise than those for individual patients, it is nevertheless interesting to physicians who care for patients to be able to answer questions from the patient or his family concerning the probable course of his disease. It is probably for this reason more than any other that physicians are interested in studies of prognostic factors. The physician's use of this information in the past has been largely informal—he knows that if a patient has no bad prognostic factors then his disease is likely to be relatively benign, but if he has many bad prognostic factors, then the opposite is likely to be true. With the development of the statistical models mentioned above, it is now possible to make more accurate predictions by considering the joint effects of the prognostic factors, even when applied to prediction for individual patients. One approach is to develop risk groups (see the section entitled 'An illustration') which may assist the clinician in making more precise predictions.

Intervening in the course of a disease

As Armitage and Gehan (1974) have pointed out, it is sometimes possible to use a knowledge of prognostic factors to alter the course of a disease by remedial action, particularly if the prognostic factors are elements of lifestyle such as diet, exercise, or habits. For example, if it were known that the prognosis for patients with chronic obstructive emphysema was worse for smokers than for non-smokers, then a smoker might reasonably expect to improve his prognosis by giving up smoking.

Whereas prognostic factors are related to the course of a disease, risk factors are characteristics which increase the probability of developing the disease in the first place. However, if we regard developing disease as the end-point, then risk factors are conceptually analogous to prognostic factors. The study of risk factors has given rise to a new kind of clinical trial in which the treatments are called 'interventions'. An excellent example is provided by the large-scale study sponsored by the National Heart, Lung and Blood Institute of the National Institutes of Health in the USA called 'MRFIT', an acronym for 'Multiple Risk Factor Intervention Trial'. In this randomized trial involving some 12 500 study subjects, one-half are encouraged to give up smoking, lower their blood pressure, and reduce their serum cholesterol by diet modification in the hope of decreasing their risk of death from heart disease, because studies have shown greater risk of myocardial infarction for people who smoke, have increased cholesterol, and/or have diastolic blood pressure exceeding normal levels.

Explaining variation and detecting interactions

In addition to the six main reasons discussed briefly above, the study of prognostic factors may also be justified from a statistical point of view. We recognize that in any medical study, the patients are heterogeneous and, therefore, the outcome of their disease or the response to treatment is likely to be extremely variable. The identification and quantification of prognostic factors may thus be viewed as the statistician's attempt to explain as much of this variation as possible. Those with a philosophical inclination might wonder if, even in principle, prognosis might become deterministic, that is, lose all elements of chance, if enough factors were known and recorded.

Finally, if convincing treatment–covariate interactions are found (as discussed above), the study of prognostic factors may permit more appropriate selection of treatment for individual patients or permit the definition of more precise hypotheses to be tested in future studies.

KINDS OF PROGNOSTIC FACTORS

In considering the kinds of prognostic factors in the field of cancer, different classifications are appropriate depending on one's interests. For thinking about the biological meaning of prognostic factors, a natural classification includes (1) host factors, (2) tumour characteristics, and (3) the effects of the tumour on the host. Such a classification may not be meaningful for other diseases (for example, arteriosclerosis) which, unlike cancer, are not regarded as foreign to the body. This classification has recently been used to describe known prognostic factors for malignant gliomas (Byar, Green, and Strike 1982). For this cancer, the age of the patient was the only clearly prognostic host factor, while the histological type of the tumour, the presence of giant cells, and the extent of surgical removal were important variables classified as tumour characteristics. Important variables related to the effect of the tumour on the host were overall performance status, the duration of symptoms, a history of seizures, and certain neurological signs and symptoms.

For statisticians it is useful to classify prognostic factors by the point in time at which they are recorded. In most studies there is a time which can be thought of as time zero, the point from which prognosis or times to response are measured. For statistical models incorporating covariates (or prognostic factors) it is generally assumed that the values of the covariates are known at time zero. In cancer studies these variables may be fixed characteristics of the patient (for example sex or race), observations or measurements made just before treatment is begun (for example information required for staging the disease), or results of medical examinations or tests required to diagnose a disease when time zero is taken as the date when the diagnosis is first established. However, other important prognostic variables which are known at time zero may be related to preceding events such as the duration of symptoms or a history of other prior illnesses. For example, a history of epileptic seizures in patients eventually diagnosed as having malignant gliomas has been shown (Gehan and Walker 1977; Scott and Gibberd 1980) to confer a favourable prognosis, presumably because tumours so located as to produce this symptom are detected earlier thus leading to a longer interval between diagnosis and death. In patients with prostatic cancer, a history of previous cardiovascular disease has been shown to be an important prognostic factor for predicting untoward toxic effects of estrogen therapy, a treatment which may otherwise confer considerable benefit (Byar and Green 1980).

The effect of a prognostic variable may change in time. Brown (1975) has studied the time-dependence of prognostic factors in patients with cancer of the stomach. For example, regional node involvement was a grave prognostic sign, but given that the patient had lived, say 3 years after diagnosis, was the prognostic importance of nodal involvement the same?

Another important class of prognostic variables consists of those measured *after* time zero which have recently been called 'time-dependent covariates'. Often such variables are measured regularly as part of a study because it is believed that changes in their values may be important in managing the patient's treatment, monitoring the toxicity of treatment, or may in themselves be of prognostic significance. Such variables include the white blood cell and platelet counts usually obtained in chemotherapy studies, values of presumed cancer markers such as α-feto protein or carcinoembryonic antigen (CEA), or serial measurements of the patient's performance status using, for example, the Karnofsky scale (Karnofsky, Abelmann, Craver, and Burchenal 1948). In studies whose only goal is to assess prognosis, study of these time-dependent covariates allows us to answer important clinical questions. The Cox proportional hazards survival model (Cox 1972) allows incorporation of these time-dependent covariates and permits estimation of their effects. Crowley and Hu (1977) have analysed the Stanford heart transplant data using time-dependent covariates. Prentice, Kalbfleisch, Peterson, Flournoy, Farewell, and Breslow (1978) used time-dependent covariates in a competing risk problem in an effort to study whether graft-versus-host disease was beneficial or harmful in leukaemia patients treated by marrow transplantation. Gail (1981) has used the Cox model with time-dependent covariates to study the prognostic value of serial CEA measurements as cancer markers in patients treated by surgery and chemotherapy for cancer of the colon.

Although the study of time-dependent covariates offers the possibility of answering many important biological questions, their use in adjusting treatment comparisons is clearly incorrect because it is possible to adjust away the very effects one is trying to study. For example, imagine that before death, patients with a serious cancer always experience a deterioration in performance status. Now suppose that treatment A is much better for treating this cancer than is treatment B, and, therefore, is much less often associated with a deterioration in performance status. If we were to compare the two treatments while adjusting, with the Cox model for example, on the time-dependent covariate 'performance status', we might find that the two treatments appeared equivalent, when in fact treatment A was distinctly superior. The reason is that we are adjusting for a variable strongly correlated with the response variable so that, in effect, we are trying to study the response while adjusting for the response itself! A general rule in deciding which variables to use in performing adjusted treatment comparisons is that the adjustment variables should never include variables which may themselves be affected by treatment. Simon (1983) provides a general discussion of the use of time-dependent variables in regression models.

Age is a host factor whose relationship to time is special because, although it changes with time, this change is perfectly regular, so that knowing the age of the patient at any point in time, say at diagnosis, is equivalent to knowing it at all preceding or subsequent times.

SCREENING VARIABLES FOR PROGNOSTIC SIGNIFICANCE

In a typical clinical trial, many variables of possible prognostic significance are recorded. During the writing of the protocol for a new study it is very likely that a sort of 'one-up-manship' game will take place in which each academic clinician will insist on including on the study forms all the factors which he believes may affect the outcome of the disease. The result is that when it comes time to analyse the results of the study, there are often as many as 20 to 30 or even more possibly prognostic variables to be taken into consideration, even though the total sample size for a study, involving say two treatments, may only be about 200 patients. How then should the statistician proceed with his analysis?

I shall refer to this problem, following the terminology used by Armitage and Gehan (1974) as that of *screening* the variables for prognostic significance. This use of the term 'screening' is to be distinguished clearly from trying to identify individuals in an apparently normal population who are at greater risk of contracting some disease, or who have an early form of it, such as 'screening' for cancer of the breast or cervix.

For this discussion I shall assume that the variables under consideration are only those which could have been known at time zero, that is, at the time of diagnosis or at the initiation of therapy. Such variables can always be viewed either as measurements (like blood pressure, white blood cell count, the values of serum enzymes, etc.), as orderable categorical variables (such as perform-ance status or stage of disease), or as unorderable categorical variables (such as race or sex). The first step in screening is to categorize the measured variables, for example age in 5-year categories or serum cholesterol into convenient intervals, and to treat them as categorical variables. The essential statistical question then becomes whether the categories, natural or arbitrarily formed, differ with respect to the outcome variable of interest.

This statistical question can be approached in many ways which differ greatly in convenience and ease. One could of course construct Kaplan–Meier (Peto *et al.* 1977) or actuarial survival curves for each category and compare them for statistical significance using for example the logrank test. We have found that a convenient and efficient procedure for routine use, where there are many potentially prognostic variables under study, is to compute an event rate for each category and then test these rates for heterogeneity, or for trend if the variable is naturally ordered. If the outcome of interest is death, then these rates are simply the death rates, and they are easily calculated by dividing the number of deaths in each category by the total follow-up time for all patients in that category, whether alive or dead when last seen. This is an old idea, used by actuaries at least since the beginning of this century, and it corresponds in fact to using the maximum likelihood estimates of the event rates when the event times are exponentially distributed (which is the same as saying that the event rates are constant over time). It has been shown by extensive examples (Metcalf 1974) that when survival for patients with cancer arising in a wide variety of sites is studied in reasonably homogeneous prognostic groups, the data are often well described by the exponential distribution. However, even if one fails to accept this generalization in particular instances, the exponential distribution may still be viewed as playing a central role in the analysis of cancer survival data as far as demonstrating a relationship between group membership and survival is concerned, in much the same way as simple linear regression is viewed as providing power against alternatives characterized by some sort of progressive association between a measurement treated as a design variable and some outcome treated as a response variable. In the early stages of an analysis, when we are screening large numbers of variables for possible prognostic significance, it is not so important that we have the best model to describe a possible association, as that we have a general test procedure with reasonable power to detect associations between potentially prognostic variables (or their categorized forms) and the outcome of interest.

In order to judge the extent to which random fluctuations and small sample sizes may produce apparently striking differences in death or event rates, it is helpful to use statistical tests of significance to assess the probability of differences as great as those observed if, in fact, the event times in the categories followed exponential distributions with identical event rates, provided that we do not take these p values too literally. Fortunately, there are easily calculated score tests (Byar 1982) which may assist us in this regard. Suppose we have defined k categories with estimated event rates $\hat{\lambda}_i$, $i = 1, 2, \ldots, k$. We may test these rates for heterogeneity by considering the observed numbers of deaths (or other events) in each category, which we denote d_i, and their expectations under the null hypothesis, which we denote e_i. If we let t_i represent the total follow-up time for all patients in category i, then the estimates of the event rates are given by $\hat{\lambda}_i = d_i/t_i$. Letting T and D represent the sums over all categories of the t_i and d_i respectively, then $e_i = t_i(D/T)$ since the quantity D/T is an estimate of the common event rate under the hypothesis that the rates are the same in all k categories. The score test for heterogeneity is given by

$$\chi^2_{k-1} = \sum_{i=1}^{k} (d_i - e_i)^2/e_i. \tag{24.1}$$

Under the null hypothesis that all the event rates are the same, this statistic is distributed approximately as a chi-square variate with $k-1$ degrees of freedom if there are k categories being compared.

If the variable is naturally ordered, it is then appropriate to test for a trend in the event rates. We may assign scores S_i to the k categories representing the increases in event rates we anticipate for patients in higher and higher categories. The score test for trend is then given by

$$\chi^2_1 = \left(\sum_{i=1}^{k} S_i(d_i - e_i) \right)^2 \bigg/ \left(\sum_{i=1}^{k} S_i^2 e_i - \left(\left(\sum_{i=1}^{k} S_i e_i \right)^2 \bigg/ \sum_{i=1}^{k} e_i \right) \right), \tag{24.2}$$

which is approximately distributed under the null hypothesis as a chi-square variate with one degree of freedom. If we do not have reason to use a particular set of S_i, we may test for a simple linear trend by replacing the S_i's in equation (24.2) by the consecutive integers $1, 2, \ldots, k$. Since the one degree of freedom chi-square statistic for trend is a formal partition of the $k-1$ degree of freedom chi-square for heterogeneity, the chi-square for trend will always be less than ɔr equal to that for heterogeneity, and it is easy to show that formulae (24.1) and (24.2) give the same result when there are only two categories. These tests help us determine which variables, when examined one at a time, may possibly be related to the outcome variable of interest.

A two-tailed test of the hypothesis of heterogeneity is appropriate, but the test for trend may be assessed with one-tailed probabilities if we have strong reasons to believe that if a trend is present, it can only be interpreted sensibly in one direction. The appropriate one-tailed probabilities are simply one-half of those usually tabled for the chi-square distribution. Using these one-tailed probabilities is less conservative than using two-tailed values and, therefore, it should be done very thoughtfully.

We may find, after examining these crude event rates, that adjacent categories for orderable variables may have similar rates and, therefore, we may choose to combine such adjacent categories in order to achieve a simpler analysis. Even if the variables are intrinsically unorderable (for example single, married, widowed, divorced), we may still choose to combine categories with similar rates in order to reduce the number of parameters we need to estimate in the final stages of analysis. One may be guided in this activity by a desire for reasonable simplicity combined when possible with a detailed substantive knowledge of the data being analysed.

This approach to screening, considering only one variable at a time, may of course fail to detect prognostic variables whose effects depend on the values of other variables (covariate–covariate interactions), but more elaborate approaches, while easy to imagine conceptually, are often unwieldy in practice. Some authors have suggested that the routine use of such techniques as 'automatic interaction detection', AID (Sonquist, Baker, and Morgan 1971) or its equivalent for categorical data CHAID (Perreault and Barksdale 1980; Kass 1980), may provide some protection from missing important co-variate–covariate interactions, but only with extensive further practical experience could one assess the value of such proposals for analysis of prognostic variables in cancer studies.

After having identified the possibly important prognostic factors from analysis of the data at hand and from knowledge of the appropriate literature concerned with the disease under study, the next step is to examine the effects of the variables when more than one is evaluated simultaneously. We may anticipate that since these variables are correlated with the outcome of interest, they are likely to be correlated with each other, although this need not be the case. The regression techniques described in this book by Simon (1983) provide a convenient way of examining the joint effects of the prognostic variables we have previously identified by studying them one at a time. Such statistical models are helpful because it is likely that we have identified more individual variables than are needed (because of their probable inter-correlations) to explain adequately the outcome variable, and because such methods allow us to assess the joint effects and possible interactions among the variables. Systolic and diastolic blood pressure might represent two variables so highly correlated that both are not needed. The idea of interactions may be illustrated by a study of malignant gliomas where we noted that although both age at diagnosis and the histological category of the tumour were important prognostic variables, the effect of age in altering prognosis was substantially less in patients having the most malignant form of the tumour (*glioblastoma multiforme*) compared with its effect in patients with less malignant histological forms (other malignant gliomas). An example of two other such covariate–covariate interactions is presented in the section entitled 'An illustration'. Recognition of such covariate–covariate interactions is important in making appropriate adjusted treatment comparisons, especially in non-randomized studies.

FORMATION OF RISK GROUPS

A knowledge of the combined effects of prognostic variables allows us to form groups of patients whose risk of death (or of suffering some other end-point, such as tumour recurrence or progression) are comparable. Such groups may be called 'risk groups' and they are characterized by patients whose covariates are such that the patients in a given risk group have comparable risk. Details of forming such groups using the Weibull survival model are given in Byar, Green, Dor, Williams, Colon, van Gilse, Mayer, Sylvester, and Van Glabbeke (1979) and Byar (1982), but the concept is a general one and can be applied to analyses based on any survival model incorporating covariates. Formation of such risk groups may be useful in several ways. Firstly, membership in a risk group provides prognostic information for individual patients or for groups of patients under consideration for future treatment studies. Secondly, risk group membership can be used as a summary prognostic variable in adjusted treatment comparisons. Although there are unresolved statistical questions about whether treatment should be included in the regression model when forming risk groups, stratification or adjustment on a summary risk score is nevertheless a reasonable procedure to use when the number of important prognostic variables is unmanageably large. Finally, risk group membership may be used as the basis for stratified randomization in future studies.

AN ILLUSTRATION

To illustrate some of the ideas discussed above I want to present a new analysis of a set of data I have presented twice before (Byar *et al.* 1979; 1982). The data were obtained from a registry sponsored by the European Organization for Research on Treatment of Cancer (EORTC) of patients with a relatively rare disease, cancer of the thyroid gland. Data collection began in 1966 on study forms which were improved at least three times during the course of the study, mainly by adding more questions or redefining existing ones. The information collected included a large number of variables such as possible risk factors for thyroid cancer (for example previous irradiation or history of goiter), a long list of possibly prognostic variables, details of the treatment given to the patients, and information about follow-up and eventual outcome. The goals of setting up the registry were not clearly stated at the outset, but it was thought that this could be a good first step before undertaking randomized clinical trials. In retrospect it seems that the collection of information on risk factors was likely to be of very limited value for testing any new epidemiological hypotheses since no control information was collected. The fact that data on the details of treatment were collected suggests that the founders of the registry may have enjoyed the naïve hope that meaningful treatment comparisons might be possible, but information in data banks is usually not suitable for this purpose (Byar 1980; 1981). Data on some 1183 patients from some 23 hospitals in various European countries were collected until 1977 and an analysis was requested. For the reasons just mentioned it appeared that the only sensible analysis which could be performed was one designed to evaluate the importance of prognostic factors.

After discarding questions with too many inconsistent or missing values and patients with unknown information on variables otherwise suitable for study, a group of 507 patients was selected for further analysis. The variables eventually selected as prognostic when examined one at a time (marginally) are shown in Table 24.1 along with the summary data for their categories, estimates of λ_i (the death rates), and the results of chi-square tests for heterogeneity and trend. Consecutive integer scores were used in computing the trend tests (eqn 24.2). Note that age, a continuous variable, has been divided into convenient categories. Except for the first and last category, deciles of age have been used, but the extreme deciles were combined (0–30 and 71 +) in order to obtain reasonably large numbers in the categories so that the corresponding λ_i could be reliably estimated. When all the variables were eventually studied in a Weibull survival model it was found that the data were slightly better fit when age was entered as a continuous rather than a categorical variable.

The categories used for cell type illustrate the concept of grouping unorderable categories on the basis of similar death rates observed in preliminary analyses. In fact there were five cell types recognized (PAP = papillary, FWD = follicular well-differentiated, FLD = follicular less-differentiated, MED = medullary, and ANAP = anaplastic) and for each tumour a principal and an associated cell type were recorded unless the tumour showed only one histological pattern (which is always true for MED tumours). It was noted that the death rate was always high if a tumour contained an anaplastic pattern, whether it was principal or associated, so this group was designated as a separate category. Death rates were similar for medullary tumours and for those with FLD as the principal pattern, so these two groups were combined. The 'Other' category contains all tumours whose

Table 24.1. *Prognostic variables for thyroid carcinoma found to be significant when examined one at a time*

Variable	Levels	Number of patients	Number of deaths	Total months* follow-up	Death rate†	Chi-squares‡ Heter	Trend
Age	0–30	91	4	5077.5	0.79		
	31–40	79	9	4176.5	2.15		
	41–50	84	25	3746.0	6.67		
	51–60	87	30	3666.5	8.18	224.3	173.0
	61–70	119	69	3637.5	18.97		
	71+	47	38	933.5	40.71		
Sex	Female	342	103	15 428.0	6.68	16.7	16.7
	Male	165	72	5809.5	12.39		
Cell type§	ANAP	77	68	760.5	89.41		
	MED-FLD	121	45	4769.5	9.43	644.1	340.4
	Other	309	62	15 707.5	3.95		
Tumour category	T0, T1, T2	401	106	18 242.5	5.81	92.7	92.7
	T3	106	69	2995.0	23.04		
Metastatic sites	None	421	122	19 041.5	6.41	149.9	98.4
	Single	78	46	2142.0	21.48		
	Multiple	8	7	54.0	129.63		
All patients		507	175	21 237.5	8.24		

* Because only completed months were recorded, 0.5 has been added to all follow-up times.
† Death rates are expressed in deaths per 1000 patient months.
‡ 'Heter' is the test for heterogeneity computed with eqn (24.1) and 'Trend' is the test for trend computed with eqn (24.2).
§ ANAP stands for anaplastic pattern, whether principal or associated. MED-FLD represents the group with medullary or follicular less-differentiated principal patterns. 'Other' includes patients whose tumours had papillary or follicular well-differentiated principal patterns.

principal patterns were either PAP or FWD unless the associated pattern was ANAP.

The extent of the primary tumour (T category) illustrates the lumping of adjacent categories of an orderable variable when those categories have similar death rates (see the survival curves displayed in Byar *et al.* 1979).

The joint effects of the variables were studied using a Weibull survival model where the effects of the covariates are assumed multiplicative. In particular, the hazard at time t was taken as $kt^{k-1} \exp(\boldsymbol{\beta}'\mathbf{X})$ where k is the Weibull shape parameter, $\boldsymbol{\beta}$ represents the vector of regression coefficients, and $\mathbf{X}$ represents the variables in the model. With the exception of age and cell type, all prognostic factors were entered as single variables with consecutive integer values assigned to the categories, starting with 0 for the category with the lowest death rate. Cell type was represented by two variables, one for ANAP and one for MED-FLD illustrating the technique of using $g-1$ indicator variables (coded 0 or 1) for factors having g categories (see Simon 1983).

The analysis presented here differs from the earlier one because, using new techniques (Byar 1982), we found that interactions were needed for age and sex and for age and metastatic site. Testing for the need for these two interaction terms in a model containing all the main effects, the likelihood ratio χ^2 was 24.57 with two degrees of freedom ($p < 0.0001$), so we decided to retain the interactions. The results of the fit (Table 24.2) revealed that these two covariate–covariate interactions have negative signs, indicating that the multiplication model without interactions overestimates the joint effects of these pairs of variables, so that the interaction terms have to correct these overestimates by reducing the estimated hazards. Further analysis using an

Table 24.2. *Estimated parameters and their standardized values for the variables fitted in the Weibull survival model*

Variable	Parameter	Estimated value	Standardized value†
Intercept	β_0	-9.2731	-14.493
Shape	k	0.8189	-3.735‡
Age	β_1	0.0755	8.368
Sex	β_2	2.9158	4.042
ANAP	β_3	2.1643	10.610
MED+FLD	β_4	0.4658	2.327
Tumour category	β_5	0.3226	1.912
Metastases	β_6	2.8862	4.508
Age–sex	β_7	-0.0393	-3.368
Age–metastases	β_8	-0.0345	-3.422

† The estimated parameter divided by its standard error.
‡ This is not $k/\text{s.e.}(k)$ but $(k-1)/\text{s.e.}(k)$ computed to test departure of the data from exponentiality since $k=1$ is an exponential model.

additive model where the hazard is given by $kt^{k-1}\boldsymbol{\beta}'\mathbf{X}$ revealed that when only age (represented by three indicator variables), sex, and metastatic site were considered, the interactions were not needed, but inclusion of the remaining variables required other interactions.

On the basis of the final model with six main effects and the two interactions, we formed risk groups using the same cut points as in the original article (predicted percentage survival at 3 years > 90, 80–90, 60–80, 20–60, and < 20). A plot of the actuarial survival curves and the curves predicted by the model (Fig. 24.1) showed a slightly better fit than that published before. The risk

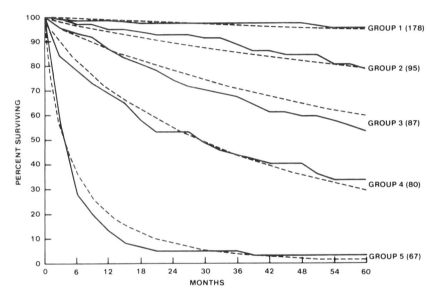

Fig. 24.1. Actuarial curves (———) and curves predicted by the Weibull model (– – – –) for five risk groups of patients with thyroid cancer. Numbers of patients in parentheses.

groups presented here caused 68 patients (13.4 per cent) to be reclassified compared with the previous analysis, but only three of these moved by more than one risk group. A tabulation of the characteristics of the patients in the five risk groups (Table 24.3) reveals some interesting points. Note that the first risk group contains only 16.3 per cent males but the remaining four risk groups have about 40 per cent males. The percentage of MED-FLD tumours rises through groups 1 to 4 but then declines in group 5 because ANAP tumours become more common. This kind of pattern is usually seen when two variables are mutually exclusive. In group 5, 97 per cent of the patients have anaplastic tumours and the survival of this group is accordingly very poor. The percentage with T3 (tumours extended beyond the thyroid gland) increases

Table 24.3. *Characteristics of the risk groups*

Risk group	Number of patients	Mean age (range)	Male (%)	MED-FLD (%)	ANAP (%)	T3 (%)	Single metastatic site (%)	Multiple metastatic sites (%)	5-Year survival rate*
1	178	30.8 (6–53)	16.3	10.7	0.0	3.9	0.6	0.0	95
2	95	48.8 (20–64)	42.1	28.4	1.1	6.3	4.2	0.0	79
3	87	61.0 (41–76)	37.9	36.8	1.1	20.7	16.1	0.0	53
4	80	61.5 (12–81)	45.0	52.5	12.5	38.8	53.8	3.8	34
5	67	66.5 (37–90)	40.3	1.5	97.0	65.7	23.9	7.5	4
All groups	507	48.9 (6–90)	32.5	23.9	15.2	20.9	15.4	1.6	64

* Computed by the actuarial method using 6-month intervals.

steadily across the risk groups and the percentage with single or multiple metastatic sites showed an inversion similar to that for cell type because the categories are again mutually exclusive. Although presented in two columns, metastatic site was used as a single variable in the model with levels coded 0, 1, and 2, as pointed out above.

Unfortunately the data in this study were not suitable for illustrating how prognostic factors can be used in adjusting treatment comparisons, but this subject is treated in some depth by Simon (1983).

SUGGESTIONS FOR FURTHER READING

There is an abundant statistical literature describing how to analyse multiple variables which in the present setting might consist of the treatment indicators, a set of covariates, and the response variable. In many problems the treatments and the responses are well defined in advance, but considerable latitude exists in choosing the covariates and often the results of an analysis depend on these choices. Unfortunately there does not appear to have been much written on the subject of how to select the covariates, and that has been the subject of this chapter. The reason for the lack of discussion of this important topic may be that the approaches used for identifying prognostic factors are usually informal and may even depend heavily on a substantive knowledge of the data being analysed. For these reasons it is difficult to formulate general strategies that lend themselves to publication in statistical journals whose editors and reviewers place a higher premium on formalism and rigour. Nevertheless there are a few articles which deserve mention. Zelen (1975) has discussed various kinds of prognostic factors, illustrated why stratification by prognostic factors is important in analysing clinical trials, and suggested a method of dynamic stratification to ensure balance of prognostic factors over treatment groups. Feinstein has written four essays concerned respectively with the purpose (1972a), process (1972b), evaluation (1972c), and further tactics for prognostic stratification (1972d). These essays were originally published in 1972 in the *Journal of Clinical Pharmacology and Therapeutics* as part of a series of some 40 essays on clinical biostatistics. They have been republished along with 24 other essays in a book (Feinstein 1977). Although Feinstein argues for 'the scientific necessity' of stratified allocation (a view that has been disputed by Peto *et al.* 1976), the essays present a thoughtful and sometimes provocative introduction to the subject with special emphasis on the biological point of view, particularly when it comes into conflict with the statistical one.

Armitage and Gehan (1974) have written an excellent expository paper on the identification and use of prognostic factors, supplemented with three examples taken from published papers concerned with breast cancer, prostate cancer, and Hodgkin's Disease. Peto (1982) has discussed various types of interactions and the extent to which medical beliefs influence their interpretation.

The recent book by Kalbfleisch and Prentice (1980) is relevant to the use of prognostic factors in survival analysis. This excellent book presents, along with other topics, a full account of the statistical literature which has appeared since the seminal paper of Cox (1972) on the proportional hazards model. The authors are in a good position to summarize this literature because they have contributed substantially to it themselves. Similar material is presented in the even more recent book by Miller (1981). Yet another recent book of interest is that of Lee (1980) who has compiled a broad summary of literature on the analysis of survival data. Her presentation is less theoretical than that in the preceding two books, and she includes abundant worked examples, most of which are taken from published papers.

Simon (1983) has provided a more concise summary in Chapter 25 of this book, and Byar has discussed the general topic of analysis of survival data in heterogeneous populations in two papers (Byar 1977; 1982), the most recent of which concentrates on the Weibull and Cox models and presents a convenient technique for identifying covariate–covariate or treatment–covariate interactions.

REFERENCES

Armitage, P. and Gehan, E. A. (1974). Statistical methods for the identification and use of prognostic factors. *Int. J. Cancer* **13,** 16–36.

Brown, C. (1975). On the use of indicator variables for studying the time-dependence of parameters in a response time model. *Biometrics* **31,** 863–72.

Byar, D. P. (1977). Analysis of survival data in heterogeneous populations. In *New developments in statistics* (ed. J. R. Barra) pp. 51–65. North Holland Publishing Company, Amsterdam.

—— (1979). The necessity and justification of randomized clinical trials. In *Controversies in cancer: design of trials and treatment* (eds H. J. Tagnon and M. J. Staquet) pp. 75–82. Masson Publishing Company, New York.

—— (1980). Why data bases should not replace randomized clinical trials. *Biometrics* **36,** 337–42.

—— (1981). Possibilities and limitations of observational studies and evaluation of medical data bases. In *Therapiestudien. 26 Jarhrestagung der GMDS* (eds N. Victor, J. Dudeck, and E. P. Broszio) pp. 528–37. Springer–Verlag, New York.

—— (1982). Analysis of survival data: Cox and Weibull models with covariates. In *Statistics in medical research: methods and issues with applications in cancer research* (eds V. Miké and K. Stanley) pp. 365–401. John Wiley and Sons, New York.

—— and Green, S. B. (1980). The choice of treatment for cancer patients based on covariate information: application to prostate cancer. *Bull. Cancer* **67,** 477–90.

—— Green, S. B., and Strike, T. A. (1982). Prognostic factors for malignant glioma. In *Oncology of the nervous system* (ed. M. D. Walker) Vol. I. Martinus Nijhoff, The Hague. In press.

—— Simon, R. M., Friedewald, W. T., Schlesselman, J. J., DeMets, D. L., Ellenberg, J. H., Gail, M. H., and Ware, J. H. (1976). Randomized clinical trials. Perspectives on some recent ideas. *New Engl. J. Med.* **295,** 74–80.

—— Green, S. B., Dor, P., Williams, E. D., Colon, J. van Gilse, H. A., Mayer, M., Sylvester, R. J., and Van Glabbeke, M. (1979). A prognostic index for thyroid carcinoma. A study of the E.O.R.T.C. Thyroid Cancer Cooperative Group. *Eur. J. Cancer* **15**, 1033–41.

Cox, D. R. (1972). Regression models and life tables (with discussion). *Jl R. Soc. Statist. Series B* **34**, 187–220.

Crowley, J. and Hu, M. (1977). Covariance analysis of heart transplant survival data. *J. Am. statist. Ass.* **72**, 27–36.

Dales, L. G. and Ury, H. K. (1978). An improper use of statistical significance testing in studying covariables. *Int. J. Epidemol.* **7**, 373–5.

Feinstein, A. R. (1972*a*). Clinical biostatistics. XIV. The purposes of prognostic stratification. *Clin. Pharmac. Ther.* **13**, 285–97.

—— (1972*b*). Clinical biostatistics. XV. The process of prognostic stratification (Part 1). *Clin. Pharmac. ther.* **13**, 442–57.

—— (1972*c*). Clinical biostatistics. XVI. The process of prognostic stratification (Part 2). *Clin. Pharmac. Ther.* **13**, 609–24.

—— (1972*d*). Clinical biostatistics. XVII. Additional tactics in prognostic stratification. *Clin. Pharmac. Ther.* **13**, 755–68.

—— (1977). *Clinical biostatistics.* C. V. Mosby Company, St. Louis.

Gail, M. H. (1981). Evaluating serial cancer markers studies in patients at risk of recurrent disease. *Biometrics* **37**, 67–78.

Gehan, E. A. and Freireich, E. J. (1974). Non-randomized controls in cancer clinical trials. *New Engl. J. Med.* **290**, 198–203.

—— and Walker, M. D. (1977). Prognostic factors for patients with brain tumors. *Natn. Cancer Inst. Monograph* **46**, 189–95.

Green, S. B. (1981). Randomized clinical trials: design and analysis. *Sem. Oncol.* **8**, 417–23.

—— and Byar, D. P. (1978). The effect of stratified randomization on size and power of statistical tests in clinical trials. *J. chron. Dis.* **31**, 445–54.

James, J. (1977). *The origin of consciousness in the breakdown of the bicameral mind.* Houghton Mifflin Co., Boston.

Kalbfleisch, J. D. and Prentice, R. L. (1980). *The statistical analysis of failure time data.* John Wiley and Sons, New York.

Karnofsky, D. A., Abelmann, W. H., Craver, L. F., and Burchenal, J. H. (1948). The use of nitrogen mustards in the palliative treatment of carcinoma, with particular reference to bronchogenic carcinoma. *Cancer* **1**, 634–6.

Kass, G. V. (1980). An exploratory technique for investigating large quantities of categorical data. *Appl. Statist.* **29** (2), 119–27.

Lee, E. T. (1980). *Statistical methods for survival data analysis.* Lifetime Learning Publications, Belmont, California.

Metcalf, W. (1974). Analysis of cancer survival as an exponential phenomenon. *Surgery Gynec. Obstet.* **138**, 731–40.

Miller, Jr, R. G. (1981). *Survival analysis.* John Wiley and Sons, New York.

Perreault, J. R. and Barksdale, H. C. (1980). A model-free approach for analysis of complex contingency data in survey research. *J. market. Res.* **17**, 503–15.

Peto, R. (1980). Statistical aspects of cancer trials. *Chemioterapia Oncologica* **4**, 303–7.

—— (1982). Statistical aspects of cancer trials. In *Treatment of cancer* (eds K. E. Halnan), pp. 867–71. Chapman and Hall, London.

—— Pike, C., Armitage, P., Breslow, N. E., Cox, D. R., Howard, S. V., Mantel, N., McPherson, K., Peto, J., and Smith, P. G. (1976). Design and analysis of randomized clinical trials requiring prolonged observation of each patient. I. Introduction and design. *Br. J. Cancer* **34**, 585–612.

—— —— —— —— —— —— —— —— —— —— (1977). Design and analysis of randomized clinical trials requiring prolonged observation of each patient. II. Analysis and examples. *Brit. J. Cancer* **35**, 1–39.

Prentice, R. L., Kalbfleisch, Peterson, Jr, A. V., Flournoy, N., Farewell, V. T., and Breslow, N. E. (1978). The analysis of failure times in the presence of competing risks. *Biometrics* **34,** 541–54.

Scott, G. M. and Gibberd, F. B. (1980). Epilepsy and other factors in the prognosis of gliomas. *Acta neurol. scand.* **61,** 227–39.

Simon, R. (1977). Adaptive treatment assignment methods and clinical trials. *Biometrics* **33,** 743–9.

—— (1983). Use of regression models: statistical aspects. In *Cancer clinical trials: methods and practice* (eds. M. Buyse, R. Sylvester, and M. Staquet) pp. 444–66. Oxford University Press, Oxford.

—— and Pocock, S. J. (1975). Sequential treatment assignment with balancing for prognostic factors in the controlled clinical trial. *Biometrics* **31,** 103–15.

Sonquist, J. A., Baker, E. L., and Morgan, J. N. (1971). *Searching for structure.* Survey Research Center, University of Michigan, Ann Arbor, Michigan.

Taves, D. R. (1974). Minimization: a new method of assigning patients to treatment and control groups. *Clin. pharmac. Ther.* **15** (5), 443–53.

Zelen, M. (1975). Importance of prognostic factors in planning therapeutic trials. In *Cancer therapy: prognostic factors and criteria of response* (ed. M. J. Staquet). Raven Press, New York.

25 Use of regression models: statistical aspects

Richard Simon

INTRODUCTION

A major objective of phase III clinical trials is the reliable determination of relative efficacy of the treatments studied for well-defined types of patients. Statistical analysis has traditionally consisted of describing the distribution of observed outcomes for each treatment and end-point of interest, demonstrating 'comparability' of the treatment groups with regard to prognostic factors, and performing significance tests (or calculating confidence intervals) to compare the treatments. This approach of comparing outcomes among balanced heterogeneous sets of patients can be ineffecient in its utilization of the available information.

In the past decade there has been a considerable increase in the utilization of statistical regression models for the analysis of clinical trials in oncology. This has resulted from the development of new methods, the increased involvement of statisticians in therapeutic studies, and the availability of fast, relatively inexpensive computing. Powerful and flexible regression models have been introduced. They permit the data analyst to evaluate relative treatment efficacy while accounting for the influence of prognostic factors, to develop predictive equations based upon multiple prognostic factors, and to address more complicated questions not easily dealt with by more rudimentary methods.

It is the purpose of this chapter to describe the basic features of some statistical regression models that are commonly used in clinical oncology. As with many technological tools, these methods can be misused and the results misinterpreted. There are many potential pitfalls in the naïve use of these methods and there are many open questions concerning how they should be employed. Though a thorough review of regression methods is not feasible, we will emphasize the assumptions and basic concepts underlying the use of statistical regression methods, provide some tools, and propose some guidelines for their use.

SOME REGRESSION MODELS

Some commonly used regression models will be introduced here and serve as a basis for subsequent discussions. The *linear regression model* is of the form

$$Y = \beta_1 x_1 + \beta_2 x_2 + \cdots + \beta_m x_m + \varepsilon, \tag{25.1}$$

where Y is an observable response, $\mathbf{x} = (x_1, x_2, \ldots, x_m)$ is a column vector of observable covariates (explanatory variables) measured without error, $\boldsymbol{\beta} = (\beta_1, \beta_2, \ldots, \beta_m)$ is a row vector of unknown regression coefficients, and ε is an unobservable 'random error'. An intercept term can be incorporated by defining $x_1 = 1$ for all observations. In vector notation this model can be written $Y = \boldsymbol{\beta}\mathbf{x} + \varepsilon$.

The *logistic model* (Cox 1970) is often used when the outcome Y is binary. In the logistic model, the probability of response $(Y = 1)$ for an individual with covariate vector $\mathbf{x}$ is

$$p(\mathbf{x}) = \Pr[Y = 1; \text{ given } \mathbf{x}] = \exp(\boldsymbol{\beta}\mathbf{x})/[1 + \exp(\boldsymbol{\beta}\mathbf{x})]. \tag{25.2}$$

This is mathematically equivalent to

$$\log \frac{p(\mathbf{x})}{1 - p(\mathbf{x})} = \beta_1 x_1 + \beta_2 x_2 + \cdots + \beta_m x_m. \tag{25.3}$$

All logarithms in this chapter are natural logarithms. More general models for categorical data are discussed by Bishop, Feinberg, and Holland (1975) and Grizzle, Starmer, and Koch (1969).

Models for failure time data are often stated in terms of the hazard function $\lambda(t)$. This is the probability of failure in the small interval $(t, t + \Delta t)$ given that the individual has not failed by time t. The hazard function value $\lambda(t)$ may be thought of as the instantaneous failure rate at t. The *Weibull regression model* postulates

$$\lambda(t; \mathbf{x}) = \lambda p(\lambda t)^{p-1} \exp(\boldsymbol{\beta}\mathbf{x}),$$

where λ and p as well as $\boldsymbol{\beta}$ are unknown model parameters. The Weibull class of models includes an *exponential model* as a special case $p = 1$:

$$\lambda(t; \mathbf{x}) = \lambda \exp(\boldsymbol{\beta}\mathbf{x}). \tag{25.4}$$

Here the time until failure for an individual with covariates $\mathbf{x}$ is exponential with mean given by the reciprocal of the right-hand side of eqn (25.4). Exponential regression models were the earliest such models for censored data (for example Feigl and Zelen 1965; Zippin and Armitage 1966; Glasser 1967) and are characterized by a hazard function which is independent of time.

The *proportional hazards model* (Cox 1972) for failure time data assumes

$$\lambda(t; \mathbf{x}) = \lambda_0(t)\exp(\boldsymbol{\beta}\mathbf{x}), \tag{25.5}$$

where $\lambda_0(t)$ is an unknown non-negative function that does not depend upon the β's or the x's. The Weibull model is a special case of the proportional hazards model.

In many applications of regression, some explanatory x's are indicator variables. For example, $x_2 = 0$ or 1 may be used to represent two treatments. Characteristics measured on a continuous scale may also be made discrete. Three age intervals (< 20, 20–50, > 50) may be represented by two indicator variables, for example, $(x_3, x_4) = (1, 0)$, $(0, 1)$ and $(0, 0)$. Discretizing a continuous variable permits one to avoid strict assumptions about the manner in which the continuous variable is related to outcome.

Treatment 'interactions' can be examined within the regression framework by appropriate definition of variables. Suppose that there are two treatments used for both male and female patients and one wishes to examine whether relative treatment efficacy for males is the same as for females. The variables might be coded as $x_2 = 0$ or 1 for treatment A or B respectively, $x_3 = 0$ or 1 for males or females respectively, and $x_4 = x_2 x_3$ representing the interaction. The hypothesis $\beta_4 = 0$ corresponds to constant relative treatment efficacy among sexes.

Methods of 'stratified analysis' can be included in the regression framework using indicator variables. In a study of the relative efficacy of two treatments, suppose that the covariates are used to define K patient strata. Each stratum is defined by a combination of values of the covariates, and each patient is contained in exactly one stratum. This structure can be represented in regression models by defining $K - 1$ indicator variables. An individual in the kth stratum is represented by $(x_1, \ldots, x_{K-1}) = (0, \ldots, 0, 1, 0, \ldots, 0)$ where the unit is in the kth position for $k < K$. An individual in stratum K is represented by a vector of zeros. An additional variable $x_K = 0$ or 1 is appended to denote treatment administered. For the proportional hazards model (25.5), an alternative is to include only the single treatment variable and to have the underlying hazard function stratum-specific, $\lambda_{0k}(t)$. The stratified approach permits one to make inferences about relative efficacy of treatment while accounting for the effect of covariates in a manner that makes fewer model assumptions. This is very desirable in many instances. The stratified approach is essentially equivalent to performing a randomized block analysis of variance for model (25.1) with normal errors, or a Mantel–Haenszel analysis (Mantel and Haenszel 1959; Mantel 1966) for models (25.3) or (25.5).

PREDICTION AND INFERENCE

Two frequent uses of regression models are prediction and inference. Prognostic factor studies may result in predictive models that are useful for several purposes: to identify poor risk subsets of patients on which to focus future studies; to determine stratification criteria for future trials; to improve the precision of treatment comparisons for randomized trials; to compare results from different institutions; to select a non-randomized control group. Sometimes it is sufficient to have a model that makes accurate predictions rather than to determine whether or not particular characteristics are of prognostic importance. Methods of assessing the predictive ability of a model will be discussed later in the section about model selection and validation. For oncological studies however, inferences about the importance of particular variables are often of interest. As will be seen in the section dealing with inferences about 'effects', inference is generally more difficult to accomplish than the development of a model capable of accurate predictions for future data collected under unchanged conditions.

Statistical significance tests and confidence intervals are frequently used for inference about treatment effects in randomized clinical trials. The statistical meaning of many commonly used methods is based on the probability distribution induced by the randomized treatment assignment for the specific patients studied. The statistical meaning of significance levels and confidence intervals derived from regression models, however, is generally based on a hypothetical assumption that the patients constitute a stratified random sample from a larger target population. In obtaining significance levels from randomization analysis the patient responses are considered fixed and independent of treatment. In model-based inference the responses are assumed to follow distributions postulated by the model (Koch, Gillings, and Stokes 1980). Inference based on the randomization distribution requires fewer assumptions than that based on a model. If, however, the model is a good description of the population relationships of response to explanatory variables, then model-based inference may give more precise answers (Royall 1976). It must be emphasized, however, that model based inferences may be critically dependent on the adequacy of the model. Consequently, model-based inference is suspect when the data are too sparse to evaluate model adequacy.

FITTING MODELS TO DATA

The data generally consist of an observed response Y_i and a set of values for potential explanatory variables $x_{i1}, x_{i2}, \ldots x_{im}$ for each patient, $i = 1, 2, \ldots n$. For failure time studies the outcome variable Y is a pair (T, δ) where T is the observed time until failure or until the limitation of observation without failure and δ is a censoring indicator; $\delta = 1$ indicates that failure was observed and $\delta = 0$ indicates that the true time until failure is not observed but is at least as large as T. It is generally assumed that the censoring mechanism is 'non-informative' (Kalbfleisch and Prentice 1980); that is, for a given set of covariates, the distribution of survival subsequent to time t conditional upon survival until t (for any t) is the same whether or not the observation is censored at t. For some models, general multivariate outcome variables Y are required. This is the case for growth curve problems but will not be discussed here. Usually the explanatory variables x are 'baseline' values measured at the start of the study. Some important problems can be addressed by regression models in which covariates are permitted to be time-dependent as will be discussed in a later section.

For a specified type of model and set of covariates, the method of *maximum likelihood* is a general technique for estimating the model parameters (β's). In the case of the linear model (25.1) with normal errors, maximizing the likelihood function is equivalent to minimizing the sum of squares of observed minus predicted values. In general the likelihood function is the product of factors, one for each patient, where each factor is the probability (or probability density) of obtaining the observed outcome Y_i given the vector of covariate values x_i for the patient. The likelihood function is a function of the unknown model parameters. For the logistic regression model, if $Y_i = 1$ then the factor is $p(x_i)$ whereas if $Y_i = 0$ then the factor is $1 - p(x_i)$. Thus, it can be seen from expression (25.2) that the likelihood function is

$$L = \prod_{i=1}^{n} \left\{ \frac{\exp(\boldsymbol{\beta} x_i Y_i)}{1 + \exp(\boldsymbol{\beta} x_i)} \right\}.$$

Methods of estimating the β's other than maximum likelihood are sometimes used though they will not be reviewed here (Chambers 1973; Gallant 1975).

For most of the models used in oncological studies, the method of maximum-likelihood yields estimators (MLEs) with well understood properties for large sample sizes. If the postulated model (with the included covariates) is correct, then as the sample size becomes large the likelihood function will generally have a single peak and the maximum likelihood estimators ($\hat{\beta}$'s) will be approximately normally distributed with expected values equal to the true value of the model parameters. The covariance matrix of the $\hat{\beta}$'s will be the inverse of

$$J_{mxm} = -E\left[\frac{\partial^2 \log L}{\partial \beta_i \partial \beta_j} \right]. \tag{25.6}$$

The bracketed part of the right-hand side represents the matrix mixed second partial derivatives of log L with regard to the m model parameters, and E denotes the expectation operator. This covariance matrix can be estimated by replacing the unknown true values of the model parameters by their MLEs. In complex cases, observed data values are used instead of taking expected values. Hence the large sample variance of any MLE $\hat{\beta}_j$ can be estimated as the jth diagonal element of this covariance matrix.

For finite samples, MLEs are generally biased and this bias can be considerable if the number of observations is small. The bias may persist even as the sample size increases for some non-standard models.

For fully parametric failure time models, the contribution to the likelihood function for a patient i who fails at time t is $f(t; x_i)$ where f denotes the density function of the failure time distribution given covariate vector x_i. The likelihood factor for a patient i censored at t is $Pr[T > t; x_i]$.

The proportional hazards model (25.5) has the advantage that assumptions concerning the form of the failure time distribution for a given covariate vector are not required since $\lambda_0(t)$ may be any non-negative function (suitably standardized). Estimation of the unknown parameters β is usually presented via a modified type of likelihood function. Suppose that no two failures occur at the same time and let $t_1, t_2, \ldots t_d$ denote the distinct uncensored failure times. Assume that the patients are indexed in such a way that patient i fails at time t_i, and let S_i denote the set of indices of patients who have not failed or been censored before t_i. Then the modified likelihood is a product of factors, the ith factor representing the probability that patient i fails at t_i given that exactly one patient fails at this time and that the patients still at risk are specified by S_i. Using eqn (25.5) the modified likelihood is thus

$$L = \prod_{i=1}^{d} \left\{ \exp(\beta x_i) \Big/ \sum_{k \in S_i} \exp(\beta x_k) \right\}. \qquad (25.7)$$

The unknown quantities $\lambda_0(t_i)$ have cancelled out of the numerator and denominator of each factor. Estimators of the β's are obtained by maximizing eqn (25.7). The use of this modified likelihood for the proportional hazards model in the way that ordinary likelihoods are used for other models has been justified in several ways (for example Breslow 1974; Cox 1975; Kalbfleisch & Prentice 1980; Tsiatis 1981). The value of the model is that inference about the β's is possible without making assumptions about the form of $\lambda_0(t)$. Expression (25.7) is derived assuming that no two failures occur at the same time. When failure times are grouped into intervals, this may not be the case. An approximate modification of eqn (25.7) for this case is

$$L = \prod_{i=1}^{d} \left\{ \exp(\beta z_i) \Big/ \left[\sum_{k \in S_i} \exp(\beta x_k) \right]^{d_i} \right\},$$

where d_i is the number of failures at t_i and z_i is the sum of the x vectors for patients who fail at t_i (Breslow 1974).

The values $\hat{\beta}$ that maximize a likelihood function L are the same as those that maximize log L. The log likelihood is easier to work with because it involves a sum of terms rather than a product of factors. Since neither L nor log L is generally a linear function of the parameters β, iterative numerical methods must be used to find the MLEs. If the MLE $\hat{\beta}$ occurs at an interior point of the set of possible values for the vector β, then the $\hat{\beta}$ is a solution to the system of equations

$$\frac{\partial \log L}{\partial \beta_j} = 0 \qquad (25.8)$$

for $j = 1, \ldots, m$ (the number of model parameters). This is generally a system of m non-linear equations in m unknowns. Newton–Raphson iteration can be used to find a solution to this sytem of equations. For many common models, the properties of maximum likelihood estimation imply that for large sample sizes there will be a unique solution to eqn (25.8). In general however, there may be several solutions corresponding to local extremes of the likelihood function. Consequently different starting values for the numerical methods must be employed to attempt to ensure that a global maximum is identified.

EXAMINING ADEQUACY OF FIT

Having tentatively selected a type of model and set of covariates, and obtained an estimate of the model parameters, the next step is to examine the adequacy of the fit. The validity of model-based inference about the importance of a variable is based upon an assumption that the model is correct, hence examination of model adequacy should come before inference about variables.

Consider the model:

$$\text{Nadir WBC} = \beta_1 + \beta_2(\text{initial WBC}) + \beta_3(\text{dose}) + \varepsilon, \tag{25.9}$$

where the random error term ε is assumed to be normally distributed with zero mean and unknown variance. If this model is correct, then it would remain correct if a totally spurious variable was added (the true value of the regression coefficient for the spurious variable is zero). The omission of an important variable, however, may render the model deficient in an important sense. For example, if the dose is selected based upon the initial WBC in eqn (25.9), then omission of WBC may result in a misleadingly small negative, or even positive estimated regression coefficient for dose. Also the model could be inadequate for other reasons. For example, the effect of dose may not be linear, the effects of dose and initial WBC may not be separately additive (for example dose effect may depend upon initial WBC), the distribution of random error may not be approximately normal, or the variance may be smaller for low initial WBC or high dose patients. In the next three subsections we will outline some general approaches to assessing goodness-of-fit for regression models.

Graphical analysis of residuals

After fitting a linear model (25.1), one can calculate for each individual i the predicted $\hat{Y}_i = \hat{\beta}x_i$. The ith *residual* is defined as $R_i = Y_i - \hat{Y}_i$. Since if the model is correct $Y_i = \beta x_i + \varepsilon_i$, the distribution of residuals should be roughly similar to the distribution of the random errors (ε_i) when the data is sufficiently extensive that $\hat{\beta}$ approaches β. Plotting the residuals R_i against the values of a variable not included in the model gives information about the relevance of the omitted variable. If the omitted variable is not important, then the plot should give a roughly horizontal scatter of points. Plots of residuals against each variable included in the model and against the fitted $\hat{Y}_i$ are useful also for detecting model inadequacies and outlying (possibly erroneously recorded) data values. For the normal linear model the distribution of residuals should be approximately normally distributed with mean zero. The residuals are correlated and the mean forced to be zero by the fitting process, but the shape of the distribution can be assessed by half-normal plotting as described by Daniel (1959). Details and examples of the graphical analysis of residuals for linear models are described by Draper and Smith (1981), Daniel and Wood (1971), and Henderson and Velleman (1981).

If there are many patients and few covariates then a graphical analysis of residuals for the logistic model can be done similarly to that for the normal linear model. In some cases these conditions can be accomplished by grouping patients with similar covariate values. Let the patients be grouped into strata in which all patients in a stratum have the same (or similar) covariate values. Suppose that there are n_k patients in the kth covariate stratum, that s_k responses $(Y = 1)$ are observed for this stratum and that the estimated success probability for this stratum is $\hat{p}_k$. Then the residual for the kth stratum can be defined as

$$R_k = \frac{s_k/n_k - \hat{p}_k}{\sqrt{\hat{p}_k(1 - \hat{p}_k)/n_k}}, \qquad (25.10)$$

where the residuals have been scaled to have approximately unit variance (Cox 1970). These residuals can then be plotted as described above. Non-normality of the distribution of residuals must be interpreted cautiously, however, because the expected closeness to normality if the model is correct depends upon the magnitude of the n_k and p_k.

The same definition of residuals (25.10) can be used for logistic models when no convenient grouping of the data is possible (that is most $n_k = 1$). The residuals should still have approximately mean zero and variance one, and trends of residuals against excluded variables can be examined. The residuals will generally have very skew distributions however, and examination of half-normal plots is not useful. Plots of residuals against fitted values may also be difficult to interpret unless the data is sufficiently extensive to sort the individuals into sets with almost constant $\hat{p}_i$ and to plot the observed proportion of successes against average $\hat{p}_i$ for the sets.

Graphical examination of residuals can also be performed for failure time models. The proportional hazards model (25.5) can be written in the form

$$\int_0^{T_i} \lambda_0(u) \, du = \varepsilon_i \exp(-\beta x_i), \qquad (25.11)$$

where the random errors ε_i are distributed as exponential random variables with mean equal to one (Kay 1977; Crowley and Hu 1977; Kalbfleisch and Prentice 1980). The left-hand side of eqn (25.11) can be thought of as a transformation of failure time, except that the transformation cannot actually be calculated when the $\lambda_0(\ )$ function is unknown. It follows from eqn (25.11) that a reasonable definition of residuals for this model is

$$R_i = \exp(\hat{\beta} x_i) \int_0^{T_i} \hat{\lambda}_0(u) \, du, \qquad (25.12)$$

where $\hat{\lambda}_0$ is an estimate of the unknown λ_0 function. Breslow (1974) approximated $\lambda_0(t)$ by a function constant between observed failure times and shifted a censored failure time to occur just following the previous observed failure time. He obtained the estimator

$$\hat{\Lambda}(T_i) = \int_0^{T_i} \hat{\lambda}_0(u)\,du = \sum_{k=1}^{i} \frac{d_k}{\sum_{j \in S_k} \exp(\hat{\boldsymbol{\beta}}\mathbf{x}_j)} \tag{25.13}$$

where T_i is the ith smallest distinct failure time, d_k is the number of failures at T_k and S_k is the risk set just before T_k. Using this estimator, the residuals can be calculated for all patients from eqn (25.12) (an observation actually censored at $T_i < t < T_{i+1}$ is considered censored at T_i). The residuals corresponding to censored failure times are themselves censored residuals $R_i +$. The residuals can be plotted against included or excluded variables, and a product-limit estimator (Kaplan and Meier 1958) $\hat{Pr}[R_i > r]$ can be calculated. The residuals should approximately follow an exponential distribution with mean equal to one, so a plot of $\log \hat{Pr}[R_i > r]$ versus r should approximately be linear with slope equal to -1.

Other graphical analyses are also possible for the proportional hazards model. An indicator variable, used to define two levels (for example male versus female), may be omitted as a covariate but used to define two strata. That is, the model becomes

$$\lambda(t; \mathbf{x}, j) = \lambda_{0j}(t)\exp(\boldsymbol{\beta}\mathbf{x}),$$

where j is the stratum of the patient and the stratum defining characteristic is omitted from $\mathbf{x}$ and $\boldsymbol{\beta}$. The regression parameters $\boldsymbol{\beta}$ are not stratum-specific and can be estimated similarly to the usual way. The $\lambda_{0j}(t)$ functions are estimated separately by stratum using the common estimator $\hat{\boldsymbol{\beta}}$ and eqn (25.13). The resulting functions $\log \hat{\Lambda}_j(t)$ are plotted. If there is approximately a constant difference between the plotted functions, then the characteristic in question can be included as a covariate rather than as a stratification variable (Kay 1977). This approach can also be used to examine a characteristic represented at more than two levels.

If there are few covariate classes (that is sets defined by combinations of the covariates) relative to the number of observations, then the logarithm of the failure time distribution predicted by the model for each covariate class $-\hat{\Lambda}(t)\exp(\hat{\boldsymbol{\beta}}\mathbf{x}_k)$ can be compared with the logarithm of the Kaplan–Meier estimate for observations in that covariate class (calculated independently of the model; Cox 1972).

Graphical approaches to evaluating goodness-of-fit for other models can be derived based upon the general definition of residuals given by Cox and Snell (1968). Nelson (1972) presents useful methods for plotting hazard functions for censored failure data with various types of underlying distributions.

Goodness-of-fit tests using nested models

Graphical examination of residuals can be illuminating, particularly when there is a large number of observations. Formal significance tests using *nested models* are often more convenient however. One model is said to be nested within another if both are in the same family of models, and one contains all the covariates of the other, plus at least one additional covariate. For example, the model specified by eqn (25.9) is nested within the model

$$\text{Nadir WBC} = \beta_1 + \beta_2(\text{initial WBC}) + \beta_3(\text{dose})$$
$$+ \beta_4(\text{prior treatment indicator}) + \varepsilon \qquad (25.14)$$

and within the model

$$\text{Nadir WBC} = \beta_1 + \beta_2(\text{initial WBC}) + \beta_3(\text{dose})$$
$$+ \beta_4(\text{initial WBC})^2 + \beta_5(\text{dose})^2$$
$$+ \beta_6(\text{initial WBC})(\text{dose}) + \varepsilon. \qquad (25.15)$$

Consider two regular nested models (that is nested models which satisfy the regularity conditions that ensure the usual nice large sample properties of maximum likelihood estimation), in which the first contains p regression coefficients while the second contains an additional q regression coefficients. Let $\hat{\beta}_p$ and $\hat{\beta}_{p+q}$ denote the MLEs for the two models and let L_p and L_{p+q} denote the values of the likelihood for the two models evaluated at $\hat{\beta}_p$ and $\hat{\beta}_{p+q}$, respectively. For large samples, the quantity

$$\Gamma_q = -2 \log(L_p/L_{p+q}) \qquad (25.16)$$

has a central chi-square distribution with q degrees of freedom if the additional variables are completely extraneous and the model with p parameters is correct. Hence, a large value of Γ_q relative to the tabulated percentiles of the chi-square distribution with q degrees of freedom is evidence that the more parsimonious model is inadequate. A likelihood ratio statistic Γ_1 could be calculated to examine whether model (25.9) gives an inadequate fit relative to model (25.14). A statistic Γ_3 could be calculated to examine whether model (25.9) gives an inadequate fit relative to model (25.15). Model (25.14) however is not nested within model (25.15). A likelihood ratio statistic Γ_2 could be calculated to examine whether a model containing only the constant term β_1 is inadequate relative to model (25.9).

This approach gives an indication of goodness-of-fit of a model relative to other models in the family. The likelihood ratio statistics may be unilluminating or even misleading if the entire family is inappropriate. Generally the family of models considered can be made sufficiently broad so that this is not a problem. The likelihood ratio tests generally do not, in themselves, provide much guidance as to what types of 'super models' to examine. Consequently this approach offers a powerful tool for conducting a careful analysis, not a standardized measure of overall goodness-of-fit.

The flexibility of the above approach is readily apparent. One less obvious example of its use relates to analysis of failure time data using the proportional hazards model (25.5). For simplicity consider the case where there is only one explanatory variable and that it takes on only values -1 and 1 (for example treatment A or B). The proportional hazards model assumes that $\lambda(t; x_1 = 1)/\lambda(t; x_1 = -1) = e^{2\beta}$ for all times t. A super model of interest could be obtained by partitioning the time axis into intervals $0 < W_1 < W_2 < W_3 < \ldots$ and defining time-dependent covariates $x_k(t) = x_1 Z_k(t)$ where $Z_k(t)$ is 1 for t in the interval (W_{k-1}, W_k) and zero elsewhere (for $k = 2$, $3, \ldots$). This super model permits the hazard ratio for the two types of patients to change over time. With K intervals, $K - 1$ time-dependent covariates are introduced and a likelihood ratio statistic Γ_{k-1} can be computed to examine the adequacy of the original simple model. Obviously, this approach is not limited to cases of only a single initial covariate. Cox (1972), Brown (1975), and Crowley and Hu (1977) provide further discussion and examples of the use of time-dependent covariates for evaluating model adequacy.

Other goodness-of-fit tests

There are other approaches to goodness-of-fit testing that warrant mention. For the linear model (25.1) in which the errors are independently distributed with mean zero and variance σ^2, the residual mean square value

$$\text{RMS} = \frac{1}{n-m} \sum_{i=1}^{n} R_i^2 \qquad (25.17)$$

has expected value σ^2 if the model is correct and expected value $\sigma^2 + \Sigma B_i^2/(n-m)$ (where B_i is the bias $E[Y_i] - \beta x$) if the model is not correct. Though the residuals are correlated, if the errors are normally distributed and the model is correct, then $(n-m)\text{RMS}/\sigma^2$ has a central chi-square distribution with $n-m$ degrees of freedom. Consequently if σ^2 is known or if an independent estimate of σ^2 can be obtained (for example from replicate independent observations at the same x value) then a goodness-of-fit test for the model can be performed. This approach to goodness-of-fit testing can be used for the logistic model when there are a reasonable number of replicate observations at each x value. Defining the residuals as in eqn (25.10), if the model is correct, the sum of the squares of residuals is distributed in large samples approximately as a central chi-square random variable with $n-m$ degrees of freedom. Cox and Snell (1971) have studied the construction of goodness-of-fit tests based upon residuals for general non-linear models.

'Omnibus' goodness-of-fit tests are tests that are directed at detecting several types of departures from the postulated model. The tests described above based upon eqn (25.17) are omnibus tests. Schoenfeld (1980) has described an omnibus test for the proportional hazards model, and Tsiatis (1980) has presented one for the logistic model. The following omnibus test for non-failure time models is based on that of Tsiatis, but requires no special computer program. Let the space of covariate vectors ($\mathbf{x}$) be partitioned into K subsets, and let $\mathbf{u}$ denote a vector of K indicator variables that specify to which subset a given $\mathbf{x}$ belongs. That is, $\mathbf{u}$ is a vector containing zeros and a single 1. Then an omnibus goodness-of-fit test is obtained by comparing the goodness-of-fit of the original model based on $\boldsymbol{\beta}\mathbf{x}$ to the nested model based on $\boldsymbol{\beta}\mathbf{x} + \boldsymbol{\gamma}\mathbf{u}$. This comparison can be assessed by calculating a likelihood ratio statistic which will have an asymptotic chi-square distribution with K degrees of freedom if the original model is adequate. This approach requires no additional computational procedures beyond those already needed to determine the MLEs.

Regression diagnostics

In some cases maximum likelihood estimates of the model parameters may be critically dependent on one or a very few observations. Such information may be of considerable interest in interpreting results of the model. Also, the model may be appropriate except for contamination of the data by a few 'outlying' observations and the outliers may dominate the MLEs. The identification of such data points has traditionally been problematical, because they may not be associated with large residuals. In fact a few outlying observations that dominate the fit will generally be associated with small residuals.

A body of techniques has been developed recently to identify outlying or pivotal observations for the normal linear model (Belsley, Kuh, and Welsch 1980). These methods have also been extended to the logistic model (Pregibon 1981). Although agreement on the most useful summary measures has not yet emerged, many informative and easily calculated diagnostic statistics have been derived. These are generally measures of the effects on the estimator $\boldsymbol{\beta}$ of deleting or perturbing individual or sets of observations.

The potential sensitivity of maximum likelihood estimators to small perturbations in the data has led also to the development of alternative methods of estimation such as robust regression, ridge regression, and principal components regression (Huber 1973; Hocking 1976). These approaches have been focused primarily on the linear model (25.1). The approach in robust regression is to use an estimation method that does not permit any individual observation to have such a large influence, as it may have in least-squares fitting. For the types of non-linear models commonly used in clinical oncology, however, it seems likely that standard maximum likelihood methods will continue to be used. Consequently, regression diagnostics may play an increasing role for evaluating model adequacy.

MODEL SELECTION AND VALIDATION

Generally there will be several models that adquately fit the data, and criteria beyond goodness-of-fit must be used for model selection. Suppose that the normal linear model

$$Y = \beta x + \gamma z + \varepsilon \qquad (25.18)$$

is correct where β is a set of p regression coefficients corresponding to covariates x, and γ is a set of r regression coefficients corresponding to covariates z. If $\gamma = 0$, then the normal linear model

$$Y = \beta x + \varepsilon \qquad (25.19)$$

is also correct. The first model will give a somewhat better fit but the variance of the MLE of a regression coefficient in β will be smaller for the second model. Also the variance of the predictor $\hat{Y}$ will be smaller for the second model. Hence, overly complicated models may give very good fits, but lead to poor estimates of regression coefficients and poor predictions.

Suppose that model (25.18) is correct but $\gamma \neq 0$ so that model (25.19) is erroneous. Let $\tilde{\beta}$ and $\tilde{\sigma}^2$ denote the MLE of β and residual mean square for model (25.19). Generally under these conditions $\tilde{\beta}$ is biased and $\tilde{\sigma}^2$ is upwardly biased. The latter fact can serve as a tool for selecting a specific model among the linear family (25.18). This is discussed by Gorman and Toman (1966) and by Daniel and Wood (1971) in the context of the C_p statistic

$$C_p = \frac{\tilde{\sigma}^2(n-p)}{\hat{\sigma}^2} + 2p - n, \qquad (25.20)$$

where $\hat{\sigma}^2$ is an estimate of σ^2 derived from the full model (25.18) or from replicate observations. Models are considered for which C_p approximately equals p or for which C_p is small. This is equivalent to considering models with the smallest estimated residual mean square. Alternatives to C_p are discussed by Hocking (1976) and Thompson (1978). Akaike (1973) proposed a generalization of C_p for selecting models from any nested family. He proposes considering models which produce small values of

$$CP^* = \log L(\hat{\beta}) - p \qquad (25.21)$$

where $L(\hat{\beta})$ is the value of the likelihood function for the model containing p parameters β evaluated at the MLE $\hat{\beta}$. Other generalizations are possible however (Schwartz 1978; Stone 1979).

With numerous potential covariates, stepwise regression procedures are often used to select a model. Sometimes a pre-screening is employed to eliminate covariates with no substantial univariate association with outcome. Stepwise procedures are reviewed by Hocking (1976). Although they may be useful, they are essentially *ad hoc* in that the criteria for adding or deleting variables are somewhat arbitrary. Different stepwise procedures may give different sets of selected models. Claims concerning relative 'importance' of covariates based upon the order of inclusion by step-up procedures are tenuous because of dependence of the procedures upon the selection criterion. Often there will be several sets of covariates that predict equally well. This is particularly true when the covariates are closely associated among themselves. A preferable approach is to identify the several best or almost best fitting p variable models of a given family for each $p = 1, 2, \ldots, m$. A relatively efficient algorithm to accomplish this for non-linear families is described by Lawless and Singhal (1978). Other criteria can then be used to select among the identified models, and the identification itself may be illuminating. Biased estimation methods such as ridge regression and principal components regression have been developed in attempts to determine improved prediction models without the need to select and reject subsets of variables. Such methods are receiving intense study (Hocking 1976, Draper and Van Nostrand 1979), but their role is currently controversial.

Clearly, model selection may be subjective. The only fully adequate approach to model validation is testing the selected model against an independent set of data. This simple fact is often forgotten. When the available data are sufficiently extensive, independent validation can be approximated by dividing the observations into two subsamples. One subsample is used for model development and the other for model validation. This idea has been employed many times and it is well established that 'predictions' are more accurate for the data on which the model was derived than for independent data (Stone 1974). This is particularly true for complicated models with many parameters.

The technique of *cross-validation* to assess the predictive ability of a model (Mosteller and Wallace 1963; Lachenbruch and Mickey 1968) has recently received increased attention (Stone 1974; Geisser 1975). This technique is based upon the concept of data splitting, but the model is developed on a subset of $n - 1$ observations and tested on the single remaining observation. Then this is repeated n times, each time selecting a different single observation for the test subset. Geisser has also considered intermediate types of cross-validation where the test subsets consist of a relatively small number of observations. Let $D(Y_i, \hat{Y}_i)$ denote some measure of the accuracy of prediction of Y_i based upon a model developed using the remaining $n - 1$ observations. Then the cross-validatory assessment of accuracy of prediction is

$$D^* = \sum_{i=1}^{n} D(Y_i, \hat{Y}_i). \tag{25.22}$$

Any single term is an intuitively reasonable assessment of predictability of the developed model for the remaining observation. The terms of the summation are correlated, however, and the model used to predict Y_i may not be the same as the model used to predict some other Y_j. That is, even if the included covariates are fixed, the estimates of the regression coefficients are re-calculated for each observation set aside. Consequently, the summation represents a measure of predictability for the method of model selection based upon the data.

The statistical properties of D^* are not well understood, except for special cases. D^* does seem to be a better assessment of predictive power than that obtained by selecting a model once based on all n observations and measuring accuracy of 'predictions' for the same set of n observations. For linear models (25.1), with $D(Y_i, \hat{Y}_i) = (Y_i - \hat{Y}_i)^2$ and the method of model selection being simply maximum likelihood estimation of a prespecified set of regression coefficients, D^* is equivalent to the PRESS measure introduced by Allen (1974). In this case D^* is easy to calculate as

$$\text{PRESS} = \sum_{i=1}^{n} R_i^2/v_i^2$$

where R_i is the ith residual for the model fitted to the full set of n observations and v_i is the variance of R_i (Hocking 1976). Cross-validation has been used also as a criterion for model selection. For example, a subset of covariates might be selected as that subset which gives the smallest value of D^*. Stone (1974) gives some interesting examples of this. Stone (1979) has also demonstrated a large sample equivalence between cross-validation and Akaike's criterion (eqn 25.21) for model selection.

INFERENCES ABOUT 'EFFECTS'

Many studies are conducted to assess the 'causative' role of a characteristic on outcome. For therapeutic studies in oncology, the characteristic is generally treatment and the outcome survival or duration of tumour control. Regression models are employed to account for the presence of other variables. Model-based inference about the importance of the characteristic in question is addressed as inference about the magnitude and sign of the regression coefficient associated with the characteristic.

When maximum likelihood estimation is used, three general approaches to inference about regression coefficients are commonly employed. For generality, suppose that the characteristic of interest is represented by a set of q (possibly one) regression coefficients γ and that the remaining p regression coefficients are denoted β. As described in the section on goodness-of-fit using nested models, a large sample statistical significance test of the hypothesis $\gamma = 0$ can be performed using the likelihood ratio statistic (25.16). The second approach is generally attributed to Wald. Under the hypothesis $\gamma = 0$ the MLE $\hat{\gamma}$ has an asymptotic multivariate normal distribution with mean zero and covariance matrix V estimated as the appropriate $q \times q$ submatrix of the inverse of (25.6) evaluated at $\hat{\gamma}$ and $\hat{\beta}$. Consequently the test statistic

$\hat{\gamma} V^{-1} \hat{\gamma}'$ has an asymptotic chi-square distribution with q degrees of freedom if the hypothesis $\gamma = 0$ is correct. A third approach to testing this hypothesis is via the score vector $\mathbf{u} = (u_1, \ldots, u_q)$ where $u_j = \partial \log L / \partial \gamma_j$ is evaluated at $\gamma = 0$ and $\boldsymbol{\beta}_0$. The vector $\boldsymbol{\beta}_0$ is the MLE calculated under the restricted model with $\gamma = 0$. Under certain conditions the statistic $\mathbf{u} V_0^{-1} \mathbf{u}'$ has an asymptotic chi-square distribution with q degrees of freedom where V_0 is the submatrix of (25.6) corresponding to the components of γ evaluated at $\gamma = 0$ and $\boldsymbol{\beta}_0$. The test of $\gamma = 0$ based on the score vector is generally of a somewhat more complex form (Cox and Hinkley 1974). Tests based on the likelihood ratio, asymptotic normality of MLEs or scores are asymptotically equivalent and no one is uniformly superior (Peers 1971). Hauck and Donner (1977) have pointed out a troublesome characteristic of Wald's test for logistic regression models. Peto and Peto (1972) and Day and Byar (1979) have pointed out useful relationships between score tests and rank tests for relatively simple situations. Kalbfleisch and Prentice (1980) have recommended the use of likelihood ratio tests.

All three approaches described above can be used to obtain large sample confidence limits for γ. For example, the set of vectors $\mathbf{c}$ not rejected at significance level α by the likelihood ratio test of $\gamma = \mathbf{c}$ constitutes an approximate $1 - \alpha$ confidence set for γ. If $q = 1$, then an approximate $1 - \alpha$ confidence interval for γ is $\hat{\gamma} \pm z_{1 - \alpha/2} \sqrt{V_1}$ where $z_{1 - \alpha/2}$ is an upper percentile of the standard normal distribution and V_1 is the estimated asymptotic variance of $\hat{\gamma}$.

The validity of these methods for drawing inferences about regression coefficients depends upon the 'correctness' of the model. Generally, the numerical value of an estimator, say $\hat{\beta}_1$, will depend upon what other variables are included in the model. In extreme cases the magnitude and even the sign of $\hat{\beta}_1$ may be very unstable based upon the inclusion or exclusion of other variables. If two variables are highly correlated, then their associated regression coefficients cannot be individually estimated with good precision. For the linear model (25.1) fitted by the method of least squares, it can be shown (Mosteller and Tukey 1977) that

$$\text{Var}(\hat{\beta}_j) = \sigma^2 / \sum_{i=1}^{n} (x_{ij} - \hat{x}_{ij})^2, \tag{25.23}$$

where x_{ij} is the value of variable j for the ith observation, and $\hat{x}_{ij}$ is the predictor of x_{ij} based on a linear regression model with variable j as response and the other x's as predictors. It follows that if x_j can be accurately predicted from the other x's then the denominator of (25.23) is small and the precision by which β_j can be estimated is poor. We cannot hope to assess independently the 'importance' of two variables (for example stage and histology) that are closely associated. In analysing a clinical trial of two treatments, 'adjustment' for a suspected prognostic factor highly imbalanced between the two treatment groups may yield an estimator of treatment effect having very low precision.

There is generally no unique interpretation that can be given to a regression coefficient independently of specifying the other variables included in the model. In fact, for the linear model (25.1) using least-squares estimation, the value $\hat{\beta}_j$ can be expressed as the estimated regression coefficient for a related univariate model. In the related model the response is the residual when Y is regressed on all the x's other than x_j, and the single explanatory variable is the residual when x_j is regressed on all the other x's (Mosteller and Tukey 1977).

It should be clear from the above discussion that conclusions about 'causality' derived from regression analyses may be quite tenuous. Assertions about causality may be reasonable for a controlled variable such as treatment whose values are assigned to patients by a mechanism which ignores all variables not included in the model. This is the case for a randomized (or stratified randomized) clinical trial. When treatment is assigned based on less well-determined mechanisms, such as in observational studies (Starmer, Lee, Harrell, and Rosati 1980), the regression coefficient for treatment may just be a surrogate for the excluded and poorly understood characteristics that determine treatment assignment. In comparing consecutive series of patients treated by different investigators, treatment assignment depends upon what patients present to different investigators. One can never be sure in this case that the characteristics determining referral, and consequently treatment, are entirely represented in the model. A good discussion of proxy phenomena is given by Mosteller and Tukey (1977). They present an example of an analysis of bombing accuracy in flights over Europe during the Second World War. The nine explanatory variables included in the regression model included altitude, type of aircraft, speed of bombing group, size of bombing group, and amount of fighter opposition. Amount of fighter opposition appeared as a strong term in the fitted regression model; the more opposition the better the accuracy. They point out that this strange result is generally regarded as a proxy phenomenon, arising because the model had no variable for amount of cloud cover. If clouds obscured the target the fighters usually did not come up and the aiming errors were generally very large.

For uncontrolled variables, it is generally more tenuous to interpret regression coefficients causatively, or to predict what the results would be if one variable (for example treatment) is changed while the others are unchanged. The fitted model can be used to predict outcomes for data collected under the same conditions as those for which the model was developed, but changing the inter-relationships among the covariates (included and excluded) generally invalidates the model. George Box (1966) said: 'The only way to find out what will happen when a complex system is disturbed is to disturb the system, not merely to observe it passively.' Mosteller and Tukey (1977) added: 'Regression is probably the most powerful technique we have for analysing data. Correspondingly, it often seems to tell us more of what we want to know than our data possibly could provide. Such seemings are, of course, wholly misleading.'

SOME USES OF REGRESSION MODELS IN CLINICAL ONCOLOGY

Regression models have been very useful in clinical oncology. In this final section some of the most common applications will be briefly listed and commented upon.

Prognostic factor studies

Determination of prognostic factors is discussed in detail in the previous chapter. It is an area of application where new regression models have had an important impact. Prognostic factor studies permit a focusing of therapeutic research on relevant subsets of patients and can lead to improvements in basic understanding of tumour biology.

Improvements in the conduct of prognostic factor studies are still possible, however. Many unreliable studies are reported based upon small numbers of patients, and there is generally too little attempt to assess the predictive ability of a model by data splitting or cross-validation. 'Statistical significance' and goodness-of-fit are often the only evidence presented supporting claims that outcomes can be accurately predicted by the model.

Treatment comparisons

Regression models are commonly used to compare treatments while accounting for the influence of prognostic factors. This is done in an attempt to improve the precision of treatment comparisons, or to remove the distortions caused by imbalances between the treatment groups with regard to prognostic factors. For randomized studies some people take the position that randomization generates a valid significance level regardless of any imbalances that arise. It is not prudent, however, to ignore imbalances in important prognostic factors. Adjusting for chance imbalances in numerous baseline variables not originally thought to be of major prognostic importance is also problematic, however. In the section on models and validation we emphasized how model selection may be difficult and, when discussing inference and 'effects', we emphasized how interpretation of specific regression coefficients depends upon the totality of variables included. Consequently problems of subjectivity in the interpretation of results can be diminished by restricting the primary analysis to a model containing a few major prognostic factors known at the outset.

For purposes of treatment comparisons, the cross-classification models described in the section on regression models are attractive because they entail the fewest assumptions. Gordon (1974) has expressed this point of view forcefully: 'The logistic model we have used assumes a linear combination of the independent variables. This assumption is not always warranted ... The

safest way to explore questions of this sort is to revert to cross-classification . . .
The multivariate logistic function proposed may produce a powerful synthetic
'predictor' but lead to completely misleading analytical conclusions . . . Where
data are too skimpy for such a categorical approach, we must forebear
drawing analytical conclusions based on the apparent general adequacy of the
fit.' Many statisticians do not accept this strong point of view, but analysis
based upon cross-classification is certainly desirable when possible. In any
case, discretization of continuous variables is recommended. A good example
of the careful use of regression models for comparing treatments is given by
Breslow (1974).

Treatment by subset interactions

Most therapeutic studies do not include sufficient numbers of patients to
definitively assess efficacy of treatments for subsets. For some small studies in
which many prognostic factors are known or suspected there may be more
definable subsets than there are patients. Ransacking the data by comparing
treatments within all subsets is likely to yield spurious conclusions. With a
reasonable number of well-defined subsets, however, a regression model can
be used to help assess whether there appears to be a substantial difference in
relative efficacy among subsets. A model with a separate treatment parameter
for each subset can be compared with a nested model with a single treatment
parameter using a likelihood ratio test. Indication of a substantial interaction
is followed by additional analyses attempting to clarify the pattern of variation
in relative efficacy. The power of interaction tests is limited by the number of
patients, but the resulting quantification of evidence for variation in
therapeutic efficacy helps temper the potential for spurious conclusions arising
from the use of multiple significance tests on a modest body of data (Simon
1982). Byar and Corle (1977) have described and illustrated a model based
approach to defining 'treatment of choice' for individual patients based on a
large body of data derived from a randomized clinical trial.

Time-dependent covariates

The development of time-dependent covariate failure time models was
stimulated by attempts to evaluate the efficacy of heart transplantation based
on a non-randomized study. In this study there was a potential bias resulting
from the fact that a transplant recipient must live long enough for a heart to be
found (Gail 1972; Mantel and Byar 1974; Turnbull, Brown, and Hu 1974).

Particular care must be taken in interpreting results from regression studies
with time-dependent variables. Problems arise in making inferences about a
characteristic after adjusting for a time-dependent variable which can itself be
influenced by the characteristic. For example, suppose that the time-
dependent variable is performance status in a model-based analysis of the

effect of treatments on survival. Since effective treatment may improve performance status, introduction of this variable may 'adjust away' a real treatment effect on survival. Kalbfleisch and Prentice (1980) define the concept of 'external' time-dependent covariates and for such variables the above dangers do not occur. Though 'internal' time-dependent covariates, such as performance status in the above example, must be dealt with carefully, the proportional hazards model can be very useful for assessing their prognostic importance on outcome. Suppose, for example, one wishes to examine the prognostic effect of obtaining a complete remission (CR) on survival. This is generally done by comparing the survivals for all patients attaining a CR to those for all patients who do not attain a CR. Such a comparison is biased by the fact that early death precludes attaining a CR. One can use the proportional hazards model with an indicator time-dependent covariate which initially has value zero for all patients and becomes one when a patient attains a CR. The resulting inference about the relevance of CR status will not contain the bias mentioned above, and other covariates can also be included in this analysis. Hubbard, Chabner, DeVita, Simon, Berard, Jones, Garvin, Canellos, Osborne, and Young (1982) have reported use of the proportional hazards model with time-dependent covariates to assess the prognostic importance of histological progression on survival for nodular lymphoma patients. Time-dependent covariates were used to indicate when first re-biopsy was performed and whether histological progression was found. Gail (1981) has reported an approach for using time-dependent covariates to assess the prognostic value of proposed biochemical tumour markers, and Prentice, Kalbfleisch, Peterson, Flournoy, Farewell, and Breslow (1978) have used a similar approach for evaluating the anti-leukemic effect of graft-versus-host disease in bone marrow transplant patients. Many problems that are conventionally addressed by *ad hoc* methods can be effectively studied in the time-dependent covariate framework.

Data description for mixed populations

As a supplement to regression analysis, the fitted model can often be useful for summarizing data. Assume, for example, that a porportional hazards model is used to evaluate the relative efficacy of two treatments and that there are important differences between the treatment groups in the distribution of covariates. Suppose that variable $z = 0$ or 1 is a treatment indicator, the covariates are specified by the vector $\mathbf{x}$, and that the associated regression coefficients are γ and $\boldsymbol{\beta}$, respectively. An estimator of the survival function $\Pr[T > t$ given $z, \mathbf{x}]$ is

$$S(t; z, \mathbf{x}) = \exp[-\hat{\Lambda}(t)\exp(\gamma z + \boldsymbol{\beta}\mathbf{x})],$$

where $\hat{\Lambda}(t)$ is estimated as in (25.13). An estimator of the probability of surviving beyond time t for a mixed population with covariate vectors $\mathbf{x}_1, \mathbf{x}_2,$

..., x_n (n being the total number of patients) receiving treatment A is thus $(1/n)\sum_{i=1}^{n} S(t; 0, x_i)$ and the corresponding estimator for treatment B is $(1/n)\sum_{i=1}^{n} S(t; 1, x_i)$. These can be plotted as functions of t to give a display of the difference in estimated treatment effect for a standardized population of patients. This approach is described and illustrated by Makuch (1982). The method is not applicable if there are 'internal' time-dependent covariates. A similar approach was presented by Lee (1981) for the logistic model.

REFERENCES

Akaike, H. (1973). Information theory and an extension of the maximum likelihood principle. *Second international symposium on information theory* (eds. B. N. Petrov and F. Czaki). Akad Kiado, Budapest.

Allen, D. M. (1974). The relationship between variable selection and data augmentation and a method of prediction. *Technometrics* **16**, 125–7.

Belsley, D. A., Kuh, E., and Welsch, R. E. (1980). *Regression diagnostics: identifying influential data and sources of collinearity.* Wiley, New York.

Bishop, Y. M. M., Feinberg, S. E., and Holland, P. W. (1975). *Discrete multivariate analysis.* MIT Press, Cambridge, Massachusetts.

Box, G. E. P. (1966). Use and abuse of regression. *Technometrics* **8**, 625–9.

Breslow, N. (1974). Covariance analysis of censored survival data. *Biometrics* **30**, 89–100.

—— (1975). Analysis of survival data under the proportional hazards model. *Int. Statist. Rev.* **43**, 45–58.

Brown, C. C. (1975). On the use of indicator variables for studying the time dependence of parameters in a response time model. *Biometrics* **31**, 863–72.

Byar, D. P. and Corle, D. K. (1977). Selecting optimal treatment in clinical trials using covariate information. *J. chron. Dis.* **30**, 445–59.

Chambers, J. M. (1973). Fitting non-linear models: numerical techniques. *Biometrika* **60**, 1–13.

Cox, D. R. (1970). *The analysis of binary data.* Methuen, London.

—— (1972). Regression models and life tables (with discussion). *Jl R. statist. Soc.* (B) **34**, 187–220.

—— (1975). Partial likelihood. *Biometrika* **62**, 599–607.

—— and Hinkley, D. V. (1974). *Theoretical Statistics.* Chapman and Hall, London.

—— and Snell, E. J. (1968). A general definition of residuals. *Jl R. statist. Soc.* (B) **30**, 248–75.

—— and Snell, E. J. (1971). On test statistics calculated from residuals. *Biometrika* **58**, 589–94.

Crowley, J. (1974). Asymptotic normality of a new nonparametric statistic for use in organ transplant studies. *J. Am. Statist. Ass.* **69**, 1006–11.

—— and Hu, M. (1977). Covariance analysis of heart transplant survival data. *J. Am. statist. Ass.* **72**, 27–36.

Daniel, C. (1959). Use of half-normal plots in interpreting factorial two-level experiments. *Technometrics* **1**, 311–41.

—— and Wood, F. S. (1971). *Fitting equations to data.* Wiley, New York.

Day, N. E. and Byar, D. P. (1979). testing hypotheses in case-control studies—equivalence of Mantel Haenszel statistics and logit score tests. *Biometrics* **35**, 623–30.

Draper, N. R. and Smith, H. (1981). *Applied regression analysis*, 2nd edn. Wiley, New York.

—— and Van Nostrand, R. C. (1979). Ridge regression and James-Stein estimation: Review and comments. *Technometrics* **21**, 451–66.

Feigl, P. and Zelen, M. (1965). Estimation of exponential survival probabilities with concomitant information. *Biometrics* **21**, 826–38.

Gail, M. H. (1972). Does cardiac transplantation prolong life? A reassessment. *Ann. intern. Med.* **76**, 815–17.

—— (1981). Evaluating serial cancer marker studies in patients at risk of recurrent disease. *Biometrics* **37**, 67–78.

Gallant, A. R. (1975). Nonlinear regression. *Amer. Statist.* **29**, 73–81.

Geisser, S. (1975). The predictive sample reuse method with applications. *J. Am. statist. Ass.* **70**, 320–8.

Glasser, M. (1967). Exponential survival with covariance. *J. Am. statist. Ass.* **62**, 561–8.

Gordon, T. (1974). Hazards in the use of the logistic function with special reference to data from prospective cardiovascular studies. *J. chron. Dis.* **27**, 97–102.

Gorman, J. W. and Toman, R. J. (1966). Selection of variables and fitting equations to data. *Technometrics* **8**, 27–51.

Grizzle, J. E., Starmer, F., and Koch, G. G. (1969). Analysis of categorical data by linear models. *Biometrics* **25**, 489–504.

Hauck, W. W. and Donner, A. (1977). Wald's test as applied to hypotheses in logit analysis. *J. Am. statist. Ass.* **72**, 851–3.

Henderson, H. V. and Velleman, P. F. (1981). Building multiple regression and models interactively. *Biometrics* **37**, 391–411.

Hocking, R. R. (1976). The analysis and selection of variables in linear regression. *Biometrics* **32**, 1–49.

Hubbard, S. M., Chabner, B. A., DeVita, Jr, V. T., Simon, R., Berard, C. W., Jones, R. B., Garvin, J. G., Canellos, G. P., Osborne, K., and Young, R. C. Histologic progression in non-Hodgkin's lymphoma. *Blood* **59**, 258–64.

Kalbfleisch, J. D. and Prentice, R. L. (1980). *The statistical analysis of failure time data.* Wiley, New York.

Kaplan, E. L. and Meier, P. (1958). Non-parametric estimation from incomplete observation. *J. Am. statist. Ass.* **53**, 457–81.

Kay, R. (1977). Proportional hazard regression models and the analysis of censored survival data. *Appl. Statist.* **26**, 227–37.

Koch, G. G., Gillings, D. B., and Stokes, M. E. (1980). Biostatistical implications of design, sampling and measurement to health science data analysis. *A. Rev. pub. Health* **1**, 163–225.

Lachenbruch, P. and Mickey, M. (1968). Estimation of error rates in discriminant analysis. *Technometrics* **10**, 1–11.

Lawless, J. F. and Singhal, K. (1978). Efficient screening of nonnormal regression models. *Biometrics* **34**, 318–27.

Lee, J. (1981). Covariance adjustment of rates based on the multiple logistic regression model. *J. chron. Dis.* **34**, 415–26.

Makuch, R. W. (1982). Adjusted survival curve estimation using covariates. *J. chron. Dis.* **35**, 437–43.

Mantel, N. (1966). Evaluation of survival data and two new rank order statistics arising in its consideration. *Cancer Chemother. Rep.* **50**, 163–70.

—— and Byar, D. P. (1974). Evaluation of response time data involving transient states: an illustration using heart transplant data. *J. Am. statist. Ass.* **69**, 81–6.

—— and Haenszel, W. (1959). Statistical aspects of the analysis of data from retrospective studies of disease. *J. nat. Cancer Inst.* **22**, 719–48.

Mosteller, F. and Tukey, J. W. (1977). *Data analysis and regression.* Addison–Wesley, Reading, Massachusetts.

—— and Wallace, D. L. (1963). Inference in an authorship problem. *J. Am. statist. Ass.* **58**, 275–309.

Nelson, W. (1972). Theory and applications of hazard plotting for censored failure data. *Technometrics* **14**, 945–66.

Peers, H. W. (1971). Likelihood ratio and associated test criteria. *Biometrika* **58**, 577–87.

Peto, R. and Peto, J. (1972). Asymptotically efficient rank invariant test procedures. *Jl R. statist. Soc. Series A* **135**, 185–206.

Pregibon, D. (1981). Logistic regression diagnostics. *Ann. Statist.* **9**, 705–24.

Prentice, R. L., Kalbfleisch, J. D., Peterson, Jr, A. V., Flournoy, N., Farewell, V. T., and Breslow, N. E. (1978). The analysis of failure times in the presence of competing risks. *Biometrics* **34**, 551–54.

Royall, R. M. (1976). Current advances in sampling theory: implications for human observational studies. *Am. J. Epidemiol.* **104**, 463–73.

Schoenfeld, D. (1980). Chi-squared goodness-of-fit tests for the proportional hazards regression model. *Biometrika* **67**, 145–53.

Schwartz, G. (1978). Estimating the dimension of a model. *Ann. Statist.* **6**, 461–64.

Simon, R. (1982). Patient subsets and variation in therapeutic efficacy. *Br. J. clin. Pharmac.* **14**, 473–82.

Snee, R. D. (1977). Validation of regression models: methods and examples. *Technometrics* **19**, 415–28.

Starmer, C. F., Lee, K. L., Harrell, F. E., and Rosati, R. A. (1980). On the complexity of investigating chronic illness. *Biometrics* **36**, 333–5.

Stone, M. (1974). Cross-validatory choice and assessment of statistical predictions (with discussion). *Jl R. statist. Soc. Series B* **36**, 111–47.

—— (1977). An asymptotic equivalence of choice of model by cross-validation and Akaike's criterion. *Jl R. statist. Soc. Series B* **39**, 44–7.

—— (1979). Comments on model selection criteria of Akaike and Schwarz. *Jl R. statist. Soc.* (B) **41**, 276–8.

Thompson, M. L. (1978). Selection of variables in multiple regression. *Int. Statist. Rev.* **46**, 1–19, 129–46.

Tsiatis, A. A. (1980). A note on a goodness of fit test for the logistic regression model. *Biometrika* **67**, 250–1.

—— (1981). A large sample study of Cox's regression model. *Statist.* **9**, 93–108.

Turnbull, B. W., Brown, Jr, B. W., and Hu, M. (1974). Survivorship analysis of heart transplant data. *J. Am. statist. Ass.* **69**, 74–80.

Zippin, C. and Armitage, P. (1966). Use of concomitant variables and incomplete survival information with estimation of an exponential survival parameter. *Biometrics* **22**, 665–72.

Index

Page numbers in **bold** refer to pages on which illustrations/tables appear.